Diabetes in Old Age

Supported by an education grant from Bayer plc

Diabetes in Old Age

Edited by

PAUL FINUCANE
Flinders University of South Australia, Adelaide, Australia

ALAN J. SINCLAIR
University of Birmingham, UK

John Wiley & Sons
Chichester · New York · Brisbane · Toronto · Singapore

Other Wiley Editorial Offices

John Wiley & Sons, Inc., 605 Third Avenue,
New York, NY 10158-0012, USA

Jacaranda Wiley Ltd, 33 Park Road, Milton,
Queensland 4064, Australia

John Wiley & Sons (Canada) Ltd, 22 Worcester Road,
Rexdale, Ontario M9W 1L1, Canada

John Wiley & Sons (SEA) Pte Ltd, 37 Jalan Pemimpin #05-04,
Block B, Union Industrial Building, Singapore 2057

Library of Congress Cataloging-in-Publication Data

Diabetes in old age / edited by Paul Finucane and Alan Sinclair.
    p.   cm.
  Includes bibliographical references and index.
  ISBN 0-471-95344-X
  1. Diabetes in old age.   I. Finucane, Paul, 1955–
II. Sinclair, Alan.
  [DNLM: 1. Diabetes Mellitus—in old age.   WK 810 D5375253 1995]
  RC660.D4485   1995
  618.97'6462—dc20
  DNLM/DLC
  for Library of Congress   94-39718
                                                                 CIP

British Library Cataloguing in Publication Data

A catalogue record for this book is available from the British Library

ISBN 0 471 95344 X

Typeset in 10/12pt Palatino by Mathematical Composition Setters Ltd, Salisbury, Wiltshire
Printed and bound in Great Britain by Biddles Ltd, Guildford, Surrey

*This book is printed on acid-free paper responsibly manufactured
from sustainable forestation, for which at least two trees are
planted for each one used in paper production.*

Contents

List of Contributors

ANTHONY H. BARNETT
Professor of Diabetic Medicine, University Department of Medicine, Birmingham Heartlands Hospital, Bordesley Green East, Birmingham B9 5SS, UK

ANDREW J. M. BOULTON
Reader in Medicine and Honorary Consultant Physician, University Department of Medicine, Manchester Royal Infirmary, Oxford Road, Manchester M13 9WL, UK

PAUL FINUCANE
Professor of Rehabilitation and Aged Care, Flinders University of South Australia, Bedford Park, SA 5042, Australia

JEFF R. FLACK
Endocrinologist, Diabetes Centre, Bankstown-Lidcombe Hospital, Sydney, NSW, Australia

GEOFFREY V. GILL
Consultant Physician and Endocrinologist, The Diabetes Centre, Walton Hospital, Rice Lane, Walton, Liverpool L9 1AE, UK

P. JEAN HO
Research Scholar, Department of Medicine, University of Sydney, Sydney, NSW 2006, Australia

JOHN E. MORLEY
Professor of Geriatric Medicine, Geriatric Research Education and Clinical Center, St Louis University Medical School, 1402 S, Grand Rm M239, St Louis, MO 63104, USA

ALAN J. SINCLAIR
Charles Hayward Professor of Geriatric Medicine, University of Birmingham, Selly Oak Hospital, Raddlebarn Road, Birmingham B29 6JD, UK

ROBERT W. STOUT
Professor of Geriatric Medicine, Department of Geriatric Medicine, The Queen's University of Belfast, Whitla Medical Building, 97 Lisburn Road, Belfast BT9 7BL, UK

PETER R. W. TASKER — *Doomsday House, Hall Lane, South Wootton, King's Lynn, Norfolk, PE30 3LQ, UK*

CHRISTOPHER J. TURNBULL — *Consultant Geriatrician, Arrowe Park Hospital, Upton, Wirral, Merseyside L49 5PE, UK*

JOHN R. TURTLE — *Professor of Medicine, Department of Medicine, University of Sydney, Sydney, NSW 2006, Australia*

DENNIS T. VILLAREAL — *Geriatric Research Education and Clinical Center, St Louis University Medical School, 1402 S, Grand Rm M239, St Louis, MO 63104, USA*

PETER J. WATKINS — *Consultant Physician, King's College Hospital, Denmark Hill, London SE5 9RS, UK*

MATTHEW J. YOUNG — *Consultant Physician, Department of Diabetes, The Royal Infirmary, Edinburgh EH3 9YW, UK*

DENNIS K. YUE — *Associate Professor, Head of Diabetic Services, Royal Prince Alfred Hospital, Camperdown, NSW 2050, Australia*

Preface

Many problems in clinical medicine are relatively straightforward in their clinical presentation and management. As such, no great level of expertise is required in dealing with them. Other problems are inherently more complex, such that most clinicians are inclined to leave them to the 'expert'. Occasionally, clinical problems which used to be regarded as straightforward become complex, with a corresponding increase in the level of expertise required to deal with them. This change tends to coincide with a rapid expansion in the body of knowledge relating to the problem.

Diabetes mellitus is a classic case in point. The increase in our knowledge and understanding of the disease in recent years has been truly remarkable. With this has come better management strategies, which in turn have been translated into a better outcome for patients. The clinician responsible for the care of diabetic patients now needs to be familiar with the epidemiology, pathogenesis, diagnosis and management of the disease *per se* as well as its myriad complications. Yet, because diabetes is so common in the elderly population, it can never become the total preserve of the 'expert'.

This text aims to provide the generalist with an understanding of diabetes mellitus in old age which is both up-to-date and comprehensive. Among the international team of contributors are those who in recent years have been to the fore in research into diabetes in elderly people. These authors have diverse backgrounds in geriatric medicine, diabetology and general practice, and thus bring together different but complementary perspectives on the disorder.

Above all, this book aims to be as relevant to the physician as to the nurse, podiatrist or other allied health worker with an interest in diabetes. The emphasis is on providing information and advice which is both appropriate and practical. We hope that those who read it gain a greater insight into the condition, so that as a result they can enhance the quality of care which they deliver to their patients.

Paul Finucane
January 1995
Alan J. Sinclair

Dedications

To my parents, Molly and the late Frank Finucane, to whom I owe everything. Though both developed diabetes in later life, neither could be considered 'a diabetic'; they are not defined by the condition.

Paul Finucane

For my parents, Radovan and Ivy, who gave me the opportunity and for my wife, Caroline, whose love and support kept me going.

Alan J. Sinclair

1

Abnormal Glucose Tolerance in Old Age: The Scale of the Problem

PAUL FINUCANE

Flinders University of South Australia, Bedford Park, Adelaide, Australia

INTRODUCTION

Abnormal glucose tolerance is a composite term for diabetes mellitus and impaired glucose tolerance (IGT). Until relatively recently, the incidence (the number of new cases occurring within a population over a specified period of time) and prevalence (the proportion of people in a population with the condition at a given time) of abnormal glucose tolerance was a source of confusion. The tools used in many epidemiological studies were unsatisfactory. Some surveys simply asked participants whether or not they had diabetes, while others relied on general practitioner or hospital records as the principal means of detection. When laboratory tests were used, some studies relied on urinalysis or random blood sugar measurements to establish the diagnosis. When a glucose challenge was given, the methodologies used were variable. There was no consensus on the criteria for diabetes mellitus and the entity of IGT was little recognized. The net result was that comparing and combining results from different studies was likely to be misleading.

Sanity and clarity began to appear in the late 1970s when the National Diabetes Data Group in the United States proposed clear and unambiguous guidelines for the classification and diagnosis of diabetes mellitus and other forms of abnormal glucose tolerance[1]. With minor modifications,

Diabetes in Old Age. Edited by P. Finucane and A. J. Sinclair
© 1995 John Wiley & Sons Ltd

these proposals were accepted by the World Health Organisation's Expert Panel on Diabetes in 1980[2] and revised by the same group in 1985[3]. Since then, a number of epidemiological studies, using appropriate and standardized methodologies and definitions, have allowed a far clearer picture of the scale of the problem of abnormal glucose tolerance to emerge.

Much of what is known about the extent of abnormal glucose tolerance comes from cross-sectional prevalence studies. This is because incidence studies require follow-up of cohorts of patients or repeated cross-sectional analyses and are therefore time consuming and expensive. Many studies of the prevalence of non-insulin-dependent diabetes (NIDDM) have focused on relatively young adult populations and a few have even excluded old people. Such studies are still of value as the young adult diabetic population of today will form part of tomorrow's elderly diabetic population. Only a few studies have specifically addressed the prevalence of abnormal glucose tolerance in elderly people.

In summarizing what is currently known about the prevalence of abnormal glucose tolerance, it is important to consider IGT in addition to diabetes mellitus. This is because subjects with IGT are at increased risk of developing diabetes mellitus and its macrovascular complications. For example, a study of Pima Indians with IGT who were followed up for a median of 3.3 years found that 31% developed NIDDM, 26% continued to have IGT, while 43% reverted to normal glucose tolerance[4]. The cumulative incidence of NIDDM was 25% at 5 years and 61% at 10 years.

THE NEED TO UNDERSTAND THE SCALE OF THE PROBLEM

Clinicians, educators, researchers, and health planners alike need to appreciate the current status and future trends in the epidemiology of abnormal glucose tolerance. This will promote:

1. Rational health planning. The magnitude of the clinical work-load relevant to diabetes can be determined together with the resources required to meet it.

2. Placement of the disease in a proper perspective. Its importance relative to other disorders can be determined and this in turn can facilitate the equitable allocation of resources.

3. The identification of individuals, groups or communities who are at high risk for the development of diabetes. This offers possibilities for

research into the aetiology of the disease, and for health promotion and disease prevention programmes.

4. Awareness of any change in the nature of diabetes over time. Furthermore, it will facilitate the evaluation of intervention programmes.

ABNORMAL GLUCOSE TOLERANCE: AN EMERGING PUBLIC HEALTH PROBLEM

In Western and developing countries alike, prevalence rates for diabetes have been on the increase since the early part of the twentieth century. For example, an upward trend in the prevalence rates of diagnosed diabetes in the United States between the 1930s and 1980 has been noted by Harris[5] (Figure 1.1). Prevalence rates in the United States are increasing in all age groups and in both sexes, with the number of known diabetics doubling between 1960 and 1980[6]. The annual review of 40 000 households comprising 120 000 US residents conducted by the National Health Interview Survey (NHIS) revealed a 17% increase in the number of Americans with

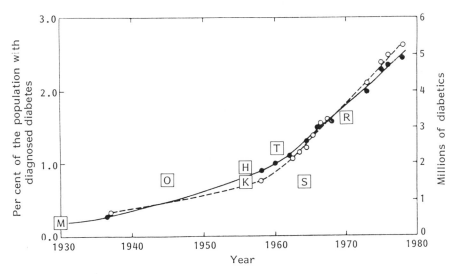

Figure 1.1. Trends in the prevalence and rate of diagnosed diabetes in the USA. Open and closed circles represent data from National Health Interview Surveys of the US Public Health Service. Rates from seven community-based surveys are included for comparison. M̄ Maryland (State); Ō Oxford, Massachusetts; H̄ Hagerstown, Maryland; K̄ Kansas City, Kansas; T̄ Tecumseh, Michigan; S̄ Sudbury, Massachusetts; R̄ Rochester, Minnesota

self-reported diabetes between 1980 and 1987[7]. Over the 15-year period 1966–81, the prevalence of diabetes in one Australian community was shown to increase by 50%[8].

To some extent, increased prevalence rates can be explained by a broadening of the diagnostic criteria for diabetes. For the most part, however, the increase has been real rather than apparent. The prevalence of any condition is the product of its average incidence and its average duration. At different times, both an increased incidence and an increased duration have contributed to the increasing prevalence of diabetes, at least in Western countries. For example, in the USA between 1960 and 1970, a greater awareness of diabetes coupled with better diagnostic methods led to better surveillance and in turn to earlier diagnoses of milder cases[5]. Since the early 1970s, however, increased duration of the disease due to enhanced survival rates have largely accounted for the continuing rise in prevalence rates in the USA. About two-thirds of diabetics die from cardiovascular disease, and diabetics and non-diabetics alike are benefiting from a general reduction in cardiovascular mortality.

The increasing prevalence of diabetes is also attributable to an ageing society, particularly in Western countries. Nowadays individuals have a longer life span during which to develop diabetes, to live with the condition and to develop its complications[9]. The population with diabetes is increasingly elderly. Even 20 years ago, 40% of newly diagnosed diabetics in a US sample were aged over 65 years[10]. Undoubtedly, this proportion has since risen. The NHIS survey already cited has documented a greater than 100% increase in the number of diabetics aged over 75 years in the USA between 1980 and 1987[7].

Diabetes is now becoming a significant problem in some developing countries where previously it was little recognized. This can be explained in part by all of the factors mentioned above: increased detection, improved survival and an ageing society. More importantly, however, people in many developing countries are switching from a traditional to a Western life-style and in the process adopting diets and exercise patterns which promote the development of diabetes.

FACTORS INFLUENCING THE PREVALENCE OF ABNORMAL GLUCOSE TOLERANCE

The prevalence of diabetes and IGT varies considerably in different populations and in different subgroups within populations. The most important variables (Table 1.1) are now discussed more fully. Some factors, for example life-style and obesity, are both closely associated and difficult to measure precisely. This makes it difficult to disentangle one from the

Table 1.1. Factors which influence the prevalence of abnormal glucose tolerance

Age
Sex
Country of residence
Place of residence
Race and ethnicity
Socio-economic status and life-style
Obesity

other when analysing their relative contribution to the development of diabetes[11].

AGE

Age is the single most important variable influencing the prevalence of abnormal glucose tolerance. Almost all epidemiological studies, whether cross-sectional or longitudinal, show that the prevalence of both diabetes and IGT initially increases with ageing, reaches a plateau and subsequently declines. However, the time of onset of the increase, the rate of increase, the time of peak prevalence and rate of subsequent decline differ in the various groups studied.

There is general agreement that the rise in prevalence begins in early adulthood. For example, Pima Indians aged 25–34 years are 10 times more likely to have diabetes than those aged 15–24 years[12]. In Americans aged 45–55 years, diabetes is over four times more common than in those aged 20–44 years[13]. The subsequent rate of increase with ageing is variable, being greatest in societies with the highest prevalence of glucose intolerance[14].

In Pima Indians, the prevalence of abnormal glucose tolerance peaks at 40 years for men and 50 years for women and declines in men after the age of 65 years and in women after the age of 55 years[12]. In other populations, prevalence rates peak in the sixth decade and subsequently decline[14]. However, in a study of elderly Finnish men, prevalence peaked in those aged 75–79, falling off in 80–84 year olds[15]. In some populations, however, the highest prevalence rates are found in the oldest age groups[8,14].

Figure 1.2 shows the prevalence rates of diabetes and IGT in different age groups, taken from the second National Health and Nutrition Examination Survey (NHANES II) carried out by the National Diabetes Data Group in the USA[13]. This survey involved 15 000 Americans aged 20–74 years and was carried out between 1976 and 1980. While these prevalence rates may

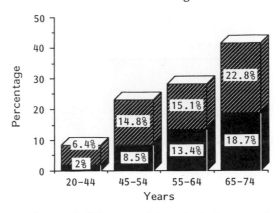

Figure 1.2 The prevalence of diabetes and impaired glucose tolerance (IGT) with ageing in the NHANES II study of 15 000 Americans IGT (▨); diabetes (■). (Modified from Harris *et al.*[13])

apply to the US population at that time, they do not necessarily reflect current rates in the USA and tell us nothing about rates in other countries.

SEX

There is evidence to suggest that diabetes was once more common in females than males. In recent years, however, a disproportionate increase in the number of males known to have diabetes has resulted in equal prevalence rates being found in some societies while males predominate in others. Possible explanations for this change include a disproportionate increase in the incidence of diabetes in males, increased detection in males and reduced mortality in diabetic males.

Between 1980 and 1987, the NHIS in the United States noted a 33% increase in the prevalence of self-reported diabetes among white males but no increase among white females[7]. Although there was a 16% increase among black males and a 24% increase among black females, this is of lesser significance as non-whites constitute only 15% of the US population. When interpreting these data, one should remember the limitations of self-reporting which the NHIS used as a measure of the prevalence of diabetes. Recent studies involving predominantly non-elderly people have found the prevalence of NIDDM in males to exceed that in females in Australia[8,16] and Finland[17], while similar rates have been reported from New Zealand[18] and Japan[19]. The NHANES II survey from the USA already cited[13] found no difference in the prevalence of NIDDM between the sexes. However, in that survey, the subgroup aged over 65 years had a slight male excess. This represented a change from previous surveys in which elderly females had predominated. There was no sex difference in the prevalence of IGT.

A review of the prevalence of diabetes from 75 communities in 32 countries, found the sex ratio for diabetes to vary widely[14]. Some studies found a male excess while females predominated in others. A regional trend was apparent, whereby in Africa/Asia and the Americas, there was a trend to male excess, whereas in the Pacific regions, females predominated. IGT was found to be generally more common in women.

The few studies that have focused on prevalence rates in elderly populations have either not reported sex differences, or found either a male[20] or female excess[21].

COUNTRY OF RESIDENCE

King and Rewers have collated data on the prevalence of abnormal glucose tolerance in over 150 000 people from 75 communities in 32 countries[14] (Figure 1.3). As diabetes is an age-related disorder, its prevalence in individual countries depends on the age structure of that society. Thus Western countries with a large elderly population have high prevalence rates; conversely, low rates are found in developing countries with few elderly people. To allow valid comparisons of countries to be made, age-standardized rather than true prevalence rates are used. As King and Rewers used a truncated age range of 30–64 years, their findings cannot be automatically extrapolated to elderly populations.

Diabetes was found to be absent or rare (less than 3% of people affected) in some traditional communities in developing countries. Prevalence rates in Europe ranged from 3 to 10% while some Arab, Asian Indian, Chinese and Hispanic American populations had rates of 14–20%. The highest rates were found in natives of the South Pacific island of Nauru and Pima/Papago Indians in the USA who had prevalence rates as high as 50%.

Migrant populations are at particular risk of developing diabetes. A study of Japanese-American men who had retained their racial and cultural identity, found that 56% had abnormal glucose tolerance and that a third had diabetes[22]. This rate is far higher than among white Americans with a similar socio-economic profile in terms of education, occupation and income. It is also higher than the rate among the native population of Japan. Chinese and Indian migrants have a particularly high prevalence of abnormal glucose tolerance when compared with indigenous communities[14]. These studies emphasize the importance of environmental factors, largely absent in the indigenous population but acquired in the migrant setting, in the development of diabetes.

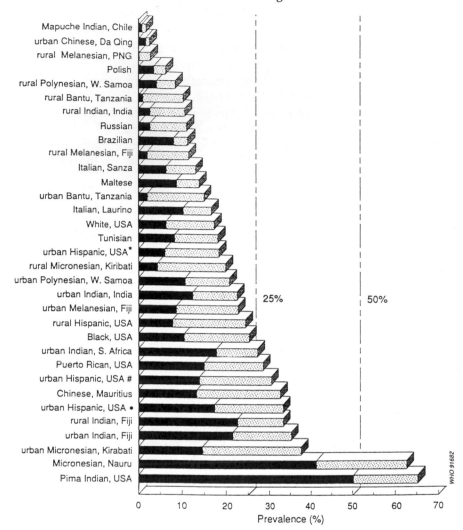

Figure 1.3. Prevalence (%) of abnormal glucose tolerance (diabetes and impaired glucose tolerance) in selected populations in the age range of 30–64 years, age standardized to the world population of Segi, sexes combined. *, Upper income; #, middle income; •, low income; ■ diabetes mellitus; ⊞ impaired glucose tolerance (from King and Rewers[14] with permission)

PLACE OF RESIDENCE

There is evidence to suggest that within countries, the prevalence of diabetes differs between regions. In the USA, for example, the prevalence of self-reported diabetes is greatest in Hawaii and in states east of the

Mississippi river[23]. Even when differences in age, sex and racial/ethnic differences between states were taken into account, a greater than threefold difference existed between the state with the highest rate and that with the lowest.

A study of people aged 18–50 years and living in nine towns in England and Wales, chosen to represent different latitude and socio-economic status, found a greater than twofold difference in the numbers receiving hospital treatment for newly diagnosed NIDDM[24]. NIDDM was found more frequently in towns with the poorest socio-economic environment, irrespective of latitude. Caution must be exercised when using such 'surrogate' markers of prevalence and incidence, as illustrated by a Finnish study which found that the prevalence of known diabetes in a cohort of elderly men was 11% in the east of the country and 5% in the west. When a glucose challenge and WHO criteria were used to measure the true prevalence rate, it was identical at 24% in both regions[15]. Regional differences are not always found. For example, a study of over 6000 Tanzanian men showed that prevalence rates for diabetes, which were generally low, were similar in six villages despite having geographical, socio-economic and dietary differences[25].

One clear trend emerging from a number of studies is the urban–rural divide in the prevalence of diabetes[14]. Diabetes is considered to be a disease of modernization and urbanization[26], with significantly higher rates being found in urban environments. Comparisons of migrant populations living in rural and urban settings in the same country also show a consistent excess of diabetes and IGT in urban migrants.

Finally, it should be remembered that particular subgroups of the population, such as those living in institutional care, will have a particularly high prevalence of diabetes[27]. This is not surprising, given that such people are chronologically old and that diabetic complications place them in need of residential care.

RACE AND ETHNICITY

Studies from multicultural societies provide compelling evidence that racial background impacts on the incidence and prevalence of abnormal glucose tolerance. For example, the prevalence of self-reported diabetes in black female Americans is twice that in whites, while in black males it is a third higher than in white males[7]. This difference is increasing. Between 1980 and 1987, the annual incidence of self-reported diabetes rose for black males and females, while at the same time, there was a small fall in incidence among white males and females.

The pitfalls in interpreting rates of self-reported diabetes have already been highlighted. More concrete evidence for racial differences in the prevalence of diabetes comes from the NHANES II study which found that in Americans aged 65–74 years, 17.9% of white and 26.4% of black people were diabetic[13]. In a large multiracial New Zealand work-force the relative risk of having diabetes was four to six times greater in Maori, Pacific Islanders and Asians, than in people of European backgrounds[18]. This increased risk remained significant after controlling for age, income and body mass index (BMI).

Attention has already been drawn to the high prevalence of abnormal glucose tolerance among the Pima Indians of Arizona in the USA[12]. For indigenous North Americans, susceptibility to NIDDM is related to the degree of racial admixing; thus Americans of mixed ethnicity have rates of NIDDM intermediate between those of full native Americans and of Caucasians[28].

In a survey of the Southall district of London which has a large Asian population, the overall age-adjusted prevalence of self-reported diabetes was almost four times higher in Asians than in Europeans[29]. It is also of interest that the excess prevalence of diabetes among Asians was greatest in the older age groups. However, this survey also relied on self-reporting to measure the prevalence of diabetes. Another study which for methodological reasons fails to shed much light on the absolute prevalence of abnormal glucose tolerance in the UK, also showed that diabetes was four times higher in Asian than white men and twice as high in Asian as white women[30].

SOCIO-ECONOMIC STATUS AND LIFE-STYLE

It is difficult to disentangle the effect of socio-economic status and life-style on the prevalence of diabetes from confounding factors, such as country, place of residence and racial origin. The evidence suggests, however, that these are independent risk factors. Certain ethnic groups are parti-cularly susceptible to developing abnormal glucose tolerance when they forsake a traditional for an urbanized life-style[31]. This has been documented among North American Indians, Mexican-Americans, Australian Aborigines, Micronesian and Polynesian Pacific Islanders and Asian Indians. For example, urban dwellers on the Pacific island of Kiribati have rates of NIDDM three times greater than those living in a rural setting; in the over 65 population, there is a fourfold urban–rural difference[32]. Urbanized Australian Aborigines also have high prevalence rates of NIDDM[33]. Migration is a potent stimulus to life-style change; the higher prevalence of NIDDM in migrant communities when compared with those left behind has been explained by socio-economic advantage, which migration tends to confer[11].

Socio-economic deprivation, which is associated with poor diet and other adverse life-style factors is also linked to high rates of NIDDM. In the USA, the 1973 National Household Interview Survey documented an inverse relationship between income and the prevalence of known diabetes[34]. A study of nine towns in England and Wales chosen to represent different latitude and socio-economic status, found that the detection rate for newly diagnosed NIDDM was greatest in towns with a 'poor' socio-economic profile and least in towns with 'good' profiles[24]. In a survey of a large multiracial New Zealand work-force, the relative risk for abnormal glucose tolerance was inversely related to income but not to other markers of socio-economic status[18].

A study of over 1100 Hindu Indians living in Dar-es-Salaam, Tanzania, looked at the prevalence of glucose intolerance in seven subcommunities of different caste. The age- and sex-adjusted prevalence of diabetes differed more than fivefold[35]. Similar differences were noted in the prevalence of IGT. These subcommunities differed in socio-economic characteristics and life-style and may also have differed genetically and in their diet. Studies such as this highlight the danger of regarding people from a single geographical area or with similar racial origins as homogeneous and of grouping them under a single label (e.g. 'Asians').

The effect of physical exercise on the pathogenesis of NIDDM is discussed in Chapter 2; there is epidemiological evidence that exercise influences prevalence rates. For example, migrant Indians in Fiji who were physically active had half the risk of diabetes than those who were inactive[36]. Physical activity was also implicated as an environmental risk factor for diabetes mellitus in a multiracial community in Mauritius[31].

OBESITY

This section outlines the epidemiological evidence for obesity as a risk factor for abnormal glucose tolerance; its importance in the pathogenesis of NIDDM is discussed in more detail in Chapter 2. There is clear evidence that diabetes is an independent risk factor for diabetes. In the NHANES II study cited earlier, obesity doubled the probability of having diabetes and was also an independent risk factor for IGT[13]. The Framingham Study had broadly similar findings, with people overweight by >40% having twice the prevalence of diabetes than others[9]. A study of 1300 Finns aged 65–74 years found an association between NIDDM and obesity and between NIDDM and central obesity[21]. Central obesity, recognized by a high waist–hip girth ratio correlates with intra-abdominal visceral fat mass. The importance of central obesity in the pathogenesis of NIDDM is explained in Chapter 2. In a study of elderly Hong Kong Chinese, diabetes was more common in overweight and obese subjects[37].

In other studies, the association between obesity and abnormal glucose tolerance has been less impressive. In a study of elderly New Zealanders, a positive association was found in newly diagnosed diabetics but not in those with known diabetes[20]. Racial factors may play a part, though the evidence is somewhat confusing. For example, in a survey of a large multiracial New Zealand work-force, the increased prevalence of glucose intolerance in Maoris and Pacific Islanders over people of European origin was partly attributable to obesity[18]. Obesity has been implicated in the high prevalence of diabetes in Pima Indians; furthermore, in those with IGT, obesity predicts subsequent deterioration to NIDDM, though it is not an independent risk factor[4]. On the other hand, a study of over 6000 young Tanzanians found that diabetes rates increased only modestly with body mass[25]. Furthermore, obesity was not prevalent among elderly Finnish men, many of whom were diabetic[15]. In this study, the BMI decreased with age in those with diabetes, IGT and normal glucose tolerance alike.

PREVALENCE OF ABNORMAL GLUCOSE TOLERANCE IN OLD PEOPLE: AN OVERVIEW

From all that has been stated above, it follows that prevalence rates for abnormal glucose tolerance are specific to the population from which the study sample is drawn and are not generalizable. However, it is still possible to profile a community in which the prevalence of abnormal glucose tolerance is likely to be particularly high. It will have both a large elderly and migrant population and be located in an urban setting in a 'developed' country. Members may be either wealthy or poor, but will have a sedentary life-style. Many will be overweight or obese. In communities which lack many of these characteristics, the prevalence of glucose intolerance will be relatively low.

THE UNITED STATES

While some 8.3 million Americans aged 20–74 years (6.8% of that population) have diabetes mellitus[13], the prevalence in the 65–74 age group is 18.7%. This ranges from 17.9% for white to 26.4% for black people. Furthermore, 11.2% of Americans aged 20–74 years have IGT; 22.8% of those aged 65–74 are affected. Overall therefore, some 41.5% of Americans aged 65–74 years have abnormal glucose tolerance (either diabetes or IGT). In numerical terms, some 4 million Americans over 65 years have diabetes[6]. Almost 20% of white North Americans can expect to develop NIDDM if they survive into their seventh decade[11].

THE UNITED KINGDOM

Two studies from the UK contain extractable data which give an estimate of the prevalence of abnormal glucose tolerance in elderly people. In a London general practice population, 4% of people aged over 60 years and 9% aged over 80 had NIDDM[38]. A further 6 and 13%, respectively, had IGT. However, this study relied on a single blood sugar estimation, taken 2 h post-glucose challenge to establish the diagnosis. Similar methodology was used to estimate that 9% of people aged over 65 years in Melton Mowbray had NIDDM[39].

AUSTRALIA AND NEW ZEALAND

A 1981 Australian study found that 10% of people over 65 years had diabetes and 8% had IGT. The corresponding figures for those over 75 were 15 and 10%[8]. While this is probably an underestimate, it indicates that at least 264 000 Australians have NIDDM and another 280 000 have IGT[40]. In a random sample of some 600 New Zealanders aged over 65, the age-adjusted prevalence of diabetes was 15%[20]. However, as very few had an oral glucose tolerance test, and as people in residential care were excluded, this rate is also likely to be an underestimate.

JAPAN

Age- and sex-adjusted prevalence rates for diabetes in Japan have recently been estimated at over 10% for people over 45 years[19]—far higher than earlier estimates derived using unsatisfactory methodologies. The new rate may still be an underestimate as the study population was largely rural and higher prevalence rates are likely in urban or mixed environments. From the same study, the prevalence rate for IGT was over 15%, giving an overall rate for abnormal glucose tolerance of 26% for people aged over 45 years.

FINLAND AND SCANDINAVIA

The prevalence of abnormal glucose tolerance in elderly Finns is remarkably high, with 30% of men aged 65–84 years having NIDDM and another 32% having IGT[15]. Less impressive rates were found in a study of 1300 younger subjects (aged 65–74 years), where 16% of men and 19% of women had NIDDM and another 18 and 19%, respectively, had IGT[21]. Prevalence studies from Sweden have had major methodological deficiencies; rates of over 6% in people aged over 60 years have been suggested[41]. Prevalence rates in Denmark[42] and in Sweden[43] appear to be only half of those in Finland.

OTHER COUNTRIES

Readers with a particular interest in the world-wide prevalence of abnormal glucose tolerance are referred to the reviews by King and Zimmett[11] and King and Rewers[14]. As can be seen from Figure 1.3, some communities and countries have remarkably high prevalence rates for NIDDM and IGT. The highest recorded rates are among the Pima Indians of Arizona, USA, where 40% of those aged 65–74 years have diabetes[12]. However, new challengers for this dubious distinction are now appearing. For example, a recent study from Papua New Guinea found that the prevalence rate there is not much lower than that found in Pima Indians[44].

Countries with large populations also deserve special mention even if the prevalence of diabetes is not particularly high. In Hong Kong Chinese, 10% of those aged over 60 and 17% aged over 75 have NIDDM[37]. Demographic and socio-economic changes in mainland China suggest that a similar prevalence rate can be expected there in time.

THE ECONOMIC COST OF ABNORMAL GLUCOSE TOLERANCE

Diabetes incurs both direct and indirect costs. Direct patient costs are the sum of what is spent on diagnosing and treating diabetes itself and on managing its acute and chronic complications; it is estimated that diabetics use hospital and primary health care services two to three times as much as the general population[45,46]. Lost productivity due to short-term illness, disability and premature mortality accounts for the indirect costs. Estimates of the economic cost of diabetes are largely drawn from a few Western countries and cannot be extrapolated to other countries or health care systems.

In the United States, the National Diabetes Data Group estimated the total cost of diabetes at $13.8 billion or 4% of the US health budget in 1984[47]. The Center for Economic Studies in Medicine put the cost at $20.4 billion for 1987[48]. Both figures are probable underestimates as they either failed to include the cost of diabetic complications or underestimated the prevalence of diabetes. For similar reasons, the finding that NIDDM alone cost the US economy $19.8 billion in 1986 is also an underestimate[49]. Even if the absolute figures are inaccurate, the breakdown of the expenditure on NIDDM in the United States in 1986 is still of interest (Table 1.2). In the UK, by the late 1980s it is conservatively estimated that diabetes cost £1.2 billion per annum or 5% of the National Health Service budget[50].

Table 1.2. Breakdown of estimated $19.8 billion spent on NIDDM in the USA, 1986 (modified from Huse *et al.*[49])

Item	Cost ($ billion)	% of total cost
Total health care expenditure	11.56	58.5
NIDDM *per se*	6.83	34.6
Circulatory complications	3.85	19.5
Visual complications	0.39	2.0
Neuropathy	0.24	1.2
Skin ulcers	0.15	0.8
Nephropathy	0.10	0.5
Lost productivity		
From disability	2.6	13.2
From premature death	5.6	28.3
Overall	8.2	41.5

There are age and sex differences in the economic cost of diabetes with men aged under 65 years accounting for 35% of cost, women aged over 65 years for 30%, men aged over 65 years for 18% and women aged under 65 years for 17%[49]. It has been further estimated that per capita health expenditure on people with diabetes is two to three times greater than on non-diabetics and the loss of productivity due to disability and premature death is also sizeable[49].

THE HUMAN COST

In the United States in 1986, NIDDM was thought to account for 144 000 deaths (6.8% of total US mortality) and the total disability of 951 000 people[49]. People aged over 65 years account for 75% of these deaths[48]. Also in the USA, coronary artery disease rates are twice as common in males with diabetes and four times as common in females[51]; stroke is four times more common[52]; blindness five times more common[49]; and lower limb amputation 10–20 times more common[53].

In terms of human pain and suffering, the cost of diabetes to patients, partners, children, other family members and other carers is incalculable. As well as physical costs, diabetes incurs psychological costs in terms of the major impositions which it places on life-style. Being relatively intangible, these costs tend to receive inadequate recognition and are too often disregarded.

ABNORMAL GLUCOSE TOLERANCE—AN
UNDERDIAGNOSED PROBLEM

A consistent finding in epidemiological studies, is that a large proportion of people found to have diabetes are previously undiagnosed. For example, the NHANES II survey estimated that almost half of the 6.6% Americans with diabetes are unaware of the problem[13]. Equal numbers of known and undiagnosed diabetics were found in black and white people, in all age groups and in both sexes. Similar findings have been reported from the UK[38] and Japan[19]. In another UK study[39] and in Australia[8], about one-third of all diabetics were previously unknown. A global picture is obtained from a comparison of the prevalence of diabetes in 32 countries, which found that in most populations over 20% of people with diabetes were previously undiagnosed and in some over 50% were undiagnosed[14]. There are regional differences in the prevalence of known diabetes. For example, in a study of elderly Finnish men, 45% of people in one geographical area but only 28% in another had been aware of the diagnosis[15].

FUTURE TRENDS

Those factors which underlay the increased prevalence in diabetes during the past 60 years continue to operate and ensure that prevalence rates will continue to rise for the foreseeable future. First, surveillance and detection of diabetes is likely to improve. In the United States alone, 500 000 new diabetics are currently being identified each year[5]. Second, survival rates for diabetics will continue to improve with better glycaemic control and with life-style modifications leading to a reduction in other atherogenic risk factors. Finally, demographic trends are such that there will be more old people in society to develop diabetes.

Trends which have already occurred in some countries have yet to happen in others. For example, despite a 50% increase between 1966 and 1981, prevalence rates in Australia in 1986 were similar to those experienced by the United States in 1973. If Australian trends parallel those of the USA, a further 50% increase will occur in the 15-year interval, 1986–2001[40].

There is every indication that abnormal glucose tolerance will emerge as a major problem in countries where prevalence is currently low. For example, rates are currently low in rural Africa but high among black people of African descent living in the USA. One school of thought is that African prevalence rates will rise if and when African nations adopt Western life-styles[11].

Health organizations face a major challenge in offsetting this impending pandemic of abnormal glucose tolerance. Success will depend on maintaining traditional life-styles in some communities and in promoting the adoption of new life-styles elsewhere. As a national health objective for the year 2000, the United States has a target of reducing overall diabetes prevalence to less than 25 per 1000 and annual incidence to less than 2.5 per 1000. This means a 15% decrease from the 1987 baseline. Primary prevention (see Chapter 3) is the key.

REFERENCES

1 National Diabetes Data Group. Classification of diabetes mellitus and other categories of glucose intolerance. *Diabetes* 1979; **28**: 1039–57.
2 WHO Expert Committee on Diabetes Mellitus: Second report. *World Health Organisation Tech Rep Ser* **646**. Geneva: WHO, 1980.
3 WHO Diabetes Mellitus: Report of a Study Group. *World Health Organisation Tech Rep Ser* **727**. Geneva: WHO, 1985.
4 Saad MF, Knowler WC, Pettitt DJ, *et al.* The natural history of impaired glucose tolerance in the Pima Indians. *N Engl J Med* 1988; **319**: 1500–6.
5 Harris M. The prevalence of diagnosed diabetes, undiagnosed diabetes, and impaired glucose tolerance in the United States. Proceedings of the Third Symposium on Diabetes in Asia and Oceania. *Excerpta Medica*, 1982; 70–6.
6 Bennett PH. Diabetes in the elderly: diagnosis and epidemiology. *Geriatrics* 1984; **39**: 37–41.
7 Centers for Disease Control. Prevalence, incidence of diabetes mellitus—United States, 1980–1987. *JAMA* 1990; **264**: 3126.
8 Glatthaar C, Welborn TA, Stenhouse NS, Garcia-Webb P. Diabetes and impaired glucose tolerance. A prevalence estimate based on the Busselton 1981 survey. *Med J Aust* 1985; **143**: 436–40.
9 Wilson PWF, Anderson KM, Kannel WB. Epidemiology of diabetes mellitus in the elderly. *Am J Med* 1986; **80** (Suppl. 5A): 3–9.
10 Palumbo PJ, Elveback LR, Chu C-P, *et al.* Diabetes mellitus: incidence, prevalence, survivorship, and causes of death in Rochester, Minnesota, 1945–1970. *Diabetes* 1976; **25**: 566–73.
11 King H, Zimmet P. Trends in the prevalence and incidence of diabetes: non-insulin-dependent diabetes mellitus. *World Health Stat Q* 1988; **41**: 190–6.
12 Knowler WC, Bennett PH, Hamman RF, Miller M. Diabetes incidence and prevalence in Pima Indians: a 19-fold greater incidence than in Rochester, Minnesota. *Am J Epidemiol* 1978; **108**: 497–505.
13 Harris MI, Hadden WC, Knowler WC, Bennett PH. Prevalence of diabetes and impaired glucose tolerance and plasma glucose levels in US population aged 20–74 yr. *Diabetes* 1987; **36**: 523–34.
14 King H, Rewers M. Global estimates for prevalence of diabetes mellitus and impaired glucose tolerance in adults. *Diabetes Care* 1993; **16**: 157–77.
15 Tuomilehto J, Nissinen A, Kivela S-L, *et al.* Prevalence of diabetes mellitus in elderly men aged 65 to 84 years in eastern and western Finland. *Diabetologia* 1986; **29**: 611–15.

16 Welborn TA, Glatthaar C, Whittall D, Bennett S. An estimate of diabetes prevalence from a national population sample: a male excess. *Med J Aust* 1989; **150**: 78–81.

17 Tuomilehto J, Korhonen HJ, Kartovaara L, *et al*. Prevalence of diabetes mellitus and impaired glucose tolerance in the middle-aged population of three areas in Finland. *Int J Epidemiol* 1991; **20**: 1010–17.

18 Scragg R, Baker J, Metcalf P, Dryson E. Prevalence of diabetes mellitus and impaired glucose tolerance in a New Zealand multiracial workforce. *NZ Med J* 1991; **104**: 395–7.

19 Sekikawa A, Tominaga M, Takahashi K, *et al*. Prevalence of diabetes and impaired glucose tolerance in Funagata area, Japan. *Diabetes Care* 1993; **16**: 570–4.

20 Lintott CJ, Hanger HC, Scott RS, *et al*. Prevalence of diabetes mellitus in an ambulant elderly New Zealand population. *Diab Res Clin Pract* 1992; **16**: 131–6.

21 Mykkanen L, Laakso M, Uusitupa M, Pyorala K. Prevalence of diabetes and impaired glucose tolerance in elderly subjects and their association with obesity and family history of diabetes. *Diabetes Care* 1990; **13**: 1099–105.

22 Fujimoto WY, Leonetti DL, Kinyoun JL, *et al*. Prevalence of diabetes mellitus and impaired glucose tolerance among second-generation Japanese-American men. *Diabetes* 1987; **36**: 721–9.

23 Centers for Disease Control. Regional variation in diabetes mellitus prevalence—United States, 1988 and 1989. *JAMA* 1990; **264**: 3123–4.

24 Barker DJP, Gardner MJ, Power C. Incidence of diabetes amongst people aged 18–50 years in nine British towns: a collaborative study. *Diabetologia* 1982; **22**: 421–5.

25 McLarty DG, Kitange HM, Mtinangi BL, *et al*. Prevalence of diabetes and impaired glucose tolerance in rural Tanzania. *Lancet* 1989; i: 871–5.

26 Welborn TA. Asia-Oceania and the global epidemic of diabetes. *Med J Aust* 1994; **160**: 740.

27 Grobin W. Diabetes in the aged: underdiagnosis and overtreatment. *Can Med Assoc J* 1970; **103**: 915–23.

28 Gardner LI, Stern MP, Haffner SM, *et al*. Prevalence of diabetes in Mexican Americans: relationship to percent of gene pool derived from native American sources. *Diabetes* 1984; **33**: 86–92.

29 Mather HM, Keen H. The Southall diabetes survey: prevalence of known diabetes in Asians and Europeans. *Br Med J* 1985; **291**: 1081–4.

30 Simmons D, Williams DRR, Powell MJ. Prevalence of diabetes in a predominantly Asian community: preliminary findings of the Coventry diabetes study. *Br Med J* 1989; **298**: 18–21.

31 Dowse GK, Gareeboo H, Zimmet PZ, *et al*. High prevalence of NIDDM and impaired glucose tolerance in Indian, Creole, and Chinese Mauritians. *Diabetes* 1990; **39**: 390–6.

32 King H, Taylor R, Zimmet P, *et al*. Non-insulin-dependent diabetes (NIDDM) in a newly independent Pacific nation: the Republic of Kiribati. *Diabetes Care* 1984; **7**: 409–15.

33 Cameron WI, Moffitt PS, Williams DRR. Diabetes mellitus in the Australian Aborigines of Bourke, New South Wales. *Diabetes Res Clin Pract* 1986; **2**: 307–14.

34 US Dept of Health, Education and Welfare. Diabetes Data: Compiled 1977, DHEW Publ. No. (NIH) 78-1468. Washington: US Government Printing Office, 1978.

35 Ramaiya KL, Swai ABM, McLarty DG, *et al.* Prevalence of diabetes and cardiovascular disease risk factors in Hindu Indian subcommunities in Tanzania. *Br Med J* 1991; **303**: 271–6.

36 Taylor R, Ram P, Zimmet P, *et al.* Physical activity and prevalence of diabetes in Melanesian and Indian men in Fiji. *Diabetologia* 1984; **27**: 578–82.

37 Woo J, Swaminathan R, Cockram C, *et al.* The prevalence of diabetes mellitus and an assessment of methods of detection among a community of elderly Chinese in Hong Kong. *Diabetologia* 1987; **30**: 863–8.

38 Forrest RD, Jackson CA, Yudkin JS. Glucose intolerance and hypertension in North London: the Islington diabetes survey. *Diabetic Med* 1986; **3**: 338–42.

39 Croxson SCM, Burden AC, Bodington M, Botha JL. The prevalence of diabetes in elderly people. *Diabetic Med* 1991; **8**: 28–31.

40 Australian Diabetes Foundation. *Diabetes in Australia 1986.* Canberra: A.D. Foundation, 1986.

41 Sartor G. Prevalence of type 2 diabetes in Sweden. *Acta Endocrinol* 1984; **262**: 27–9.

42 Agner E, Thorsteinsson B, Eriksen M. Impaired glucose tolerance and diabetes mellitus in elderly subjects. *Diabetes Care* 1982; **5**: 600–4.

43 Ohlson L-O, Larsson B, Eriksson H, *et al.* Diabetes mellitus in Swedish middle-aged men. *Diabetologia* 1987; **30**: 386–93.

44 Dowse GK, Spark RA, Mavo B, *et al.* Extraordinary prevalence of non-insulin-dependent diabetes mellitus and bimodal plasma glucose distribution in the Wanigela people of Papua New Guinea. *Med J Aust* 1994; **160**: 767–74.

45 Damsgaard EM, Froland A, Green A. Use of hospital services by elderly diabetics: the Frederica Study of diabetic and fasting hyperglycaemic patients aged 60–74 years. *Diabetic Med* 1987; **4**: 317–22.

46 Damsgaard EM, Froland A, Holm N. Ambulatory medical care for elderly diabetics: The Fredericia survey of diabetic and fasting hyperglycaemic subjects aged 60–74 years. *Diabetic Med* 1987; **4**: 534–8.

47 Entmacher PS, Sinnock P, Bostic E, Harris MI. Economic impact of diabetes. In: US Department of Health and Human Services (eds), *Diabetes in America: Diabetes data compiled 1984*. Bethesda: NIH Publication No. 85-1468, 1985; **XXXII**: 1–13.

48 Fox NA, Jacobs J. *Direct and Indirect Costs of Diabetes in the United States in 1987*. Alexandria: American Diabetes Association, 1988.

49 Huse DM, Oster G, Killen AR, *et al.* The economic costs of non-insulin-dependent diabetes mellitus. *JAMA* 1989; **262**: 2708–13.

50 Laing W, Williams R. *Diabetes, A Model for Health Care Management.* London: Office of Health Economics, 1989.

51 Barrett-Connor E, Orchard T. Diabetes and heart disease. In: US Department of Health and Human Services (eds), *Diabetes in America: Diabetes data compiled 1984*. Bethesda: NIH Publication No. 85-1468, 1985; **XVI**: 1–41.

52 Kuller LH, Dorman JS, Wolf PA. Cerebrovascular disease and diabetes. In: US Department of Health and Human Services. *Diabetes in America: Diabetes data compiled 1984*. Bethesda: NIH Publication No. 85-1468, 1985; **XVIII**: 1–18.

53 Palumbo PJ, Melton LJ. Peripheral vascular disease and diabetes. In: US Department of Health and Human Services (eds), *Diabetes in America: Diabetes data compiled 1984*. Bethesda: NIH Publication No. 85-1468, 1985; **XV**: 1–21.

2

Ageing and Glucose Tolerance

ROBERT W. STOUT

The Queen's University of Belfast, Northern Ireland

Hyperglycaemia and glucose intolerance in older people was first described in 1921[1] and has been confirmed on many occasions since[2]. Diabetes is a common condition in older people and becomes increasingly common with advancing age. As the number of people in the older age groups is rising rapidly, the number of those with diabetes will correspondingly increase. Although both insulin-dependent diabetes mellitus (IDDM) and non-insulin-dependent diabetes mellitus (NIDDM) may occur at any age, the prevalence of IDDM decreases rapidly with increasing age of onset of diabetes while the prevalence of NIDDM correspondingly increases[3] so that most diabetes in older people is NIDDM (Table 2.1). As in younger people morbidity from diabetes in elderly people is high and the prevalence of cardiovascular disease, hypertension, overweight and obesity, neurological and visual disease is higher in elderly diabetic subjects than non-diabetic people of the same age[4].

There is a high prevalence of undiagnosed diabetes in older people. An English survey showing that in people aged 65–85 years, the prevalence of known diabetes was 6.0% and the prevalence of undiagnosed diabetes was 3.3%[5]. The National Health and Nutrition Examination Survey (NHANES II) of 15 357 subjects from a stratified sample of households throughout the United States found a prevalence of previously diagnosed diabetes increasing from 1.1% in those aged 20–44 to 9.3% in those aged 66–74, and of undiagnosed diabetes increasing from 0.9% in those aged 20–44 to 8.4% in those aged 65–74 (Table 2.2; Figure 2.1). The prevalence of impaired glucose tolerance rose from 2.1% in those aged 20–44 to 9.2% in those aged 65–74 and blood glucose levels correspondingly increased with age[6]. The Coventry Diabetes Study found a high proportion of undetected diabetes

Diabetes in Old Age. Edited by P. Finucane and A. J. Sinclair
© 1995 John Wiley & Sons Ltd

Table 2.1. Insulin treatment by age in diabetic patients in Oxford[4]. Reproduced with permission

Age (years)	Insulin treatment (%)
20–59	58
60–69	28
70–79	21
80+	11

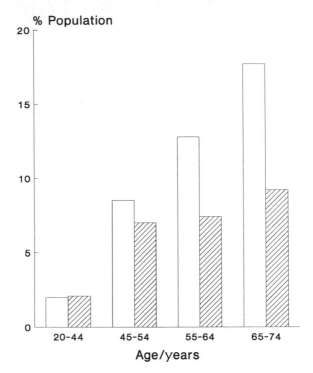

Figure 2.1. Prevalence of diabetes and impaired glucose tolerance in US population[6] (NHANES II 1976–80). □, diabetes; ▨ impaired glucose tolerance. Reproduced by permission of the American Diabetes Association Inc

in elderly subjects. It also found that the prevalence of diabetes in these older age groups was very much higher in those of South Asian origin than in Europeans[7].

While there have been many studies of the prevalence of diabetes and impaired glucose tolerance in elderly people, there have been few longitudinal studies. A Finnish study[8] of the natural history of glucose tolerance in elderly men found that 31% of the subjects with normal

Table 2.2. Prevalence of diabetes in the United States (NHANES II)[6]. Reproduced by permission of the American Diabetes Association Inc

Age (years)	Prevalence of diabetes (%)	
	Diagnosed	Undiagnosed
20–44	1.1	0.9
45–54	4.3	4.2
55–64	6.6	6.2
65–74	9.3	8.4

glucose tolerance at the initial test had either died or were otherwise unavailable after 5 years. Of the remainder, approximately 25% had either impaired glucose tolerance or diabetes during the follow-up. Higher body mass index (BMI) and blood glucose levels and a higher frequency of hypertension were present in those whose glucose tolerance deteriorated. The risk of glucose intolerance among obese subjects was about twice as high as that in non-obese subjects, but age itself had no impact on the development of glucose intolerance. Among those with impaired glucose tolerance, neither BMI nor age had an impact on the development of overt diabetes. Fifty-three per cent of the men with diabetes at baseline had either died or were otherwise unavailable after 5 years and of the remainder about one-half remained diabetic at follow-up and the other half had reverted either to impaired or to normal glucose tolerance. The development of impaired glucose tolerance is relatively common among elderly Finnish men and impaired glucose tolerance is an important risk factor for diabetes. Obesity seems to be associated with the initiation rather than the worsening of glucose intolerance while age itself did not appear to be a risk factor for diabetes in this group of elderly men.

The same Finnish study gave information on mortality of elderly diabetic men aged 65–84[9] (Table 2.3). The relative risk of death among diabetic men was 2.10, and among men with impaired glucose tolerance 1.17 compared with men with normal glucose tolerance. In those with diabetes, cardiovascular disease was the commonest cause of death, while deaths from cancer and other causes were also increased. Thus diabetes, even when mild and in elderly people, is a very important condition and increases mortality and morbidity.

Severe uncontrolled diabetes in elderly people also has a very high mortality; among the reasons for this is the presence of associated disease and the fact that elderly diabetics tend to present rather late[10]. Even in advanced old age diabetes remains a serious condition. Among people aged 85 years and over the mortality of those having previously diagnosed

Table 2.3. Age-adjusted 5-year mortality in men aged 65–84 years[9]. Reproduced by permission of Springer-Verlag GmbH & Co

	Cardiovascular deaths	All deaths
Glucose tolerance	Rate per 1000 men	
Normal	118	209
Impaired	134	234
Diabetes	184	364

diabetes was higher than that of those without diabetes. There was no difference in the mortality of those with newly diagnosed diabetes from that of non-diabetics. An unexplained finding of this study was the high mortality in non-diabetic subjects with the lowest blood sugar levels[11].

MECHANISMS OF DECREASED GLUCOSE TOLERANCE IN OLD AGE

A number of possible mechanisms for the glucose intolerance of ageing will be discussed (Table 2.4).

INSULIN SECRETION

Insulin secretion may be measured in the basal (fasting) state, or after stimulation by oral or intravenous glucose or by other secretagogues, such as arginine. There is some variation in the results of studies in insulin secretion in old age, probably related to differences in the selection of the experimental subjects, but in general there is no evidence that an absolute deficiency of insulin is responsible for the glucose intolerance of ageing[12]. Changes in the kinetics of insulin secretion have been described, and it has been suggested that insulin secretion in elderly people may be inadequate

Table 2.4. Mechanisms of decreased glucose tolerance in old age

Decreased insulin secretion
Peripheral insulin insensitivity
    insulin receptor
    postreceptor
Changes in other hormones

in comparison with the coexisting hyperglycaemia. This is discussed in more detail in the next section.

INSULIN RESISTANCE

Insulin resistance occurs when a normal amount of insulin produces a subnormal biological response[13]. It implies an impairment of insulin's action on its target tissues and may occur at different levels including insulin's interaction with its membrane receptor, or by intracellular mechanisms (postreceptor insulin resistance). Insulin resistance is often inferred when normal or slightly elevated levels of glucose occur simultaneously with high levels of insulin.

Insulin resistance may be measured directly by a number of methods, including clamp techniques, where glucose and insulin are infused, with frequent measurements of glucose levels allowing glycaemia to be maintained at a steady state, while insulin levels are maintained or changed, and measurements made of the delivery of glucose into the tissues, usually known as glucose disposal. These techniques may be used at normal levels of glucose (euglycaemic clamp) or high levels of glucose (hyperglycaemic clamp) and at different levels of insulin. Often infusion of radiolabelled glucose is also undertaken, allowing measurements to be made of insulin's action on the liver.

Another method uses computer modelling (the minimal model). This is based on a frequently sampled intravenous glucose tolerance test and a series of measurements can be made representing insulin output from the pancreas and insulin action on the periphery. Simultaneous studies of the clamp and the modelling techniques have shown that they give comparable results. Both techniques have been used in studies of insulin resistance in relation to age.

Studies Using Clamp Techniques

In general these studies have found tissue insensitivity to insulin in older people[14]. In a study of 17 elderly (mean age 69 years) and 27 younger (mean age 37 years) non-obese subjects[15], glucose and insulin levels following a 75 g oral glucose load were elevated in the elderly subjects compared with the young and this in itself suggested insulin resistance. The glucose disposal rate during a euglycaemic clamp in the elderly subjects was considerably lower than that in the younger subjects and the severity of the abnormality in carbohydrate tolerance was directly correlated with the degree of peripheral insulin resistance. As had been shown earlier[12] insulin binding to isolated fat cells and monocytes was similar in the elderly and young subjects, suggesting that the defect of insulin action was postreceptor in site. Further studies using higher levels of insulin and inspection of the dose–response curve confirmed the presence of a postreceptor defect. There was also some decrease in insulin's ability to suppress hepatic glucose output in the older subjects. The differences between the young and elderly could not be accounted for by differences in adiposity and it seemed unlikely that they were due to changes in physical activity.

In the same year a similar study[16] showed that in 17 young (age range 22–37 years) and 10 elderly (age range 63–77 years) non-obese male subjects, who had clamp studies, the dose–response curve to changing insulin concentrations was shifted to the right in the older subjects suggesting a decreased sensitivity of the tissues to insulin. Insulin binding to receptors on circulating monocytes was the same in the young and the old. These studies also suggested a postreceptor defect in insulin action. The results did not seem to be accounted for by changes in adiposity.

A contrary view came from an Italian study where insulin resistance was found in the older subjects but a decrease in the number of insulin receptors in adipose cells was also found. Thus, this study suggests that the insulin resistance of ageing is at least partly explained by a fall in the number of insulin receptors[17]. In another study[18] fasting blood glucose was similar in young and old subjects but 2 h blood glucose and glycosylated haemoglobin were higher in the older group. There was no significant difference in the groups in serum insulin or C-peptide levels at any point during the oral glucose tolerance test (OGTT). Early insulin secretion, related to the glucose stimulus, did not differ between the groups and free fatty acid (FFA) levels suppressed normally. Insulin-stimulated glucose turnover, as a measurement of peripheral tissue insulin sensitivity, was similar in both groups and insulin suppression of hepatic glucose production, reflecting hepatic sensitivity to insulin, was greater in the older group. Thus, neither decreased insulin secretion nor changes in hepatic or peripheral tissue insulin sensitivity were demonstrated as causes for the deterioration of glucose tolerance. There was a slight reduction of insulin-stimulated glucose disposal combined with a slight reduction in the late insulin response to oral glucose. It is difficult to reconcile these results with those of other studies and it is likely that selection of patients may be related to the differences between the studies that have been reported.

While the hyperinsulinaemia that occurs in older people is thought to be a compensatory phenomenon related to the need for higher concentrations of insulin to overcome the insulin resistance that occurs with ageing, other explanations have been put forward. For example, it has been suggested that there is a decrease in the metabolic clearance of insulin associated with ageing[19] or that there may be a defect in the feedback inhibition of insulin secretion from the pancreas in older people[20].

The possibility that the mechanism of the glucose intolerance of ageing is insulin resistance at a postreceptor level resulting in both reduced glucose uptake and impaired intracellular glucose metabolism was investigated in more detail by a study of intracellular glucose metabolism by a method which equalized glucose uptake[21]. The subjects were carefully chosen to be healthy and had identical glucose and insulin profiles to OGTTs. Thus, elderly subjects without hyperglycaemia were studied. The results showed that at equivalent basal glucose uptake, muscle glycogen synthase activity was similar in young and old but whole body rates of glucose oxidation were reduced in the elderly subjects. This could be overcome by increasing the concentration of insulin in the infusion. Plasma FFA concentrations, fat oxidation and protein oxidation were similar under all study conditions. When glucose uptake was normalized, glucose oxidation was reduced in the submaximal but not maximal range of glucose uptake. In other words, the glucose oxidation capacity was unimpaired and skeletal muscle glycogen synthase activity was similar to that of controls. Thus, impaired intracellular glucose metabolism contributes to the insulin resistance of ageing independent of a defect in glucose uptake through decreased sensitivity of whole body glucose oxidation to insulin stimulation. In contrast, skeletal muscle glycogen synthase activity was normal and did not contribute to the insulin resistance of ageing.

Although insulin resistance is a common feature in old age, it may not be universally distributed among all tissues. A detailed study showed that the age-related impairment of glucose disposal persists at low levels of insulin, similar to those found physiologically[22]. The reduction of the hepatic glucose output in response to insulin does not differ with age but occurs more rapidly in elderly people and the effects of insulin on suppression of lipolysis are unaltered in elderly adults. The resistance to the action of insulin in lowering blood glucose levels also occurred in relation to branched-chain amino acids[23]. The relationship of ageing to insulin action, which is found in the disposal of glucose, is not present in amino acid metabolism[24].

Glucose uptake occurs by two mechanisms. Insulin-mediated glucose uptake, which occurs primarily in muscle and fat, and non-insulin-mediated glucose uptake which occurs in both insulin sensitive and insulin insensitive tissues, primarily the central nervous system. In states of insulin deficiency non-insulin-mediated glucose uptake was impaired in elderly subjects; insulin secretion was suppressed and blood glucose levels were maintained at normal levels[25]. However, during conditions of hyperglycaemia, non-insulin-mediated glucose uptake was similar in young and elderly subjects. The age-associated impairment of non-insulin-mediated glucose uptake in the basal state may explain in part the increase in fasting glucose with age. It has been suggested that the effects of age on energy metabolism are different in males and females, with impaired stimulation of non-oxidative glucose metabolism by insulin with age only observed in males[26].

An alternative explanation for impaired insulin action in elderly people has recently been suggested[27]. In a group of subjects aged 75 years and over a euglycaemic hyperinsulinaemic clamp study revealed a significant reduction in glucose disappearance rate, total body glucose disposal and non-oxidative glucose metabolism. In the elderly subjects all of these changes correlated with one another, and the production of free radicals had a significant relationship with total body glucose disposal and non-oxidated glucose metabolism. There is a considerable amount of interest in the possibility that free radicals may be associated with many of the changes which occur physiologically with advancing age and this study suggests that the glucose intolerance found in elderly people may also be related to free radical production.

Modelling Techniques

A study of the factors responsible for the glucose intolerance of ageing used 10 young (aged 18–36 years old) and 10 older (57–82 years old) men of normal body weight[28]. Frequently sampled intravenous glucose tolerance tests were performed and the data analysed by a computer program using the minimal model approach. Beta-cell responsiveness was also assessed by measuring plasma insulin responses to arginine injections at three levels of glycaemia. Compared with the younger men the older men were glucose intolerant and this was due to both a beta-cell defect and insulin resistance. These changes were unrelated to differences in body fat. On the other hand there was little evidence for changes in insulin clearance or insulin-independent glucose disappearance. Further studies by the same group found that the changes that occurred in elderly men could be decreased by increasing the amount of carbohydrate in the diet[29].

An Italian study using the minimal model technique found no differences between fasting levels of glucose and insulin in young and elderly subjects[30]. The C-peptide concentration was lower in elderly people suggesting a reduction in insulin secretion. Insulin levels seemed to be maintained by a reduction in the hepatic extraction of insulin.

Other Methods

A number of studies have looked at insulin activity in relation to ageing by different techniques. The uptake of radiolabelled glucose into forearm muscle was found to be lower in elderly subjects aged 70–83 years than in younger or middle-aged subjects at similar insulin concentrations[31]. There was no difference in the binding of insulin to peripheral monocytes in respect of either receptor numbers or affinity in elderly and middle-aged subjects. This study, therefore, is further evidence for postreceptor resistance to insulin's effects in old age. Another isotope study came to similar conclusions[32].

The effect of ageing on glucose-mediated glucose disposal and transport was studied in young and elderly subjects using a clamp technique and also by studying glucose metabolism in isolated fat cells from the same subjects[33]. Whole body glucose disposal was decreased by about one-third in the elderly subjects in the presence of similar concentrations of insulin. Similarly, insulin-stimulated glucose transport in isolated fat cells was reduced in the elderly subjects. The results suggest that the insulin resistance in ageing is due to a reduction in the capacity of the glucose uptake system while the affinity of glucose utilization is unchanged. The greatest decrease in glucose transport in isolated fat cells occurred in the subjects with the greatest decrease of insulin-stimulated glucose disposal using the clamp studies[34].

The effect of age on the insulin-mediated glucose handling was studied in another way by using an intravenous–oral modification of the euglycaemic insulin clamp technique[35]. This allowed the posthepatic delivery of oral glucose to be studied. It was found that normal ageing is associated with a delayed but overall equal posthepatic delivery of oral glucose and reinforces the role of impaired peripheral utilization as the primary mechanism of glucose intolerance of ageing.

In general, ageing is associated with high circulating insulin levels, both in the fasting state and after glucose stimulation, despite the fact that glucose levels are normal or slightly elevated. While this indicates a state of insulin resistance, it does not clarify whether the high insulin levels are due to increased secretion of insulin or decreased clearance of insulin or both. It is difficult to measure insulin secretion directly in humans as the portal circulation is inaccessible. However, it can be studied indirectly by measuring the secretion kinetics of C-peptide, the residual peptide from the proinsulin molecule which is not cleared by the liver. In a group of young (mean age 30) and elderly (mean age 66) subjects, who did not have diabetes, the fasting and post-glucose serum glucose and insulin levels were higher in the elderly subjects, but endogenous insulin clearance, under both basal and physiological conditions, was unchanged by ageing and insulin secretion was increased[36]. However, the fact that despite hyperinsulinaemia the blood glucose levels remained elevated, indicated an impairment of insulin secretion in relation to the glucose levels. Thus, appropriate hyperinsulinaemia as compensation for insulin resistance in elderly subjects does not occur.

Another study of the mechanism of glucose intolerance on ageing was performed by comparing the responses with the ingestion of a glucose load in young (20–23 year old) and elderly (73–80 year old) normal men using isotope techniques[37]. Although fasting glucose and insulin concentrations were similar in young and elderly subjects, there was marked glucose intolerance in the elderly and insulin levels after glucose were also somewhat higher in the elderly subjects. Suppression of hepatic glucose output after a glucose load was similar in young and elderly but delayed in the elderly subjects. Glucose absorption was also delayed with age. The biggest difference between the young and elderly was in glucose disappearance which was markedly reduced with age, the elderly demonstrating peripheral insulin insensitivity. The deficit in peripheral glucose disappearance was about twofold greater than the deficit of the fall in hepatic glucose output. Thus, there is impaired peripheral glucose utilization in the elderly while the delayed fall in hepatic glucose output may be a consequence of the delay in insulin secretion.

Young and elderly patients with impaired glucose tolerance were compared with an elderly group with normal glucose tolerance[38]. These were highly selected subjects and are not comparable with the usual studies of healthy elderly people with slightly abnormal blood glucose levels. In the young and elderly subjects with abnormal glucose tolerance there were no differences in the basal hepatic glucose output or in glucose turnover. The insulin response to oral glucose was also similar. Compared with the elderly patients with normal glucose tolerance, those with abnormal glucose tolerance were insulin resistant and also had a lower early insulin response to glucose. The suppression of hepatic glucose output in response to insulin was rather greater in the elderly than the young subjects. Thus, elderly patients with abnormal glucose tolerance are similar to younger patients with abnormal glucose tolerance, except for the fact that the older subjects have an increased sensitivity to insulin suppression of hepatic glucose output. The authors suggested that both insulin resistance and reduced early insulin secretion are important determinants of impaired glucose tolerance in elderly subjects. There was no difference in maximum oxygen uptake between the young and elderly abnormal glucose tolerance groups but the elderly subjects with normal glucose tolerance were physically fitter than the elderly group with abnormal glucose tolerance. There was a significant correlation between the measure of insulin action and the measure of physical training. There was little change in the lean body mass across the age ranges studied.

A small study of young and elderly healthy men matched for height and weight showed no difference in leg blood flow but a close negative correlation of body fat with glucose uptake and glucose oxidation[39]. In contrast age did not correlate totally with any measure of glucose metabolism.

Insulin action on lipid metabolism is also impaired[13]. There is inhibition of lipolysis, with increased FFA levels and increased FFA oxidation. This may result in decreased glucose oxidation via the so-called glucose/FFA cycle and hence contribute to hyperglycaemia.

Conclusions

These studies suggest that the abnormal glucose tolerance in elderly people is multifactorial in nature. There is general agreement that decreased insulin sensitivity in the peripheral tissues occurs and general, although not universal, acceptance is that this is due to a postreceptor defect. Whether there is a hereditary element to the insulin resistance of ageing is unknown. There are no age-related differences in receptor number or insulin binding to peripheral cells. There also appears to be a decrease or delay in insulin-induced suppression of hepatic glucose output. Although insulin levels are higher in older than younger people, there seems to be a deficit in insulin secretion from the pancreas and this is possibly compensated for by decreased metabolic clearance of insulin in the peripheral tissues. While adiposity, diet and decreased physical exercise may have exacerbated these changes, there appears to be a phenomenon related to ageing itself. This may be accentuated or brought out by the other factors.

COUNTER-REGULATORY HORMONES

A possible explanation for glucose intolerance in elderly people is that there is an increased secretion of hormones which increase glucose levels or which interact with, modify or oppose the action of insulin.

Glucagon

Glucagon secreted by the alpha cells of the pancreatic islets, has actions which are the opposite of many of those of insulin. In particular raised glucagon levels cause increases in plasma glucose by increasing glucose released from the liver. A study of 44 healthy volunteers aged 22–81 found that although there was an increase in adiposity with increasing age, there was no effect of age on fasting levels of glucose, glucagon or insulin[40]. Glucose disappearance rates following intravenous glucose were significantly lower in the elderly subjects but there was no difference in glucose-stimulated insulin release and insulin responses after arginine infusion were the same in the young and old subjects. The release of glucagon in response to an arginine infusion was also unchanged by advancing age.

A later study of glucagon in relation to ageing, in which three groups of subjects—young (24 years), middle-aged (31 years), and older (62 years)—were investigated, showed that fasting glucagon levels were unchanged in the different age groups[41]. The suppression of glucagon by both hyperglycaemia and hyperinsulinaemia was the same in younger and older subjects as was the secretion of glucagon in response to alanine infusion and the metabolic clearance rate of glucagon. However, the liver was more sensitive to glucagon in the older subjects as during a continuous glucagon infusion increases in plasma glucose concentration were greater in the older than the younger subjects as was the rise in glucose concentration measured during an infusion of labelled glucose.

There are differences in the structure of glucagon molecules secreted from the gastrointestinal tract and from the pancreas. Studies of fasting glucagon levels and glucagon responses to an OGTT in which the two species were separately measured showed no differences in the responses of the younger and older subjects[42]. In a group of subjects aged 20–42 compared with another group aged 66–77, infusion of insulin to produce a blood glucose level at or below 3.3 mmol/l resulted in no difference in either basal or maximum levels of glucagon in the young and old subjects[43].

Overall, there is little evidence that changes in the secretion or action of glucagon is responsible for the glucose intolerance of ageing.

Growth Hormone

Growth hormone is a hyperglycaemic hormone whose secretion is stimulated by hypoglycaemia. In a study comparing young and old subjects, there was no difference in either basal or stimulated growth hormone levels in response to an infusion of insulin resulting in hypoglycaemia[43]. Experiments in animals suggest that there is no change in the sensitivity to the hyperglycaemic action of growth hormone with ageing[44]. The nocturnal growth hormone response is slightly higher in the older subjects[45].

Growth hormone produces its action by means of another peptide, insulin-like growth factor 1 (IGF-1), which has some actions similar to those of insulin. A study of 107 subjects of age range 17–83 years showed a significant inverse correlation of age and IGF-1 in both males and females. IGF-1 also had a negative relationship with body weight, which was independent of the effect of age[46,47]. The significance of this finding in relation to the carbohydrate intolerance of ageing is unknown.

Gastric Inhibitory Polypeptide

While the exact role and actions of gastric inhibitory polypeptide (GIP) remain unknown, it is a possible mediator of insulin secretion. GIP is secreted from the gastrointestinal tract in response to a number of nutrients and acts on the pancreatic beta cells causing or potentiating insulin secretion in response to oral glucose. Mean fasting and post-glucose GIP levels did not differ in young and old subjects[42]. However, in the elderly subjects, post-glucose GIP levels were higher in females than males. A study of the response of GIP to oral glucose was made in a group of non-diabetic young, middle-aged and old subjects, of age range 19–84 years[48]. In the study a hyperglycaemic glucose clamp technique was used to raise glucose loads to 125 mg/dl above basal for 2 h and this was followed by oral glucose ingestion. There were no significant age-related differences in the fasting plasma GIP levels or the levels during the intravenous glucose infusion. The peak level after glucose ingestion was not different in young, middle-aged and old subjects and differences in the relative increases in plasma GIP were not statistically different. A measure of the beta-cell sensitivity to GIP in relation to insulin secretion was undertaken by using the rise in plasma insulin after glucose ingestion. In the elderly subjects beta-cell sensitivity to GIP was lower than in young or middle-aged subjects and across the entire age range there was a significant negative correlation between age and beta-cell sensitivity to GIP. In contrast there was no age difference in any insulin response to infused glucose. A reduced beta-cell sensitivity to GIP with ageing may contribute to the glucose intolerance of ageing but further work is needed to clarify this.

Catecholamines

Catecholamines can impair glucose tolerance by multiple mechanisms including inhibition of insulin secretion, stimulation of hepatic glucose production and impairment of glucose disposal[49]. Alpha- and beta-adrenergic receptor stimulation have different actions on both insulin secretion and insulin effects. Adrenaline and noradrenaline are important in glucose counter-regulation, particularly in acute hypoglycaemia. Basal adrenaline levels were similar in young and old, as were increases in adrenaline[43], in response to insulin-induced hypoglycaemia. In contrast fasting noradrenaline levels were elevated in the elderly subjects as were the levels following insulin-induced hypoglycaemia but the change between fasting and stimulated levels was the same in young and old and the levels of noradrenaline reached in the study are unlikely to result in hyperglycaemia. Night-time levels of adrenaline and cortisol were no different in young and old subjects although noradrenaline levels were slightly higher in the older subjects[45].

In a group of young and older subjects, plasma catecholamine levels were measured before and for 2 h after the administration of 100 g of oral glucose, before and after 3-day weight maintaining high or low carbohydrate formula diets[49]. The elderly men had higher fasting noradrenaline levels than the younger men and these rose slightly after oral glucose. Adrenaline levels were similar in young and old and the decrease after glucose was similar in young and old. There was no relationship between catecholamine levels and the degree of glucose tolerance, which was impaired in the older subjects. A high carbohydrate diet improved glucose tolerance in both old and young subjects but this was not associated with consistent changes in plasma catecholamine levels. It was concluded that the glucose intolerance of ageing cannot be explained by changes in plasma catecholamine levels nor are the age-related changes in plasma catecholamines caused by changes in dietary carbohydrate. The responsiveness of the pancreatic islet cells to beta-adrenergic stimulation does not appear to be altered with ageing. This contrasts with the reduced responsiveness of cardiovascular adrenergic stimulation in older people[50].

Adrenaline has both alpha- and beta-adrenergic actions and inhibits insulin secretion in both animals and humans. A study looked at the relationship between ageing and sensitivity to the effects of catecholamines on measurements of glucose tolerance and insulin secretion using the minimal model system[51]. In both young and old subjects small concentrations of adrenaline reduced glucose-mediated glucose disposal and impaired the acute phase insulin secretion in response to intravenous glucose. Older subjects had delayed recovery from the adrenergic-induced hyperglycaemia. Increased sensitivity to adrenergic activity in elderly people may be related to the increased frequency of stress hyperglycaemia and hyperosmolar hyperglycaemic non-ketotic coma in elderly patients. These may be particularly important in elderly patients with an underlying impairment of carbohydrate metabolism.

Human Pancreatic Polypeptide (HPP)

Both fasting and post-glucose HPP levels are higher in elderly than young subjects[42] although the volume and weight of PP cells does not vary with age[52]. The significance of this is unclear as the metabolic role of HPP remains uncertain.

Conclusions

There is no consistent evidence that the glucose intolerance of ageing is due to changes in the secretion of hormones, which influence carbohydrate metabolism or insulin secretion and action.

OTHER FACTORS AFFECTING GLUCOSE TOLERANCE IN OLDER PEOPLE

A number of features which commonly occur in older people may influence glucose tolerance (Table 2.5).

Table 2.5. Factors affecting glucose tolerance in older people

---

Increased body fat
Physical inactivity
Reduced dietary carbohydrate
Impaired renal function
Hypokalaemia
Increased sympathetic nervous system activity
Drugs

OBESITY

Two physiological changes, which may relate to impaired glucose tolerance, tend to occur as people grow older: obesity and a decrease in physical activity. With advancing age there is an overall increase in body weight and a change in the distribution of body fat, particularly an increased central distribution. There is controversy over the roles of obesity and decreased physical activity in the glucose intolerance and insulin resistance of ageing.

Glucose tolerance tests, measures of insulin resistance, body weight and maximal oxygen uptake as a measure of physical fitness were performed in groups of young and older subjects[53]. The young subjects had normal glucose tolerance and low insulin levels while the older subjects had glucose levels ranging from no different from those of the young subjects to progressively abnormal and reaching those diagnostic of NIDDM. Insulin levels in the older subjects ranged from elevated to deficient. Body fat content was greater in all the groups of older subjects than the young and tended to be highest in those with NIDDM. The subjects with the higher glucose levels also tended to have more central adipose tissue. The older subjects tended to have larger skinfold thicknesses and girths, particularly at central body sites but those who were insulin sensitive had no difference in the measures of adiposity than the young subjects. Maximal oxygen capacity was also higher in the younger than the older subjects. During a euglycaemic insulin clamp the glucose disposal rate in the older subjects with normal glucose tolerance and those with insulin deficiency was similar to that of the young group but was reduced in the groups with high normal and impaired glucose tolerance and by 60% in the NIDDM group. Correlations between the various measurements showed that insulin sensitivity was significantly associated with age, maximal oxygen capacity, body fat content and a number of measures of central obesity. Waist circumference alone accounted for more than 40% of the variance of insulin sensitivity among subjects studied whereas age explained only 10–20% of the variance and less than 2% of the variance when the effects of waist circumference were statistically controlled. Thus, the study showed that insulin resistance was more closely related to measures of regional adiposity than to age. Insulin sensitivity was normal in about one-third of older men and women. Older subjects with normal insulin sensitivity had either normal glucose tolerance or glucose intolerance as a result of insulin deficiency and there were little differences in measures of regional adipose tissue between the young and older insulin sensitive subjects. In contrast the insulin resistant older subjects, whose glucose tolerance ranged from high normal to mild diabetic, had larger skinfold thicknesses and circumferences than the young and older insulin sensitive subjects, particularly in the central region of the body. Regional adiposity rather than age may be the more important determinant of insulin resistance and the associated glucose intolerance in older people.

The relative contributions of ageing and obesity to the glucose intolerance of ageing were studied in a group of obese and non-obese premenopausal (age 27–32 years) and postmenopausal women (age 62–65 years)[54]. The glucose levels 30 min after oral glucose in the postmenopausal women were higher than those in the premenopausal women when both non-obese and obese groups were compared. Insulin levels were also higher in the postmenopausal women, although not significantly so in those who were obese. The peripheral glucose disappearance rates and endogenous glucose production rates were comparable in the four groups. However, higher insulin infusion rates suppressed endogenous glucose production in all groups but more so in the non-obese than obese, irrespective of age. These results show that peripheral insulin resistance occurs in both obese and in ageing women. However, some differences were identified between the response to obesity and ageing, namely that the endogenous glucose production is normally suppressed by insulin in ageing whereas suppression is impaired in obese subjects. Ageing did not appear to amplify the insulin resistance of obesity.

Another attempt to study whether ageing was an independent determinant of glucose tolerance used 742 men and women aged 17–92 years from the Baltimore Longitudinal Study of Aging[55]. Diseases or drugs known to influence glucose tolerance were carefully excluded. With increasing age both men and women showed increasing obesity, a shift in fat distribution to the abdomen from the hips, decreasing physical fitness and decreasing glucose tolerance. In multivariate analysis age accounted for 15–20% of the 2 h glucose concentration in men and women and remained independent when other characteristics were taken into account. The data were further analysed by dividing the population into three age groups: young, aged 17–39 years; middle-aged, aged 40–59 years; and old, aged 60–92 years. A progressive increase in the 2 h glucose level was found and all age differences were highly significant. However, when adjustment was made for age-related changes in the amount and distribution of body fat and in physical fitness levels, the age differences in glucose tolerance between the young and middle-aged men and women disappeared but the old men and women still showed a significant decline in glucose tolerance compared with middle-aged or young subjects.

A study of 1300 men and women aged 65–74 years in Finland looked at the relationship of obesity and a family history of diabetes to the prevalence of diabetes and impaired glucose tolerance[56]. Obesity and central adiposity doubled the prevalence of impaired glucose tolerance and NIDDM. A family history added further to the prevalence. Nevertheless they explained only 10% of the variance of the 2 h blood glucose levels on multiple regression analysis. Thus, while obesity may increase the prevalence of abnormalities of glucose tolerance in older people, it is not the main or major cause of this disorder.

In 77 men aged between 46 and 73 years there was a significant negative relationship between age and maximum oxygen capacity and with the glucose level 120 min after glucose[57]. Some subjects were put on a diet to cause weight loss and others were exercised. Weight loss produced a reduction in both glucose and insulin levels whereas exercise training raised plasma insulin levels in the fasting state but did not change insulin or glucose levels during an OGTT. Weight loss rather than exercise testing were associated with the greatest improvement in metabolic function in these obese elderly men. Body composition seemed to be a more important determinant of metabolic function than either age or exercise. Other studies quoted earlier in this chapter found no relationship between the insulin resistance of ageing and adiposity[15,16].

Conclusion

Obesity and increased abdominal adiposity are common in old age and increase both blood glucose levels and insulin resistance. Their role in the glucose intolerance of ageing appears to be to accentuate an age-related disorder.

PHYSICAL ACTIVITY

Ageing is associated with a decrease in the amount of physical activity with a further decrease in the very aged[58] and measurements of physical fitness show that this is decreased in older people[59]. Many elderly people reduce their physical activity as they get older, sometimes because of conditions such as arthritis or neurological disorders. Physical activity is closely related to carbohydrate metabolism and insulin action. A 12-month endurance training programme in 11 healthy men and women aged 63 years resulted in no change in glucose tolerance, which had been normal initially, but a considerable decrease in insulin secretion[60]. This suggests an increased sensitivity to insulin with exercise. In another study older untrained people had higher glucose levels and insulin levels than those who were trained[61]. Exercise resulted in improved glucose tolerance and insulin sensitivity.

In a study to evaluate the effect of physical activity on insulin action in healthy men aged between 60 and 75 years, 13 older subjects, not exercising regularly, were compared with seven older subjects who took at least 45 min swimming, cycling or walking at least three times per week[62]. There was no difference in either the BMI or the percentage body fat between the two groups. However, the maximum oxygen consumption (V_{O_2max}) was higher in those who exercised regularly as was insulin-stimulated glucose uptake. There was a direct relationship between maximum aerobic capacity and *in vivo* insulin action which was independent of either BMI or percentage body fat.

Although insulin resistance is a very common finding in elderly people, even in those with normal glucose tolerance, this can be partially reversed by physical training[63]. This effect is independent of changes in weight or body composition and can be seen after a moderate exercise programme lasting 12 weeks. Whether some of the insulin resistance of ageing is related to a more sedentary life-style is therefore worthy of consideration. Young athletes have the same glucose disposal rates in response to insulin as elderly athletes[64]. Thus, physical training in elderly people may improve insulin resistance at the postreceptor insulin binding site, which is normally impaired by the ageing process.

Glucose transport through cell membranes is mediated by glucose transporter proteins of which GLUT-4 appears to be the most important in muscle. In a study of middle-aged men it was found that in trained men plasma insulin levels during the glucose tolerance test were lower but there were no differences in glucose responses. However, the GLUT-4 protein content was approximately twice as high in the trained men. This suggests that the glucose transporter protein levels were increased in conjunction with insulin sensitivity in chronically exercised trained middle-aged men[65].

A long-term study in Sweden in middle-aged men who had early diabetes or impaired glucose tolerance, showed that diet resulting in weight loss and regular physical exercise resulted in considerable improvement in glucose tolerance and remission of diabetes[66]. Insulin levels were also reduced and mortality was lower in the treated group. Similar studies have not taken place in old people but it would seem likely that at least some of the glucose intolerance and mild diabetes in old age might be prevented by attention to body weight and to exercise.

FAMILY HISTORY OF DIABETES

In younger age groups, a family history of diabetes is often found, particularly in those with NIDDM[6]. There have been few studies of family history in relation to diabetes in old age, but a Finnish study[56] of subjects aged 65–74 years found an interaction between obesity, family history and an increased prevalence of impaired glucose tolerance or NIDDM. Nevertheless, obesity, central fat distribution and a family history of diabetes explained only 10% of the variance in 2 h plasma glucose levels in a multivariate analysis.

OTHER FACTORS

Reduced Dietary Carbohydrate

Although it has been shown that some of the metabolic changes that occur in older people can be reversed by a high carbohydrate diet[29], there is no evidence on the role of diet in the glucose intolerance of ageing. Magnesium administration also improved glucose and insulin abnormalities in old age[67].

Impaired Renal Function and Hypokalaemia

Renal function tends to decline with advancing age and this may contribute to carbohydrate intolerance. However, in most of the studies which show carbohydrate intolerance and insulin resistance in older people, renal impairment has been carefully excluded in the subjects studied. Electrolyte abnormalities have also been excluded.

Increased Sympathetic Nervous System Activity

The possible role of catecholamines in the glucose intolerance of ageing has been discussed elsewhere in this chapter, and a significant role excluded. Elderly people are less sensitive to the effects of insulin on sympathetic nervous system activity[68].

Drugs

Elderly people have a high level of drug ingestion[69], and of the drugs used, the commonest are diuretics. Thiazide diuretics cause glucose intolerance and insulin resistance[70]. However, the use of such drugs has been excluded in the selection of subjects for the investigations which have shown glucose intolerance and insulin resistance. Similar mechanisms are involved in the glucose intolerance precipitated by corticosteroids whether ingested therapeutically, or of endogenous origin as in Cushing's disease.

Conclusions

All of the factors discussed above may contribute to or worsen the glucose intolerance of ageing. However, they do not account for the occurrence of glucose intolerance in older people.

CONCLUSIONS

In older people a metabolic disorder consisting of glucose intolerance, peripheral insulin resistance at the postreceptor level, impaired insulin secretion and decreased hepatic insulin sensitivity occurs (Figure 2.2). This may be ameliorated by increased physical activity, and is made worse by increased body weight and abdominal adiposity. Other factors which are common in older people, including impaired renal function and ingestion of diuretic drugs, will also worsen glucose tolerance in old age.

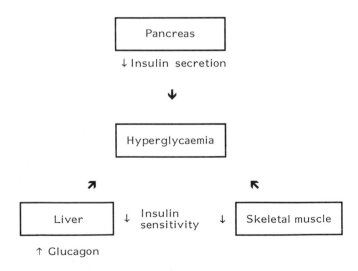

Figure 2.2. Diagram showing the influence of different factors on hyperglycaemia in old age

REFERENCES

1 Spence JC. Some observations on sugar tolerance with special reference to variations found at different ages. *QJ Med* 1921; **14**: 314–26.
2 Davidson MB. The effect of aging on carbohydrate metabolism: a review of the English literature and a practical approach to the diagnosis of diabetes mellitus in the elderly. *Metabolism* 1979; **28**: 688–705.
3 Laakso M, Pyorala K. Age of onset and type of diabetes. *Diabetes Care* 1985; **8**: 114–17.
4 Neil HAW, Thompson AV, Thorogood M, Fowler GH, Mann JI. Diabetes in the elderly: the Oxford Community Diabetes Study. *Diabetic Med* 1989; **6**: 608–13.
5 Croxson SCM, Burden AC, Bodlington M, Botha JL. The prevalence of diabetes in elderly people. *Diabetic Med* 1991; **8**: 28–31.
6 Harris MI, Hadden WC, Knowler WC, Bennett PH. Prevalence of diabetes and impaired glucose tolerance and plasma glucose levels in US population aged 20–74 yr. *Diabetes* 1987; **36**: 523–34.
7 Simmons D, Williams DRR. Diabetes in the elderly: an under-diagnosed condition. *Diabetic Med* 1993; **10**: 264–6.
8 Stengard JH, Pekkanen J, Tuomilehto J, *et al.* Changes in glucose tolerance among elderly Finnish men during a five-year follow-up: The Finnish cohorts of the Seven Countries Study. *Diabete Metab* 1993; **19**: 121–9.
9 Stengard JH, Tuomilehto J, Pekkanen J, *et al.* Diabetes mellitus, impaired glucose tolerance and mortality among elderly men: the Finnish cohorts of the Seven Countries Study. *Diabetologia* 1992; **35**: 760–5.
10 Gale EAM, Dornan TL, Tattersall RB. Severely uncontrolled diabetes in the over-fifties. *Diabetologia* 1981; **21**: 25–8.
11 Kaltiala KS, Haavisto MV, Heikinheimo RJ, Mattila KJ, Rajala SA. Blood glucose and diabetes mellitus predicting mortality in persons aged 85 years or above. *Age Ageing* 1987; **16**: 165–70.
12 McConnell JG, Buchanan KD, Ardill J, Stout RW. Glucose tolerance in the elderly: the role of insulin and its receptor. *Eur J Clin Invest* 1982; **12**: 55–61.
13 Bell PM. Insulin resistance. In: Stout RW (ed.), *Diabetes and Atherosclerosis.* Dordrecht: Kluwer Academic Publishers, 1992: 27–51.
14 De Fronzo RA. Glucose intolerance and aging. Evidence for tissue insensitivity to insulin. *Diabetes* 1979; **28**: 1095–101.
15 Fink RI, Kolterman OG, Griffin J, Olefsky JM. Mechanisms of insulin resistance in aging. *J Clin Invest* 1983; **71**: 1523–35.
16 Rowe JW, Minaker KL, Pallotta JA, Flier JS. Characterization of the insulin resistance of aging. *J Clin Invest* 1983; **71**: 1581–7.
17 Pagano G, Cassader M, Cavallo-Perin P, *et al.* Insulin resistance in the aged: a quantitative evaluation of *in vivo* insulin sensitivity and *in vitro* glucose transport. *Metabolism* 1984; **33**: 976–81.
18 Broughton DL, James OWF, Alberti KGMM, Taylor R. Peripheral and hepatic insulin sensitivity in healthy elderly human subjects. *Eur J Clin Invest* 1991; **21**: 13–21.
19 Minaker KL, Rowe JW, Tonino R, Pallotta JA. Influence of age on clearance of insulin in man. *Diabetes* 1982; **31**: 851–5.
20 Fink RI, Revers RR, Kolterman OG, Olefsky JM. The metabolic clearance of insulin and the feedback inhibition of insulin secretion are altered with aging. *Diabetes* 1985; **34**: 275–80.

21 Gumbiner B, Thorburn AW, Ditzler TM, Bulacan F, Henry RR. Role of impaired intracellular glucose metabolism in the insulin resistance of aging. *Metabolism* 1992; **41**: 1115–21.

22 Meneilly GS, Minaker KL, Elahi D, Rowe JW. Insulin action in aging man: evidence for tissue-specific differences at low physiologic insulin levels. *J Gerontol* 1987; **42**: 196–201.

23 Marchesini G, Cassarani S, Checchia GA, et al. Insulin resistance in aged man: relationship between impaired glucose tolerance and decreased insulin activity on branched-chain amino acids. *Metabolism* 1987; **36**: 1096–100.

24 Fukagawa NK, Minaker KL, Rowe JW, Matthews DE, Bier DM, Young VR. Glucose and amino acid metabolism in aging man: differential effects of insulin. *Metabolism* 1988; **37**: 371–7.

25 Meneilly GS, Elahi D, Minaker KL, Sclater AL, Rowe JW. Impairment of non insulin-mediated glucose disposal in the elderly. *J Clin Endocrinol Metab* 1989; **63**: 566–71.

26 Franssila-Kallunki A, Schalin-Jantti C, Groop L. Effect of gender on insulin resistance associated with aging. *Am J Physiol* 1992; **263**: E780–5

27 Paolisso G, D'Amore A, Di Maro G, et al. Evidence for a relationship between free radicals and insulin action in the elderly. *Metabolism* 1993; **42**: 659–63.

28 Chen M, Bergman RN, Pacini G, Porte D Jr. Pathogenesis of age-related glucose intolerance in man: insulin resistance and decreased beta-cell function. *J Clin Endocrinol Metab* 1985; **60**: 13–20.

29 Chen M, Bergman RN, Porte D Jr. Insulin resistance and beta-cell dysfunction in aging: The importance of dietary carbohydrate. *J Clin Endocrinol Metab* 1988; **67**: 951–7.

30 Pacini G, Beccaro F, Valerio A, Nosadini R, Crepaldi G. Reduced beta-cell secretion and insulin hepatic extraction in healthy elderly subjects. *J Am Geriatr Soc* 1990; **38**: 1283–9.

31 Jackson RA, Blix PM, Matthews JA, et al. Influence of ageing on glucose homeostasis. *J Clin Endocrinol Metab* 1982; **55**: 840–8.

32 Robert J-J, Cummins JC, Wolfe RR, et al. Quantitative aspects of glucose production and metabolism in healthy elderly subjects. *Diabetes* 1982; **31**: 203–11.

33 Fink RI, Wallace P, Olefsky JM. Effects of aging on glucose-mediated glucose disposal and glucose transport. *J Clin Invest* 1986; **77**: 2034–41.

34 Fink RI, Kolterman OG, Kao M, Olefsky JM. The role of the glucose transport system in the postreceptor defect in insulin action associated with human aging. *J Clin Endocrinol Metab* 1984; **58**: 721–5.

35 Tonino RP, Minaker KL, Rowe JW. Effect of age on systemic delivery of oral glucose in men. *Diabetes Care* 1989; **12**: 394–8.

36 Gumbiner B, Polonsky KS, Beltz WF, Wallace P, Brechtel G, Fink RI. Effects of aging on insulin secretion. *Diabetes* 1989; **38**: 1549–56.

37 Jackson RA, Hawa MI, Roshania RD, Sim BM, DiSilvio L, Jaspan JB. Influence of aging on hepatic and peripheral glucose metabolism in humans. *Diabetes* 1988; **36**: 119–29.

38 Broughton DL, Webster J, Taylor R. Insulin sensitivity and secretion in healthy elderly human subjects with 'abnormal' glucose tolerance. *Eur J Clin Invest* 1992; **22**: 582–90.

39 Boden G, Chen X, DeSantis RA, Kendrick Z. Effects of age and body fat on insulin resistance in healthy men. *Diabetes Care* 1993; **16**: 728–33.

40 Dudl RJ, Ensinck JW. Insulin and glucagon relationships during aging in man. *Metabolism* 1977; **26**: 33–41.

41 Simonson DC, De Fronzo RA. Glucagon physiology and aging: evidence for enhanced hepatic sensitivity. *Diabetologia* 1983; **25**: 1–7.

42 McConnell JG, Alam MH, O'Hare MJ, Buchanan KD, Stout RW. The effect of age and sex on the response to enteropancreatic polypeptides to oral glucose. *Age Ageing* 1983; **12**: 54–62.

43 Meneilly GS, Minaker KL, Young JB, Landsberg L, Rowe JW. Counterregulatory responses to insulin-induced glucose reduction in the elderly. *J Clin Endocrinol Metab* 1985; **61**: 178–82.

44 Cameron CM, Kostyo JL. Influence of age on responsiveness to diabetogenic action of growth hormone. *Diabetes* 1987; **36**: 88–92.

45 Rosenthal MJ, Woodside WF. Nocturnal regulation of free fatty acids in healthy young and elderly men. *Metabolism* 1988; **37**: 645–8.

46 Copeland KC, Colletti RB, Devlin JT, McAuliffe TL. The relationship between insulin-like growth factor-1, adiposity and aging. *Metabolism* 1990; **39**: 584–7.

47 Yamamoto H, Sohmiya M, Oka N, Kato Y. Effect of aging and sex on plasma insulin-like growth factor 1 (IGF-1) levels in normal adults. *Acta Endocrinol (Copenh)* 1991; **124**: 497–500.

48 Elahi D, Andersen DK, Muller DC, Tobin JD, Brown JC, Andres R. The enteric enhancement of glucose-stimulated insulin release. The role of GIP in aging, obesity, and non-insulin-dependent diabetes mellitus. *Diabetes* 1984; **33**: 950–7.

49 Chen M, Halter JB, Porte D Jr. Plasma catecholamines, dietary carbohydrate, and glucose intolerance: a comparison between young and old men. *J Clin Endocrinol Metab* 1986; **62**: 1193–8.

50 Morrow LA, Rosen SG, Halter JB. Beta-adrenergic regulation of insulin secretion: evidence of tissue heterogeneity of beta-adrenergic responsiveness in the elderly. *J Gerontol* 1991; **46**: M108–13.

51 Morrow LA, Morganroth GS, Herman WH, Bergman RN, Halter JB. Effects of epinephrine on insulin secretion and action in humans. Interaction with aging. *Diabetes* 1993; **42**: 307–15.

52 Rahier J, Wallon J, Loozen S, Lefevre A, Gepts W, Haot J. The pancreatic polypeptide cells in the human pancreas: the effects of age and diabetes. *J Clin Endocrinol Metab* 1983; **56**: 441–4.

53 Kohrt WM, Kirwan JP, Staten MA, Bourey RE, King DS, Holloszy JO. Insulin resistance in aging is related to abdominal obesity. *Diabetes* 1993; **42**: 273–81.

54 O'Shaugnessy IM, Kasdorf GM, Hoffman RG, Kalkhoff RK. Does aging intensify the insulin resistance of human obesity? *J Clin Endocrinol Metab* 1992; **74**: 1075–81.

55 Shimokata H, Muller DC, Fleg JL, Sorkin J, Ziemba AJ, Andres R. Age as an independent determinant of glucose tolerance. *Diabetes* 1991; **40**: 44–51.

56 Mykkanen L, Laakso M, Uusitupa M, Pyorala K. Prevalence of diabetes and impaired glucose tolerance in elderly subjects and their association with obesity and family history of diabetes. *Diabetes Care* 1990; **13**: 1099–105.

57 Coon PJ, Bleecker ER, Drinkwater DT, Meyers DA, Goldberg AP. Effects of body composition and exercise capacity on glucose tolerance, insulin, and lipoprotein lipids in healthy older men: a cross-sectional and longitudinal intervention study. *Metabolism* 1989; **38**: 1201–9.

58 Dallosso HM, Morgan K, Bassey EJ, Ebrahim SBJ, Fentem PH, Arie THD. Levels of customary physical activity among the old and the very old living at home. *J Epidemiol Community Health* 1988; **42**: 121–7.

59 Astrand I, Astrand P-O, Hallback I, Kilbom A. Reduction in maximal oxygen uptake with age. *J Appl Physiol* 1973; **35**: 649–54.

60 Seals DR, Hagberg JM, Hurley BF, Ehsani AA, Holloszy JO. Effects of endurance training on glucose tolerance and plasma lipid levels in older men and women. *JAMA* 1984; **252**: 645–9.

61 Seals DR, Hagberg JM, Allen WK, *et al.* Glucose tolerance in young and older athletes and sedentary men. *J Appl Physiol* 1984; **56**: 1521–5.

62 Hollenbeck CB, Hasskell W, Rosenthal M, Reaven GM. Effect of habitual physical activity on regulation of insulin-stimulated glucose disposal in older males. *J Am Geriatr Soc* 1984; **33**: 273–7.

63 Tonino RP. Effect of physical training on the insulin resistance of aging. *Am J Physiol* 1989; **256**: E352–6.

64 Yamanouchi K, Nakajima H, Shinozaki T, *et al.* Effects of daily physical activity on insulin action in the elderly. *J Appl Physiol* 1992; **73**: 2241–5.

65 Houmard JA, Egan PC, Neufer PD, *et al.* Elevated skeletal muscle glucose transporter levels in exercise-trained middle-aged men. *Am J Physiol* 1991; **261**: E437–43.

66 Eriksson K-F, Lindgarde F. Prevention of type 2 (non-insulin-dependent) diabetes mellitus by diet and physical exercise. *Diabetologia* 1991; **34**: 891–8.

67 Paolisso G, Sgambato S, Pizza G, Passariello N, Varricchio M, D'Onofrio F. Improved insulin response and action by chronic magnesium administration in aged NIDDM subjects. *Diabetes Care* 1989; **12**: 265–9.

68 Minaker KL, Rowe JW, Young JB, Sparrow D, Pallotta JA, Landsberg L. Effect of age on insulin stimulation of sympathetic nervous system activity in man. *Metabolism* 1982; **31**: 1181–4.

69 Nolan L, O'Malley K. Prescribing for the elderly: Part II. Prescribing patterns: differences due to age. *J Am Geriatr Soc* 1988; **36**: 245–54.

3

Prevention of Diabetes in Elderly People

DENNIS T. VILLAREAL and JOHN E. MORLEY

Geriatric Research Education and Clinical Center, St Louis University Medical
School, St Louis, MO, USA

INTRODUCTION

It is well known that the prevalence rate of diabetes rises with age. In the
United States, the prevalence of non-insulin-dependent diabetes mellitus
(NIDDM) increases from 2.0% in the 20–44 year age group to 18.7% in
65–74 year olds; an additional 22.8% of the older group have impaired
glucose tolerance (IGT)[1] (see Chapter 1). Of the 6.5 million diagnosed
diabetics in the United States, nearly 3.1 million are older than 65 years[2].
The prevalence of diagnosed diabetes in elderly people is expected to
increase 44% in the next 20 years, to an estimated population of 3.9 million
people[3].

Elderly diabetic patients utilize the health care system more than elderly
non-diabetics. About 30% of diabetics aged 65–74 years are hospitalized
each year, a rate twice that of elderly people without diabetes[3]. Diabetics
older than 65 years have a higher institutionalization rate than non-
diabetics[2,3]. More importantly, they also have an increased relative risk for
mortality: 1.7 for those aged 65–74 years and 1.3 for those 75 and older. In
these two age groups the relative risk of death from heart disease is 2.7 and
2.2, respectively[4]. Recent data suggest that age interacts with diabetes to
accelerate the onset of chronic complications including retinopathy and
peripheral neuropathy[5]. Furthermore, acute complications of hyperglycaemia, such as polyuria and visual disturbances, play a major role

Diabetes in Old Age. Edited by P. Finucane and A. J. Sinclair
© 1995 John Wiley & Sons Ltd

in increasing morbidity and decreasing the quality of life in older individuals[6].

Since diabetes is clearly a major cause of morbidity and mortality in older people who constitute a growing segment of the population, the problem of diabetes in elderly people has major economic and public health consequences. In order to control acute symptoms and to prevent or delay chronic complications, it is essential to establish good diabetic control in older diabetic persons. This aims to improve their quality of life, reduce hospital admissions and the overall utilization of health care.

Conventionally, glycaemic control of NIDDM has been achieved by diet and/or exercise alone or through the additional use of oral hypoglycaemic agents or insulin. However, the treatment of the elderly diabetic patient poses special problems (Table 3.1) that may also entail considerable use of the health care resources.

An alternative approach to the diabetic epidemic in elderly people is primary prevention. If attainable, prevention of diabetes in older people

Table 3.1. Special problems in the management of older diabetic patients

Problem	Outcome	Management solutions
Visual disturbance	Inadequate or overdosage of insulin; hyper- or hypoglycaemia	Predrawn insulin syringes; insulin syringe magnifier
Decreased activities of daily living	Decreased food intake; hypoglycaemia	Adaptive devices: 'Meals-on-Wheels'
Cognitive impairment	Decreased compliance	Memory aids
Depression	Poor compliance; death; suicide	Early detection and treatment of depression
Polypharmacy	Drug interactions; hyper- or hypoglycaemia	Periodic review of medications; discontinue non-essential drugs
Multiple disease processes	Polypharmacy; anorexia	Prioritize management decisions; treat where appropriate
Poverty	Malnutrition; poor compliance	Advise social worker; modify management plan accordingly
Altered renal and hepatic function	Hypoglycaemia	Decrease dose of hypoglycaemics
Physical inactivity	Obesity; hyperglycaemia	Exercise programme

may be preferred to treatment of established cases since this may be cost-effective. Inherent in the preventive approach is the notion that diabetes is not entirely an inevitable consequence of ageing but is consequent, at least in part, on some modifiable or preventable factors. In this chapter we will explore the interesting possibility that diabetes in the elderly may indeed be a preventable disorder in an attempt to propose practical prophylactic measures. In addition, in dealing with the prevention of diabetic complications, we will briefly discuss secondary and tertiary prevention.

PATHOPHYSIOLOGY OF GLUCOSE INTOLERANCE AND DIABETES OF AGEING

A number of previous studies have consistently reported an age-related decline in glucose tolerance, summarized as an increase of 10 mg/dl rise in the 2-h glucose level per decade[7-9]. The primary mechanism for this age-related hyperglycaemia appears to be peripheral insulin resistance as evidenced by the presence of hyperinsulinaemia and the demonstration of reduced glucose disposal rate by glucose clamp techniques[9,10]. This insulin resistance is thought to be secondary to a postreceptor defect in the insulin action since insulin receptor binding is comparable in older and young subjects[11,12]. On the other hand, although the predominant defect is insulin resistance, a few studies suggest that impaired insulin secretion with ageing may be a contributory factor[13,14].

NIDDM is characterized by defects in both insulin secretion and insulin action. Given the similar mechanisms for both the hyperglycaemia of ageing and NIDDM, and that subjects with IGT have increased risk of developing NIDDM[15], it is possible that in some cases, the age-related deterioration in glucose tolerance may represent a stage in the evolution of the diabetic syndrome. Subjects with glucose intolerance of ageing have been shown to have an increase in atherosclerotic cardiovascular disease[16]. Furthermore, hyperglycaemia of ageing may be associated with increased protein glycation, which plays a major role in the pathogenesis of microangiopathic complications[17].

A word of warning is needed concerning the diagnosis of diabetes mellitus in that it is now recognized that 'white coat' hyperglycaemia (a condition similar to 'white coat' hypertension) can result in spuriously elevated glucose levels during a visit to the physician. This is secondary to anxiety-induced catecholamine discharge. Thus pseudohyperglycaemia needs to be considered in the differential diagnosis of diabetes in older persons.

THE ROLE OF ENVIRONMENTAL FACTORS

Although several studies have shown an age-related decline in glucose tolerance, it has been repeatedly pointed out that most have failed to control for age-associated conditions which in themselves adversely affect glucose tolerance[18-20]. For example, older individuals tend to be more obese and have more body fat as well as greater upper body fat distribution, all of which are associated with insulin resistance. Furthermore, older people tend to be more sedentary and since the level of habitual physical activity is directly related to insulin-stimulated glucose uptake[21], it has been suggested that decreasing physical activity with ageing may be another factor in the impairment in glucose tolerance. Other age-associated factors that may negatively impact on glucose tolerance include the increasing prevalence of many acute and chronic conditions, the exposure to a variety of medications that may alter glucose tolerance and the alteration in dietary composition (i.e. decreased carbohydrate intake). Accordingly, it has been suggested that the worsening of glucose tolerance with increasing age may not be a primary manifestation of ageing but is, instead, secondary to these age-associated conditions[19-21]. Indeed, recent studies support this contention. In 1986, Zavaroni *et al.*[22] studied 732 factory workers aged 22–73 years in Parma, Italy and noted that after taking account of ideal body weight, leisure time activity and use of diabetogenic drugs, the variance in glucose accounted for by ageing was only 6% in men and 1% in women. In the Baltimore Longitudinal Study of Aging involving 742 males and females (aged 17–92 years), divided into three groups of young, middle-aged and old, a progressive increase in the 2-h glucose levels was noted with ageing[23]. However, after adjusting for age-associated variables such as body mass index,% body fat, waist–hip ratio and levels of physical activity, the difference between the young and middle-aged group was not significant with only the oldest group still having a significant decline in glucose tolerance. Importantly, when age was introduced only after the other variables were entered in the multiple regression analyses, the overall contribution of age to the variance in glucose was only 3–6%. Thus, it appears that age *per se* may account for less than 10% of the decline in glucose tolerance of ageing, with a number of potentially modifiable factors playing a significant role.

Recently, increasing interest has been given to the type of obesity as an important predictor of diabetes mellitus in late middle age[24,25]. For example, in a study by Kaye *et al.*[26], women with the highest tertile of waist to hip circumference ratio had a 14.4-fold increased risk for diabetes compared with women in the lowest tertiles. The increased diabetes risk with abdominal obesity has been attributed to: (i) the greater lipolytic activity in abdominal adipocytes, resulting in increased free fatty acids in the portal vein; (ii) increased metabolic clearance rate of insulin in abdominal fat; and (iii) greater concentrations of free testosterone (which increases insulin resistance) in women with abdominal obesity[26]. In a recent study of 36 healthy older men aged 47–73 years, Coon et al.[27] found that the glucose disposal rate negatively correlated with the waist to hip ratio and% body fat and positively with V_{O_2max} but not with age. Only waist to hip ratio was independently related to glucose disposal rate in the stepwise multiple regression analyses, supporting the important role of body composition as a determinant of glucose tolerance in older individuals. Although the distribution of body fat is thought to be genetically determined, current evidence suggests that it may be modifiable[28,29].

PRIMARY PREVENTION

DIETARY FACTORS

Weight Loss

A strong association between obesity and NIDDM is suggested by the fact that 80% of middle-aged persons with adult-onset diabetes mellitus are obese. Obesity is thought to affect carbohydrate metabolism by inducing tissue insulin resistance and causing a compensatory increase in circulating insulin levels[30]. Caloric restriction to induce weight loss can return glucose metabolism to normal in some patients[31].

Preliminary evidence also suggests that the resultant weight loss may be associated with a more favourable fat distribution[27,28]. In a study of elderly overweight patients with poor control despite insulin therapy, moderate weight loss was followed by a dramatic improvement in glycaemic control[32]. Thus, weight reduction through dietary restriction may represent one preventive measure against the development of diabetes in the elderly.

However, there appear to be several problems limiting the usefulness of dietary restriction in the older diabetic patient. First, while the percentage of body fat increases with ageing, concomitant with a decrease in muscle mass, ageing is generally associated with a decrease in average body weight[33]. It is not known whether elderly diabetics tend to be overweight compared with healthy non-diabetic elderly subjects. In fact, most elderly diabetic patients in nursing homes frequently have normal body weight[34]. Second, studies have shown that in spite of the ability of many to lose weight with moderate caloric restriction, there is less ability to maintain weight loss[35]. Third, dietary restriction may predispose the older person to develop malnutrition[33,36]. In view of these, it is not recommended that weight reduction be instituted in diabetic patients over 70 years of age unless weight is at least 20% above average[36]. When dietary intervention is undertaken, this should be highly individualized taking into consideration such factors as the older individual's life-style, economic status, food preferences and social needs.

Alternatively, moderate dietary restriction may be initiated in young and middle age in order to prevent obesity in later life that may increase insulin resistance and predispose to diabetes. Although it has been notoriously difficult to maintain weight loss in obese individuals, it has been suggested that the incorporation of dietary intervention into a behavioural programme including life-style changes with long-term follow-up may provide better results[37]. Although this approach may rarely be practical in all younger individuals, it seems reasonable for those who are overweight and/or have additional risk factors for diabetes such as a positive family history, a history of stress hyperglycaemia, or IGT. At present, studies are needed to determine whether long-term weight loss through dietary restriction can be maintained and whether it will ultimately prove effective in preventing the development of diabetes in later life.

Dietary Composition

Some previous dietary surveys have shown decreased total carbohydrate intake in the old as compared with the young[38,39]. Based on evidence that carbohydrate restriction worsens[40] while carbohydrate supplementation improves glucose tolerance[41,42], it has been suggested that deficient carbohydrate intake in the elderly may be partially responsible for the age-related impairment in glucose tolerance. In accordance with this hypothesis, Chen *et al.* were able to demonstrate in small studies (15 young and 16 older men) that the elderly could improve their glucose tolerance by increasing their carbohydrate intake from 45 to 85% of total calories[43]. This favourable effect was shown to be associated with improvement in β-cell responsiveness as well as insulin sensitivity. However, in a larger population sample[23], it was found that older individuals actually relied more heavily on carbohydrate than did young subjects, while decreasing their fat intake. Thus, the role of deficient carbohydrate intake in the decline in glucose tolerance with ageing remains unclear.

The optimal dietary composition for the elderly diabetic is unknown. Furthermore, considerable controversy still surrounds the recommendation of the American Diabetes Association (ADA) of a high carbohydrate (55–60% of calories) and low-fat diet (<30% of calories; with <10% of total calories coming from saturated fat and cholesterol restricted to 300 mg/day)[44]. Concerns about the high carbohydrate diet include increased insulin levels and carbohydrate-induced hypertriglyceri-daemia[45,46]. One study reported that the use of a high monounsaturated fat diet (50% fat, 35% carbohydrate) was more effective in lowering glucose and triglycerides than the high carbohydrate diet recommended by the ADA[47]. Although the limitation in total and saturated fat is based on the premise that such a diet will decrease the risk of coronary heart disease by reducing total and low-density lipoprotein (LDL) cholesterol, hyperlipidaemia is generally less common in the elderly and the role of reducing serum lipids in overall outcome in this population remains to be determined. Thus, reducing dietary fat content may be appropriate for the healthy older diabetic but not for the malnourished older person in whom emphasis should be on the total energy content of the diet. In the past, it was recommended that simple sugars be rigorously restricted but this no longer seems appropriate in as much as when taken with a mixed meal, the glycaemic effects of simple sugars are substantially reduced[48,49]. While the ambulatory elderly patient may benefit from increasing the dietary fibre content to slow carbohydrate digestion and absorption, it has been pointed out that the immobilized elderly may be at risk of bowel impaction from fibre supplementation[44]. It is also not known whether the high fibre diet may interfere with micronutrient bioavailability in elderly subjects.

Micronutrients

Although a number of micronutrients have been implicated in the pathogenesis of carbohydrate intolerance, their specific role in age-related glucose intolerance is unclear[50]. For example, tissue chromium levels decrease with age and a bioactive form of chromium–glucose tolerance factor (a complex of chromium, nicotinic acid, amino acids) may be responsible for the glycaemic alteration. Accordingly, a combination of chromium and nicotinic acid has been shown to improve glucose tolerance in older individuals statistically but the changes did not appear clinically important[51].

Vitamin E was given to 25 patients with NIDDM with a mean age of 71 years. Vitamin E was associated with a decrease in fasting glucose and glycosylated haemoglobin (Hb A_1C) and a decrease in cholesterol and triglycerides[52]. It is possible that vitamin E decreased the lipid peroxidation and free radical activity, both of which tend to be increased in diabetics and may play a role in the development of poor metabolic control and microangiopathy.

Ten to 20% of people with NIDDM develop decreased serum zinc levels secondary to reduced zinc absorption and hyperzincuria[53,54]. This mild zinc deficiency does not appear to be involved in metabolic control, but may play a role in the immune deficiency and poor wound healing in some diabetics.

Summary

Overall, until the ideal dietary composition for the ageing diabetic is determined, the best dietary approach is individualization so as not to adversely affect the older diabetic person's quality of life. It is emphasized that in some older individuals, the risk of malnutrition may potentially outweigh the benefits of a rigid dietary intervention. At present, studies demonstrating the efficacy of long-term adherence to a particular dietary composition in the prevention of diabetes in the elderly are lacking. Since the impact of differences in dietary composition on the metabolic abnormalities remain to be clarified, it is probably not justifiable to recommend a specific type of diet as part of a preventative programme against diabetes in the elderly other than moderate caloric restriction to induce weight loss in the overweight. The possible role of micronutrient deficiency in the pathogenesis of NIDDM is tantalizing but not proven.

EXERCISE

Ageing is associated with decreased physical activity, which in turn is associated with reduced insulin sensitivity and glucose intolerance. The important effect of physical activity on glucose homeostasis in ageing is supported by cross-sectional studies which demonstrate that well-trained older individuals have normal insulin sensitivity and glucose tolerance[55]. In addition, maximum voluntary oxygen consumption (V_{O_2max}), a measure of physical fitness, has been shown to be correlated with glucose disposal in older people[56]. Recently, prospective studies have investigated the effects of exercise on insulin action and glucose tolerance in the elderly. For example, insulin levels declined in 13 healthy men of mean age 69 years subjected to 6 months of endurance training, though no change in oral glucose tolerance was noted[57]. This decreased insulin response in the face of unchanged glucose response suggests that exercise resulted in improvement in insulin action. On the other hand, at present there are no prospective studies evaluating the effect of endurance exercise training in older patients with NIDDM. However, studies on exercise in middle-aged patients with NIDDM suggest modest improvement in glucose control associated with increased insulin sensitivity. In a study by Hollozy et al.[58], high intensity exercise training for 12 months was followed by normalization of the oral glucose tolerance test in subjects with NIDDM (mean age 56) or IGT (mean age 54). It is important to note, however, that most studies have demonstrated that the improvement in insulin action following exercise is a short-term effect, suggesting that repeated acute bouts of exercise may be needed to derive benefits[59,60]. In addition, as demonstrated by a study by Wing *et al.*[61], exercise may be a useful adjunct to dietary restriction in the achievement of weight loss and better glycaemic control in obese patients with NIDDM.

The precise mechanism by which exercise improves insulin action is not fully understood. As shown in previous studies[56-61], this effect may be mediated indirectly by weight loss or may be a direct effect on insulin action. During exercise, both adipose and muscle tissue substantially increase their total number of glucose transporters; this has been associated with enhanced glucose transport in response to insulin stimulation[62]. Other factors include increased capillary density in muscle and increased intracellular glucose metabolism. Recently, an interesting finding is that exercise training may significantly change the distribution of body fat to a lower body pattern in older men suggesting that the relationship of glucose metabolism to physical fitness may be due to the ability of exercise training to alter the distribution as well as the mass of body fat[63].

Given that exercise improves insulin sensitivity and that IGT and the early stages of NIDDM are primarily characterized by insulin resistance, increased physical activity appears to be an attractive approach to the prevention of diabetes in the elderly. In fact, several lines of evidence suggest that exercise can actually prevent the development of diabetes. First, physically active societies have less NIDDM than less active societies and as populations have become more sedentary, the incidence of NIDDM has increased[64]. Second, a retrospective study of 5000 college alumni found that the risk of developing diabetes was 3.4 times higher in non-athletes than in the former athletes[65]. Third, three large prospective studies from the United States with 5–8 years follow-up support the value of exercise in preventing the development of NIDDM. In the Nurse Health Study of 87 253 people aged 34–59 years, the age-adjusted relative risk of developing NIDDM for those who exercise at least once per week was 0.67[66]. For the same degree of exercise, the age-adjusted relative risk in the Physicians Health Study of 21 271 subjects aged 40–84 years was 0.64[67]. A third study involving 5990 University of Pennsylvania alumni aged 39–68 years found that exercise had a dose-dependent protective effect[68]; the occurrence of NIDDM decreased by 6% for each increment of 500 kcal/week. In all of these studies, the protective effect of exercise was independent of other risk factors for NIDDM (i.e. older age, positive family history, obesity). Moreover, the protective effect seemed to be most evident in those with multiple risk factors.

Thus, the bulk of evidence suggests that physical inactivity may be a modifiable risk factor for the development of NIDDM. Accordingly, in order to decrease the prevalence of diabetes in the elderly, older people should be encouraged to increase their physical activity. However, as previously mentioned, since it is the cumulative effect of repetitive exercise that offers the best protection against NIDDM, regular exercise should probably be undertaken as early as possible, i.e. in younger years. When started in older age, exercise should be highly individualized, taking into consideration the individual's functional capacity. In most cases, however, the recommendation is 20–30 min of brisk walking to maintain the pulse rate between 100 and 120 beats/min. The principles of exercise prescription in older people are summarized in Table 3.2. The other potential beneficial effects of exercise in the elderly include a decreased risk of cardiovascular disease, greater musculoskeletal strength and denser bones.

MEDICATIONS

Because of increasing prevalence of many acute and chronic illnesses, the older person is exposed to a variety of medications. These may include drugs that adversely affect glucose tolerance. In the epidemiological study by Zavaroni *et al.*[22], the use of potentially diabetogenic drugs (diuretics, beta blockers, oral contraceptives and cimetidine) correlated positively with age. Furthermore, the influence of age on glucose intolerance could be largely explained by diabetogenic drug use, together with other confounding variables (e.g. obesity, physical activity). In a survey of 10 most often used drugs by patients 75 years and older, two of these were diabetogenic: hydrochlorothiazide, the most commonly used medication, and propanolol[69]. Not surprisingly, these are antihypertensive drugs, reflecting the high prevalence of hypertension and the benefits of controlling blood

Table 3.2. Principles of exercise prescription in the elderly

1. Pre-exercise evaluation to identify high risk persons:
   (i) complete history and physical exam; and
   (ii) exercise testing.
2. Consider the older person's functional capacity.
3. Start slow and go slow.
4. Initial preferred types of exercise are aerobic activities (i.e. walking).
5. Training sessions should be held at least 3 days per week.
6. Each session should include 5 min warm-up, 30 min aerobic exercise, and 5 min cool-down.
7. Isometric exercise using low resistance weights can complement the aerobic exercise programme.
8. Avoid straining and breath-holding exercises.
9. Prevent injuries (e.g. proper footwear)
10. Promote compliance:
    (i) focus on specific needs and values; and
    (ii) build on previous habits.

pressure in this age group. Although the control of hypertension has been shown to decrease the overall cardiovascular mortality, it has been suggested that the inability of thiazides to specifically reduce the risk of coronary artery disease in some studies, may be related to its adverse metabolic effects, including the induction of glucose intolerance[70].

Pandit *et al.*[71] have recently reviewed several medications that influence glucose metabolism and their mechanisms of action. In particular, thiazides negatively affect glucose tolerance by reducing insulin secretion, probably mediated by diuretic-induced hypokalaemia. Other possible mechanisms include decreased insulin sensitivity, increased hepatic glucose production, direct effect on the pancreatic beta cells and alterations on the levels of catecholamines. Likewise, beta blockers may inhibit insulin release, an effect which is associated with enhanced hepatic glucose production; they may also decrease hepatic and peripheral glucose uptake. A list of commonly used drugs adversely affecting glucose tolerance in older persons is given in Table 3.3. In addition to polypharmacy, it is important to point out that the older person is at risk from adverse drug effects (including drug-induced hyperglycaemia) because of altered pharmacokinetics and pharmacodynamics. Altered pharmacokinetics may be due to changes in drug distribution (i.e. increase in body fat, low albumin),

Table 3.3. Commonly used drugs that may induce glucose intolerance in older persons

1. Antihypertensives diuretics (thiazide, furosemide) nicotinic acid beta blockers calcium-channel blockers centrally-acting alpha blockers	5. Antituberculosis 6. Miscellaneous morphine indomethacin dopamine
2. Hormones oestrogen/progesterone corticosteroids growth hormone thyroxine	ethanol nalidixic acid theophylline cyclosporin amoxapine beta-2 agonists sugar-containing medications
3. Psychotropics phenothiazines lithium	(cough syrup)
4. Antiarrhythmic drugs disopyramide encainide amiodarone	

metabolism (altered liver function), and excretion (decreased renal function) while altered pharmacodynamics may be related to the increased sensitivity of the older person to the effects of the drug. These age-related changes can also increase the potential drug interactions related to the use of multiple drugs. For example, the combination of thiazides and loop diuretics in the elderly may augment potassium loss and consequently worsen glucose tolerance. It has been shown that the rate of drug interactions rises and falls with the number of drugs prescribed[72,73].

In some older persons exposed to diabetogenic medications, the associated glucose intolerance or diabetes may therefore possibly represent a form of iatrogenic disorder. Thus, in order to minimize polypharmacy and the risk of drug side-effects, it is prudent to periodically review the medication list of all elderly persons. During each patient visit, the appropriateness of each medication should be determined and only essential drugs should be continued. In some older patients, simple discontinuation of diabetogenic medication can result in normal glucose tolerance while in others this may lead to better glycaemic control, thus contributing to a better quality of life.

'HEALTHY LIVING' AND DIABETES

A question arises whether a combination of diet and exercise ('healthy living') can prevent persons with IGT from developing NIDDM. A study in middle-aged persons has suggested that 'healthy living' does not decrease glucose levels but does lower systolic blood pressure and total cholesterol with an increase in the HDL:LDL ratio[74].

SECONDARY AND TERTIARY PREVENTION

CONTROL OF BLOOD SUGAR

Secondary prevention implies the early detection and reversal of ill health before adverse complications arise while tertiary prevention is concerned with the prevention or delay of complications in established cases. Since hyperglycaemia is the major metabolic abnormality in diabetes and since the duration of hyperglycaemia correlates with chronic complications, the focus in secondary and tertiary prevention of diabetes has been on maintaining euglycaemia. However, in older diabetics, it has been argued that glycaemic control may not be worth while on the basis that they may not live long enough to develop complications. Nevertheless, since NIDDM can have a very gradual onset, many newly diagnosed older diabetics may actually have been hyperglycaemic for some time. It has also been shown that chronic complications such as retinopathy and neuropathy increase with advancing age and that age by itself may be an independent predictor for the development of these complications[5]. These findings suggest that diabetic complications may be accelerated in elderly people. Further, as previously mentioned, acute complications such as osmotic diuresis and visual disturbances adversely affect the quality of life of the elderly diabetic. Thus, with increasing longevity of the older population, the ageing diabetic is at increased risk of acute and chronic complications unless appropriately treated.

In the past, there has been a long-standing debate on how aggressively to control blood sugar and whether tight control actually affects the development of long-term complications. Two recent large and well designed prospective studies, the Diabetes Control and Complications Trial (DCCT)[75] and the Stockholm Diabetes Intervention Study (Stockholm Study)[76] have shown that intensive insulin therapy can delay the onset and slow the progression of chronic microvascular complications in insulin-dependent diabetes mellitus (IDDM). It is now clear that normal glycaemic control is the ideal target of therapy. However, when applying the results of these studies to the care of older diabetics who predominantly have NIDDM, there are obvious limitations. These include the need for a highly motivated patient with the ability to acquire special skills, the considerable expense involved, and most importantly, the need for intensive insulin therapy with the associated risks of hypoglycaemia. Furthermore, in view of insulin resistance in NIDDM, intensive insulin therapy may predispose to hyperinsulinaemia, a condition suspected of exacerbating macrovascular complications[77,78]. Fortunately, however, insulin treatment is not necessary in all older diabetic patients because, at least in the early stages of the disease, excellent glycaemic control can be achieved with diet and exercise. These two forms of interventions are much simpler, less costly and safer (little risk of hypoglycaemia) than intensive insulin treatment. They also reduce insulin resistance and have major ancillary cardiovascular health benefits. Thus, in order that diet and exercise can be instituted at the stage when they are most successful, it may be important to diagnose the older diabetic as early as possible. Accordingly, in recognizing the benefits of early detection and appropriate treatment, the ADA has included older age as one of the risk factors for diabetes in which routine screening is recommended[79].

Most recently, there is evidence that good metabolic control is important in the elderly as it is in young and middle-aged diabetic patients in preventing chronic diabetic complications. Similar to the DCCT and the Stockholm Study, Morisaki *et al.*[80], in a 5-year prospective follow-up of 114 NIDDM patients (age >60 years) showed that lower mean glycosylated haemoglobin (Hb A_1C) was negatively correlated with the progression of retinopathy. Interestingly, a substantial proportion of subjects (38%) were treated with diet alone while the rest required oral hypoglycaemic drugs or insulin. However, no information on side-effects was provided which would be important since in both the DCCT[74] and the Stockholm Study[76,81], lower Hb A_1C was also correlated with an increased incidence of hypoglycaemia.

After failure of an adequate trial of diet and exercise, many older diabetics may require treatment with oral hypoglycaemic agents or insulin. In these cases, despite the results of the DCCT and the Stockholm Study supporting the value of tight glycaemic control, the goals of treatment should be highly individualized. The many special problems in the treatment of the older diabetic should be recognized (Table 3.1) and overcome. Specifically, the risk of poor control must be carefully weighed against the potential benefits of achieving good control including the attendant risk of serious hypoglycaemia. In many cases the balance may be in favour of less intensive management, but this is not invariably so. Much of the decision will depend on a thorough assessment of the patient's physical and mental capabilities and social circumstances. Although in most cases the information to make such a decision is readily available to the primary physician, a formal geriatric assessment using tools such as Folstein's Mini-Mental Status Exam, the Katz Activities of Daily Living Scale and the Philadelphia Geriatric Center Instrumental Scale may be useful[82]. Furthermore, as elderly diabetics may have a higher risk of depression[5] which can adversely affect compliance, it may be prudent to routinely screen for this problem using a tool such as the Yesavage Geriatric Depression Scale[83].

CONTROL OF MACROVASCULAR RISK FACTORS

Macrovascular complications (coronary artery disease, cerebrovascular disease and peripheral vascular disease) are increased two- to fourfold in diabetic patients. In the elderly diabetic in particular, they are a major cause of morbidity and mortality. However, in contrast to microvascular complications, associations between hyperglycaemia and macrovascular complications are weak. The two long-term randomized studies of intensive treatment in IDDM, the DCCT[75] and Stockholm Study[76] together with the only randomized study in NIDDM (University Group Diabetes Program)[84] did not demonstrate a beneficial effect of lower glucose levels on cardiovascular morbidity and mortality. The results of the United Kingdom Prospective Study[85] with more than 5000 newly diagnosed people with NIDDM, now in its ninth year, will be available shortly and will hopefully finally resolve the issue of the role of glycaemic control on the progress of macrovascular complications in NIDDM.

Although the presence of diabetes itself is a risk factor for macrovascular disease, most older diabetic individuals have multiple other risk factors that can potentially interact with each other to increase this risk[86]. These may include the usual cardiovascular risk factors such as smoking, obesity, hypertension and hypercholesterolaemia. Available data from the Framingham Study and Multiple Risk Factor Intervention Trial suggest that these risk factors retain the same adverse impact on the development of macrovascular disease in NIDDM individuals as in non-diabetic individuals[86]. Thus, in addition to controlling hyperglycaemia, it may be as important to control these other risk factors. For example, hypertension should be controlled, particularly since numerous studies have demonstrated that lowering blood pressure in older hypertensive persons has beneficial effects on overall cardiovascular morbidity and mortality. In the elderly, systolic blood pressure (SBP) may be more predictive of future cardiovascular events than diastolic blood pressure (DBP) and in this regard, two studies—the Systolic Hypertension in the Elderly Program (SHEP) Trial[87] and the Medical Research Council Trial[88]—have shown that control of isolated systolic hypertension (SBP >160 and DBP <90) lowers cardiovascular morbidity and mortality in non-frail older persons. On the other hand, although there are numerous studies demonstrating that control of hyperlipidaemia decreases cardiovascular risk in young and middle-aged populations, as previously mentioned, no prospective information is available about the long-term effects of such interventions on overall mortality in the elderly. However, as the risk of macrovascular complications of diabetes may be further increased by the presence of hyperlipidaemia, it seems reasonable to institute lipid-lowering interventions in the relatively healthy older diabetic when the cholesterol is >300 mg/dl. As with the control of hypertension, this should be initiated with non-pharmacological measures such as diet and exercise, particularly if the person is 30% or more overweight. In the diabetic who smokes, every attempt should be made to achieve smoking cessation which may include behavioural treatment for psychological and social dependency.

The very strong association between NIDDM and obesity, hypertension, hyperlipidaemia and premature atherosclerosis has now been referred to as 'syndrome X'. As proposed by Reaven, De Fronzo, Ferrannini and others[89-91], this syndrome recognizes that the underlying defect is insulin resistance and compensatory hyperinsulinaemia. It is suggested that the hyperinsulinaemia may exert these deleterious effects by: (i) acting as a growth factor in arterial walls; (ii) promoting renal tubular absorption of sodium and stimulating sympathetic nervous system overactivity to cause hypertension; and (iii) directly stimulating hepatic production of very low density lipoproteins[89-91]. If this hypothesis is proven, it would stress the importance of relying mainly on measures to decrease insulin resistance (diet and exercise) rather than those that promote hyperinsulinaemia (sulphonylureas and insulin). Furthermore, it is suggested that recognition of this syndrome would remind physicians to manage all cardiac risk factors in the patient and to avoid drugs that aggravate the other components of the syndrome[92]. For example, when non-pharmacological measures to control hypertension are unsuccessful, drugs such as thiazides and beta blockers would not be considered first-line since they might worsen hyperglycaemia and hyperlipidaemia. In this case, angiotensin-converting enzyme inhibitors may have a primary role since in addition to its protective effect on nephropathy[93], it may decrease insulin resistance[94].

PREVENTION OF AMPUTATION

Two-thirds of all amputations in diabetes occur in older diabetics[9]. Foot amputation can be prevented by careful attention to early foot lesions and good podiatry care (see Chapter 7). Preventive foot care is clearly a key area in maintaining the quality of life of older diabetics.

SUMMARY AND CONCLUSIONS

Not only does the prevalence of diabetes increase with age but diabetes is also a major cause of morbidity and mortality in the elderly, thus probably accounting for the higher utilization of health care by older diabetics. Accordingly, diabetes in the elderly constitutes a significant economic and public health problem.

Because the treatment of the older diabetic is limited by several problems, an alternative solution to the diabetic epidemic in the elderly may be primary prevention. Several epidemio-logical studies suggest that the age-related deterioration in glucose tolerance can be largely attributed to a number of age-related factors associated with insulin resistance, i.e. obesity and greater upper body fat distribution, physical inactivity, chronic illness and use of diabetogenic medications. All of these factors are potentially modifiable.

As suggested by the demonstration in several prospective studies of a lower incidence of diabetes in physically active people, regular exercise appears to be the most promising primary approach to diabetes in the elderly. To gain a maximum protective effect, it should probably be started as early in life as possible. Exercise mediates its positive effect by directly improving insulin sensitivity or indirectly by promoting weight loss and a more favourable distribution of body fat. On the other hand, although dietary restriction may be effective in producing weight loss and diminishing insulin resistance in obese individuals, there is a considerable risk of inducing malnutrition with dietary intervention in older people. Furthermore, the role of altering dietary composition in the prevention and treatment of diabetes is still unclear. Though diet incorporated into a behavioural modification programme initiated in younger age has been suggested, studies are needed to demonstrate the practicality and efficacy of such an approach in ultimately preventing diabetes in later life. Certainly, because of the prevalence of polypharmacy in the elderly and the susceptibility of older people to adverse drug effects as a result of altered drug metabolism, the possibility of drug-induced glucose intolerance should always be considered. Avoidance of unnecessary medications and polypharmacy is therefore a useful way of preventing diabetes in older people.

Secondary and tertiary prevention deal with improving the quality of life of older diabetics primarily through prevention and delay of complications. Since excellent glycaemic control has now been clearly shown to be the most important factor in the prevention of chronic (microvascular) complications, this should be the ideal goal of therapy. However, side-effects of aggressive treatment, particularly the risk of serious hypoglycaemia in the elderly, should also be considered and treatment, therefore, needs to be highly individualized taking into consideration a number of factors, i.e. the patient's mental capacity, economic status, family and social support, availability of social work and home care services. In addition to good metabolic control, it is important to control the usual coexistent macrovascular risk factors. The strong association of diabetes with hypertension, obesity, hyperlipidaemia and premature atherosclerosis has now been recognized as 'syndrome X', which proposes that the underlying defect is insulin resistance and compensatory hyperinsulinaemia. Recognition of this syndrome emphasizes not only the need to treat all cardiac risk factors in the older diabetic but also to rely mainly on approaches to reduce hyperinsulinaemia (such as diet and exercise) in establishing good diabetic control.

At present, there is much hope but little evidence that 'healthy living' will prevent the subsequent development of diabetes in older persons. Similarly, the appropriate use of micronutrients may have minor effects on glucose tolerance but there is little evidence that they should be used routinely in older persons. There is mounting evidence that aggressive control of hyperglycaemia once frank diabetes develops will improve the quality of life and delay microvascular complications. Regulation of hypertension, appropriate foot care and recognition of potential deleterious effects of drugs will appear to be cost-effective preventive strategies in the prevention of NIDDM. Table 3.4 summarizes some of the secondary and tertiary approaches to diabetes prevention in older persons.

Table 3.4. Secondary and tertiary prevention of diabetes in older people

1. Secondary prevention
   A. Better control of hyperglycaemia
      1. Diabetes education
      2. Dietary restriction if appropriate
      3. Regular exercise
      4. Avoidance of diabetogenic medications
      5. Oral hypoglycaemic agents or human insulin
      6. Self-monitoring of blood glucose or by caretaker
      7. Use of serum fructosamine or glycosylated haemoglobin to monitor 10–12 weeks control[*]
      8. Development of a team approach (doctor, nurse, dietitian etc)
      9. Improve compliance
         a. Screen and treat for depression
         b. Use of ancillary services (social work and home care)
   B. Better control of macrovascular risk factors
      1. Smoking cessation
      2. Control of hypertension by diet, exercise, or drugs
      3. Control of hyperlipidaemia by diet, exercise, or drugs
      4. Weight reduction by diet or exercise
      5. Avoidance of polypharmacy
2. Tertiary prevention
   A. Microangiopathy
      1. Retinopathy
         a. Regular ophthalmoscopic examination
         b. Laser photocoagulation or early vitrectomy
      2. Nephropathy
         a. Control of hypertension (especially with ACE inhibitor)
         b. Early detection of proteinuria (microalbuminuria)
         c. Early dialysis or renal transplantation
   B. Macroangiopathy
      1. Coronary artery disease
         a. Antianginal medications
         b. Angioplasty or bypass surgery
      2. Cerebrovascular disease
         a. Aspirin or anticoagulation
         b. Angioplasty
         c. Physical therapy
      3. Peripheral vascular disease
         a. Exercise
         b. Pentoxyfilline
         c. Angioplasty or bypass surgery
      4. Amputation
         a. Regular foot observation
         b. Podiatrist
   C. Neuropathy
      1. Peripheral
         a. Better podiatric care
         b. Special fitting shoes
         c. Diabetic foot education
         e. Better glycaemic control (as above)
      2. Autonomic
         a. Cisapride or metoclopromide for gastroparesis
         b. Intermittent catheterization for neurogenic bladder
         c. Fludrocortisone for orthostatic hypotension
         d. Better glycaemic control (as above)

[*] Because of falsely elevated levels of glycosylated haemoglobin in the elderly, fructosamine is preferred[95].

REFERENCES

1 Harris MI, Hadden WC, Knowler WC, *et al.* Prevalence of diabetes and impaired glucose tolerance and plasma glucose levels in US population, ages 24–74 years. *Diabetes* 1987; **36**: 523–34.
2 Centre for Economic Studies in Medicine. *Direct and Indirect Costs of Diabetes in the United States in 1987.* Alexandria, VA: American Diabetes Association, 1989.
3 Harris MI. Epidemiology of diabetes mellitus among the elderly in the United States. *Clin Geriatr Med* 1990; **4**: 703–19.
4 Waugh NR, Dallas JM, Jung RT, Newton RW. Mortality in a cohort of diabetic patients. *Diabetologia* 1989; **32**: 103–4.
5 Naliboff BD, Rosenthal M. Effects of age on complications in adult-onset diabetes. *J Am Geriatr Soc* 1989; **37**: 838–43.
6 Morley JE, Kaiser FE. Unique aspects of diabetes mellitus in the elderly. *Clin Geriatr Med* 1990; **6**: 693–702.
7 Andres R. Aging and diabetes. *Med Clin North Am* 1971; **55**: 835–46.
8 Davidson MD. The effect of aging on carbohydrate metabolism. A review of the English literature and a practical approach to the diagnosis of diabetes mellitus in the elderly. *Metabolism* 1979; **28**: 688–705.
9 Morley JE, Mooradian AD, Rosenthal MJ, Kaiser FE. Diabetes mellitus in elderly patients. Is it different? *Am J Med* 1987; **83**: 533–41.
10 De Fronzo RA, Robin JD, Andres R. Glucose clamp technique. A method for quantifying insulin secretion and resistance. *Am J Physiol* 1979; **237**: E214–23.
11 Fink RI, Kolterman OG, Griffin J, Olefsky JM. Mechanism of insulin resistance in aging. *J Clin Invest* 1983; **71**: 1523–35.
12 Rowe JW, Minaker KL, Pallotta JA, Flier JS. Characterization of the insulin resistance of aging. *J Clin Invest* 1983; **71**: 1581–7.
13 Chen M, Bergman RN, Pacini G, Portre D Jr. Pathogenesis of age-related glucose intolerance in man: insulin resistance and decreased B-cell function. *J Clin Endocrinol Metab* 1985; **60**: 13–20.
14 Pacini G, Valerio A, Beccaro F, Nosacine R, Cobelli C, Crepaldi G. Insulin sensitivity and beta-cell responsivity are not decreased in elderly subjects with normal OGTT. *J Am Geriatr Soc* 1988; **36**: 317–23.
15 Jarrett RJ, Keen H, McCartney P. The Whitehall Study: ten year follow-up report on men with impaired glucose tolerance with reference to worsening to diabetes and predictors of death. *Diabetic Med* 1984; **1**: 279–83.
16 Jarrett RJ, McCartney P, Keen H. The Bedford Survey: ten year mortality rates in newly diagnosed diabetics, borderline diabetics and normoglycaemic controls and risk indicators for coronary heart disease in borderline diabetics. *Diabetologia* 1982; **22**: 79–84.
17 Cerami A. Glucose as a mediator of aging. *J Am Geriatr Soc* 1985; **9**: 626–34.
18 Laws A, Reaven GM. Effect of physical activity on age-related glucose intolerance. *Clin Geriatr Med* 1990; **6**: 849–63.
19 Reaven GM, Reaven EP. Effects of age on various aspects of glucose and insulin metabolism. *Mol Cell Biochem* 1980; **31**: 37–47.
20 Goldberg AP, Coon PJ. Diabetes mellitus and glucose metabolism in the elderly. In: Hazzard WR, Andres R, Burman ED, *et al.* (eds), *Principles of Geriatric Medicine and Gerontology.* New York: McGraw-Hill, 1994; 825–43.
21 Rosenthal M, Haskell WL, Solomon R, *et al.* Demonstration of a relationship between level of physical training and insulin-stimulated glucose utilization in normal humans. *Diabetes* 1983; **32**: 408–11.

22 Zavaroni I, Dall'Aglio E, Bruschi R, *et al.* Effect of age and environmental factors on glucose tolerance and insulin secretion in a worker population. *J Am Geriatr Soc* 1986; **34**: 271–8.

23 Shimokata S, Muller DC, Fleg JL. Age as independent determinant of glucose tolerance. *Diabetes* 1991; **40**: 44–51.

24 Kissebah AH, Peiris AN. Biology of regional fat distribution: Relationship to non-insulin-dependent diabetes mellitus. *Diabetes Metab Rev* 1989; **5**: 83–109.

25 Peiris AN, Gistafson AB, Kissebah AH. Health and regional adiposity: Implications for the clinician. In: Bagdade JD (ed.), *Yearbook of Endocrinology*. St Louis: Mosby Yearbook, 1989: 283–95.

26 Kaye SA, Folsom AR, Sprafka JM, Prineas RJ, Wallace RB. Increased incidence of diabetes mellitus in relation to abdominal adiposity in older women. *J Clin Epidemiol* 1991; **44**: 329–34.

27 Coon PJ, Rogus EM, Drinkwater D, *et al.* Role of body fat distribution in the decline of insulin sensitivity and glucose tolerance with age. *J Clin Endocrinol Metab* 1992; **75**: 1125–32.

28 Shimokata H, Andres R, Coon PJ, Elahi D, Muller DC, Tobin JD. Studies in the distribution of body fat: II. Longitudinal effects of change in weight. *Int J Obes* 1989; **13**: 455–64.

29 Coon PJ, Bleecker E, Drinkwater D, Meyers D, Goldberg AP. Effects of body composition and exercise capacity on glucose tolerance, insulin and lipoprotein lipids in healthy older men. *Metabolism* 1989; **38**: 1202–9.

30 Kahn CR. Insulin resistance, insulin insensitivity, and insulin unresponsiveness—a necessary distinction.*Metabolism* 1978; **27**: 1893–902.

31 Rendell M, Ross DA, Drew HM, Zarriello J. Endogenous insulin secretion measured by C-peptide in maturity-onset diabetes is controllable by diet alone. *Arch Intern Med* 1981; **141**: 1617–22.

32 Reaven GM. Beneficial effect of moderate weight loss in older patients with non-insulin-dependent diabetes mellitus poorly controlled with insulin. *J Am Geriatr Soc* 1988; **33**: 93–5.

33 Morley JE. Nutritional status of the elderly. *Am J Med* 1986; **81**: 679–95.

34 Rosenthal MJ, Hartnell JM, Morley JE, *et al.* UCLA geriatric grand rounds: diabetes in the elderly. *J Am Geriatr Soc* 1987; **35**: 435–47.

35 National Institutes of Health. Consensus development conference on diet and exercise in non-insulin-dependent diabetes mellitus. *Diabetes Care* 1987; **10**: 639–44.

36 Morley JE, Perry HM III. The management of diabetes mellitus in older individuals. *Drugs* 1991; **41**: 548–65.

37 Stern MP. Kelly West lecture. Primary prevention of type II diabetes mellitus. *Diabetes Care* 1991; **14**: 399–409.

38 O'Hanlon P, Kohrs MB. Dietary studies of older Americans. *Am J Clin Nutr* 1978; **31**: 1257–69.

39 US Department of Agriculture. *Household Food Consumption Survey, 1965–66.* Report No. 11, 1972.

40 Anderson JW, Herman RH. Effect of fasting, caloric restriction and refeeding on glucose tolerance on normal men. *Am J Clin Nutr* 1972; **24**: 41–52.

41 Brunzell JD, Lerner RL, Porte D Jr, Bierman EL. Effect of a fat-free, high carbohydrate diet on diabetic subjects with fasting hyperglycemia. *Diabetes* 1974; **23**: 138–42.

42 Anderson JW, Herman RH, Zakim D. Effect of high glucose and high sucrose diets on glucose tolerance in normal men. *Am J Clin Nutr* 1973; **26**: 600–7.

43 Chen M, Halter JB, Porte D Jr. The role of dietary carbohydrate in the decreased glucose tolerance of the elderly. *J Am Geriatr Soc* 1987; **35**: 417–24.
44 Reed RL, Mooradian AD. Nutritional status and dietary management of elderly diabetic patients. *Clin Geriatr Med* 1990; **6**: 882–901.
45 Coulston AM, Hollenbeck CB, Swislocki ALM, Chen YD, Reaven GM. Deleterious metabolic effects of high carbohydrate, sucrose-containing diets in patients with NIDDM. *Am J Med* 1987; **84**: 213–20.
46 Reaven GM. Dietary therapy for non-insulin-dependent diabetes mellitus. *N Engl J Med* 1988; **319**: 862–4.
47 Gorg A, Bonanome A, Grundy SM, *et al.* Comparison of a high carbohydrate diet with a high monosaturated fat diet in patients with non-insulin-dependent diabetes mellitus. *N Engl J Med* 1988; **319**: 829–34.
48 Bantle JP, Laine DC, Castle JW, *et al.* Postprandial glucose and insulin responses to meals containing different carbohydrates in normal and diabetic subjects. *N Engl J Med* 1983; **309**: 7–12.
49 Bantle JP. Clinical aspects of sucrose and fructose metabolism. *Diabetes Care* 1989; **12**: 56–61.
50 Mooradian AD, Morley JE. Micronutrient status in diabetes mellitus. *Am J Clin Nutr* 1987; **45**: 877–95.
51 Urgerg M, Zemel MB. Evidence for synergism between chromium and nicotinic acid in the control of glucose tolerance in elderly patients. *Metabolism* 1987; **35**: 435–47.
52 Paolisso G, Guigliano D, D'Amore A, *et al.* Daily vitamin E supplements improve metabolic control but not insulin secretion in elderly type II diabetic patients. *Diabetes Care* 1993; **16**: 1433–7.
53 Kinlaw WB, Levine AS, Morley JE, Silvis SE, McClain CJ. Abnormal zinc metabolism in type II diabetes mellitus. *Am J Med* 1983; **75**: 273–7.
54 Niewoehner CB, Allen JI, Boosalis M, Levine AS, Morley JE. The role of zinc supplementation in type II diabetes mellitus. *Am J Med* 1986; **81**: 63–8.
55 Seals DR, Hagberg JM, Allen WK, *et al.* Glucose tolerance in young and older athletes and sedentary men. *J Appl Physiol* 1984; **56**: 1521–5.
56 Hollenberg CR, Haskell W, Rosenthal M, Reaven GM. Effect of habitual physical activity on regulation of insulin-stimulated glucose disposal in older males. *J Am Geriatr Soc* 1984; **33**: 273–7.
57 Kahn SE, Larson VG, Beard JC, *et al.* Effect of exercise on insulin action, glucose intolerance and insulin secretion in aging. *Am J Physiol* 1990; **258**: E937–43.
58 Hollozy JO, Schultz J, Kusnierkiewics J, *et al.* Effects of exercise on glucose tolerance and insulin resistance: brief review and some preliminary results. *Acta Med Scand* 1986; **711** (Suppl.): 55–65.
59 Burstein R, Polychronakos C, Toews CJ, *et al.* Acute reversal of the enhanced insulin action in trained athletes: association with insulin receptor changes. *Diabetes* 1985; **43**: 756–60.
60 Health GW, Gavin JR III, Hinderliter JM, *et al.* Effects of exercise and lack of exercise on glucose tolerance and insulin sensitivity. *J Appl Physiol Respir Environ Exercise Physiol* 1983; **55**: 512–17.
61 Wing RR, Epstein LH, Paternostro-Bayles M, *et al.* Exercise in a behavioural weight control programme for obese patients with type II (non-insulin-dependent) diabetes. *Diabetologia* 1988; **31**: 902–9.
62 Hirshman MF, Wardzala LJ, Goodyear LJ, Fuller SP, Horton ED, Horton EX. Exercise training increases the number of glucose transporters in rat adipose cells. *Am J Physiol* 1989; **257**: E520–30.

63 Schwartz R, Shuman W, Larson V, *et al*. The effect of intensive endurance training on body fat distribution in young and older men. *Metabolism* 1991; **40**: 545–51.

64 Zimmet P, Dowse G, Finch C, Serjeantson S, King H. The epidemiology and natural history of NIDDM—lessons from the South Pacific. *Diabetes Metab Rev* 1990; **6**: 91–124.

65 Frisch RE, Wyshak G, Albright TE, *et al*. Lower prevalence of diabetes in female former college athletes compared with nonathletes. *Diabetes* 1986; **35**: 1101–5.

66 Manson JE, Rimm EB, Stampfer MJ, *et al*. Physical activity and incidence of non-insulin-dependent diabetes mellitus in women. *Lancet* 1991; **338**: 774–8.

67 Manson JE, Nathan DM, Krolewski AS. A prospective study of exercise. *JAMA* 1992; **268**: 63–7.

68 Helmrich SP, Ragaland DR, Leung RW, *et al*. Physical activity and reduced occurrence of non-insulin-dependent diabetes mellitus. *N Engl J Med* 1991; **325**: 147–52.

69 Lamy P. The elderly and drug interactions. *J Am Geriatr Soc* 1986; **34**: 586–92.

70 Ames RP. Negative effects of diuretic drugs on metabolic risk factors for coronary heart disease: possible alternative drug therapies. *Am J Cardiol* 1983; **51**: 632–8.

71 Pandit MK, Burke J, Gustafson AB, *et al*. Drug-induced disorders of glucose tolerance. *Ann Intern Med* 1993; **118**: 529–39.

72 Nolan L, O'Malley K. Prescribing for the elderly. Part II. Prescribing patterns: differences due to age. *J Am Geriatr Soc* 1988; **36**: 245–54.

73 Montamat SC, Cusack BJ, Vestal RE. Management of drug therapy in the elderly. *N Engl J Med* 1989; **321**: 303–9.

74 Page RCL, Harnden NKN, Walravens NKN, *et al*. 'Health living' and sulpho-nylurea therapy have different effects on glucose tolerance and risk factors for vascular disease in subjects with impaired glucose tolerance. *QJ Med* 1993; **86**: 145–54.

75 The Diabetes Control and Complications Trial Research Group. The effect of intensive treatment of diabetes on the development and progression of long-term complications in insulin-dependent diabetes mellitus. *N Engl J Med* 1993; **329**: 977–86.

76 Reichard P, Nilsson B-Y, Rosenqvist U. The effect of long-term intensified insulin treatment on the development of microvascular complications of diabetes mellitus. *N Engl J Med* 1993; **329**: 304–9.

77 Genuth S. Insulin use in NIDDM. *Diabetes Care* 1990; **13**: 140–1264.

78 Donahue RP, Orchard TJ. Diabetes mellitus and macrovascular complications: an epidemiological perspective. *Diabetes Care* 1992; **15**: 1141–55.

79 Position Statement of the American Diabetes Association: Screening for diabetes. *Diabetes Care* 1989; **12**: 588–90.

80 Morisaki N, Watanabe S, Kobayashi J, *et al*. Diabetic control and progression of retinopathy in elderly patients: five year follow-up study. *J Am Geriatr Soc* 1994; **42**: 142–5.

81 Reichard P, Pihl M. Mortality and treatment of side-effects during long-term intensified conventional insulin treatment in the Stockholm Diabetes Interven-tion Study. *Diabetes* 1994; **43**: 313–17.

82 Applegate WB, Blass JP, Williams TF. Instruments for the functional assessment of older patients. *N Engl J Med* 1990; **322**: 1207–14.

83 Yesavage JA, Brink TL, Rose TL. Development and validation of a geriatric depression screening scale: a preliminary report. *J Psychiatr Res* 1983; **17**: 37–49.

84 The University Group Diabetes Program. A study of the effects of hypoglycemic agents on vascular complications in patients with adult-onset diabetes. II. Mortality results. *Diabetes* 1970; **19** (Suppl. 2): 787–830.
85 UK Prospective Diabetes Study Group. UK Prospective Diabetes Study (UKPDS). VIII. Study design, progress and performance. *Diabetologia* 1991; **34**: 877–90.
86 Consensus Statement. Role of cardiovascular risk factors in prevention and treatment of macrovascular disease in diabetes. *Diabetes Care* 1990; **13** (Suppl. 1): 53–9.
87 The Systolic Hypertension in the Elderly Program (SHEP) Cooperative Research Group: Prevention of stroke by hypertensive drug treatment in older patients with isolated systolic hypertension. Final results of SHEP. *JAMA* 1991; **265**: 3255–64.
88 MRC Working Party. Medical Research Council of trial treatment of hypertension in older adults: Principal results. *Br Med J* 1992; **304**: 405–12.
89 De Fronzo RA, Ferrannini E. Insulin resistance: A multifaceted syndrome responsible for NIDDM, obesity, hypertension, dyslipidemia and atherosclerotic cardiovascular disease. *Diabetes Care* 1991; **14**: 173–8.
90 Reaven GM. Role of insulin resistance in human disease. *Diabetes* 1988; **37**: 1595–607.
91 Reaven GM. Resistance to insulin-stimulated glucose uptake and hyperinsulinemia. Role of non-insulin-dependent diabetes, high blood pressure, dyslipidemia and coronary heart disease. *Diabetes Metab* 1991; **17**: 78–86.
92 Karam JH. Type II diabetes and syndrome X. Pathogenesis and glycemic management. *Endocrinol Metab Clin North Am* 1992; **21**: 329–50.
93 Lewis EJ, Hunsicker LG, Bain RP, *et al*. The effect of angiotensin-converting-enzyme inhibition on diabetic nephropathy. *N Engl J Med* 1993; **329**: 1456–62.
94 Pollare T, Lithell H, Berne C. A comparison of the effects of hydrochlorthiazide and captopril on glucose and lipid metabolism in patients with hypertension. *N Engl J Med* 1989; **321**: 868–73.
95 Negoro H, Morley JE, Rosenthal MJ. Utility of serum fructosamine as a measure of glycemia in young and old diabetic and non-diabetic subjects. *Am J Med* 1988; **85**: 360–4.

4

Establishing the Diagnosis

P. JEAN HO and JOHN R. TURTLE
Department of Medicine, University of Sydney, NSW, Australia

WHY DIABETES IS A PROBLEM IN ELDERLY PEOPLE

Diabetes is one of the most common chronic diseases which can lead to complications that seriously affect quality of life and life span. It has an incidence and prevalence which increase greatly with age[1] and is therefore particularly relevant to the elderly age group, defined here as persons who are 65 years of age or older. Diagnosed diabetes is present in 7–10% of the elderly population, making up approximately 40% of persons with known diabetes in the general population[2,3]. In addition, 10% of elderly persons have undiagnosed diabetes[4], are untreated and at an even higher risk from the morbidity and mortality of diabetes. Another 20% of elderly persons have impaired glucose tolerance (IGT)[3,5], and are at increased risk of developing macrovascular disease and diabetes. Thus, nearly one in five of the elderly population have diabetes, diagnosed or undiagnosed. When IGT is included, 40% of the elderly population have some degree of impaired glucose homeostasis[3].

With increasing longevity, this 65 years and over age group which currently represents 11% of the United States population will increase to approximately 20% by the year 2021[5]. Elderly diabetic persons have much higher hospitalization rates and use of ambulatory services than those without diabetes[6]. With the ageing population, more people will live long enough to develop diabetes. The number of persons with diabetes among this age group will rise and continue to place increasing demands on health care resources.

Diabetes in Old Age. Edited by P. Finucane and A. J. Sinclair
© 1995 John Wiley & Sons Ltd

MORBIDITY FROM DIABETES

The main argument in favour of detection of diabetes in its early stages is to reduce or prevent its complications, which otherwise would lead to further morbidity. Poor vision and blindness due to diabetic eye disease, lower limb amputation due to peripheral vascular disease, neuropathy and infection, ischaemic heart disease, cerebrovascular accidents and chronic renal failure can all severely limit an elderly person's mobility, independence and quality of life.

Chronic complications of diabetes are often present in elderly people with newly diagnosed diabetes; at diagnosis 10% have established retinopathy[7] and there is a two- to threefold excess of cardiovascular complications adding to the effect of other cardiovascular risk factors[8]. The prevalence of some diabetic complications such as retinopathy, peripheral neuropathy, and proteinuria increase with age, although duration of diabetes and glycaemic control were more important predictors than age in some studies[9-11]. Chronic diabetic complications can be more devastating to the patient's well-being when they first occur at an elderly age. By diagnosing diabetes early, complications may be prevented or even reversed. The current life expectancy for Australians aged 65 years is 15 years for men and 19 years for women, thus prevention of long-term diabetic complications is important even in this age group.

The elderly diabetic person is prone to certain acute complications of the disease. Hyperglycaemia leads to osmotic diuresis. With the decreased sense of thirst, the elderly diabetic person is less able to ingest sufficient fluids and therefore is at risk of sodium and water depletion, hypotension, hyperosmolarity, hypokalaemia (especially if the patient is taking diuretics), reduction in insulin secretion, and thrombotic events. Following myocardial infarction or septicaemia, elderly patients are more likely to develop shock, which may lead to lactic acidosis particularly in patients with poorly controlled diabetes. Such acute complications can become life-threatening but many can also be prevented by early diagnosis of diabetes and appropriate management.

MORTALITY FROM DIABETES

The majority (86–92%) of elderly people with diabetes have non-insulin-dependent diabetes (NIDDM). Patients with NIDDM have an overall 10-year mortality rate as high as 44%. With advancing age of onset of NIDDM, overall mortality increases although the increment from diabetes falls. Although there may be no further increase in mortality due to diabetes when the diagnosis is made after the age of 75 years[12], one study suggested that there may still be a higher cohort mortality in diabetic than non-diabetic persons above the age of 80 years[13]. Cardiovascular disease is the major cause of death among people with diabetes, and ischaemic heart disease may account for half the number of deaths in this group[14]. Persons with diabetes, have 1.5 times the in-hospital mortality rate and 1.4 times the post-discharge mortality rate after acute myocardial infarction compared with non-diabetic persons[15]. It is imperative therefore that diabetes is diagnosed early to reduce, delay or prevent the associated morbidity, mortality and cost in this age group.

With increasing life expectancy, the opinion that people who get diabetes in the older age group do not live long enough to develop complications and so do not need treatment for mild to moderate hyperglycaemia, is no longer valid. Early detection of diabetes may be of benefit in other ways. A physician may consider the possibility of diabetes-related problems more promptly in an emergency. The offspring of a person with diabetes can be induced into screening and preventative measures themselves.

WHEN DIABETES SHOULD BE SUSPECTED

Early diagnosis of diabetes requires a high degree of vigilance on the part of the physician. Many people with diabetes, especially the elderly are asymptomatic. At the time of diagnosis of diabetes, long-term complications of diabetes are often present but the patient may be asymptomatic. Elderly patients may present with non-specific symptoms only, which may be dismissed as 'normal ageing' by themselves and their physicians. Elderly patients are generally more likely to present at a later stage of illness. This leads to underreporting of illness, confusion as to the cause of the illness and atypical presentation. Multiple pathology is usually present in the elderly patient, and may further complicate the diagnosis.

Even a typical mode of presentation of diabetes may be missed in an elderly person. Mild to moderate weight loss and fatigue may be unnoticed, unreported or dismissed. Even the classical symptoms of hyperglycaemia, namely polyuria, thirst, polydipsia and polyphagia may be absent. Polyuria may be misinterpreted as dribbling, incontinence from mechanical bladder problems, or as urinary tract infection. Polydipsia is often mild or absent due to the increased renal threshold for glucose and reduced thirst mechanism with ageing[16]. Polyphagia is difficult to elicit, as the elderly usually present with anorexia when ill. Infection, usually of mild severity, is often present but may be asymptomatic until a very late stage.

Some clinical manifestations of hyperglycaemia which should lead a physician to suspect diabetes are presented in Table 4.1; however, it must be emphasized that like many other diseases in the elderly, diabetes often mimics, coexists with and complicates other diseases.

Table 4.1. Clinical features of hyperglycaemia in elderly people. Reprinted by permission of Blackwell Scientific Publications, Inc

Primary effect	Secondary effect
Osmotic diuresis	Increased urination, nocturia, poor sleep, nocturnal falls, incontinence, dehydration, excessive thirst, polydipsia, weakness
Fluctuating refraction	Poor vision, decreased mobility, falls, impaired ability to drive
Poor red cell deformability and platelet adhesiveness	Intermittent claudication, thrombotic stroke, myocardial infarction
Recurrent infections	
Poor wound healing	
Non-specific complaints e.g. weight loss, fatigue	
Alteration in mentation	Poor memory, poor compliance
Depression	
Decreased pain threshold	Increased symptoms of pain
Impaired recovery from stroke	
Hyperosmolar non-ketotic hyperglycaemia	Severe dehydration, decreased consciousness, coma, visual disturbances, seizures, cerebral thrombosis
Diabetic ketoacidosis	

(Adapted from Rosenthal MJ, Morley JE. Diabetes and its complications in older people. In: Morley JE, Korenman SG (eds), *Endocrinology and Metabolism in the Elderly*. Boston: Blackwell Scientific Publications, 1992: 373–87.)

Some elderly patients may present with symptoms of chronic complications of diabetes such as visual loss, peripheral nerve abnormalities, ischaemic heart disease, congestive cardiac failure, peripheral vascular or cerebrovascular disease. Even when there are no symptoms suggestive of hyperglycaemia, a survey for risk factors for diabetes mellitus in every elderly patient is warranted (Table 4.2) because of the high prevalence of undiagnosed diabetes in this age group, and the large proportion of diabetic elderly who are asymptomatic. Such a survey is simple to perform and highlights the relevance of various aspects of routine primary care of the elderly patient.

Most elderly persons who develop diabetes have NIDDM. Obesity may be the most important factor related to NIDDM[1]. An elderly diabetic person is more likely to be obese than a non-diabetic person[13]. In the Framingham Study, men and women with Metropolitan relative weights exceeding 140%

Table 4.2. Risk factors for diabetes mellitus in elderly people

---

1. Obesity—body mass index >25 (weight in kg/height in m^2) or percentage ideal weight equal to or greater than 115%.

2. Abdominal obesity—waist circumference >95 cm in women and >100 cm in men.

3. Positive family history of non-insulin-dependent diabetes in direct relatives.

4. Ischaemic heart disease.

5. Hypertension.

6. Cerebrovascular disease.

7. Peripheral vascular disease.

8. Dyslipidaemia.

9. Positive history of glucose intolerance.

10. Morbid obstetrical history or a history of babies over 4 kg at birth.

11. Certain racial groups, e.g. Asian migrants[17], Hispanic Americans[18].

12. Use of diabetogenic drugs, e.g. corticosteroids, oestrogens, thiazides, beta blockers and phenytoin.

---

had twice the prevalence of diabetes compared with those with relative weights less than 119%[1]. Abdominal obesity is positively associated with insulin resistance and increased risk of diabetes[19,20]. Although its mode of inheritance is unknown, NIDDM occurs in identical twins with high concordance[21,22] and its high prevalence in certain racial groups is decreased by foreign genetic admixture[23]. In comparison with the general population, the risk of NIDDM is four times higher in the siblings of cases and eight times higher in the offspring of two parents with NIDDM[24]. Cardiovascular disease, intermittent claudication, increased very low-density lipoprotein cholesterol, and decreased high-density lipoprotein (HDL) cholesterol have also been identified as possible precursors of diabetes[1]. Both isolated systolic and diastolic hypertension are more prevalent in diabetic than non-diabetic persons[1]. Considering the morbidity associated with diabetes and its high prevalence in the elderly, all elderly persons should be screened for diabetes. Elderly persons with one or more risk factors (other than advanced age) should have the diagnosis of diabetes ruled out definitively.

ESTABLISHING THE DIAGNOSIS OF DIABETES IN ELDERLY PEOPLE

If a patient has classic symptoms of hyperglycaemia (polyuria, polydipsia and weight loss) with gross and unequivocal elevation of plasma glucose level ($\geqslant$11.1 mmol/l; $\geqslant$200 mg/dl), the diagnosis of diabetes mellitus is established. No biochemical confirmation is required[25,26].

SCREENING OF ASYMPTOMATIC ELDERLY PATIENTS WHO HAVE NO RISK FACTORS FOR DIABETES OTHER THAN AGE

What is the justification for screening for diabetes in the population who are 65 years or older? The prevalence of the disease is increased in these individuals. It has a significant impact on quality of life and life span. There is an asymptomatic period, during which effective treatment reduces morbidity, mortality and financial cost due to the disease. Tests are available at reasonable cost to detect diabetes in the asymptomatic period.

In one study, yearly screening of venous plasma glucose levels post-prandially or post oral glucose loading in elderly nursing home residents (average age 82 years) revealed progressive deterioration in glucose tolerance[13]. Almost one-half of those subjects with abnormal screening levels were diabetic on oral glucose tolerance testing (OGTT), indicating how easily diabetes can be missed in this group without screening, noting that the disease was present in 14.5% of nursing home residents[12]. Currently, the National Health and Medical Research Council of Australia recommends that elderly people 65 years of age or older be screened annually for diabetes during routine visits to their general practitioners[27]. This should be done in all persons in this age group whether or not there are symptoms of hyperglycaemia, or any other high risk factors for diabetes mellitus.

Screening Procedure

The primary purpose of screening is to identify those elderly persons who have a high probability of meeting the diagnostic criteria for diabetes. Screening is simply done by measuring a random venous plasma glucose level. The fasting plasma glucose level or the OGTT have higher sensitivity, specificity and positive predictive value for diagnosing diabetes[28] but require more organization. Glycosylated haemoglobin is not suitable for screening purposes due to its poor sensitivity and predictive value[29]. Several factors other than plasma glucose concentration commonly present in older persons may alter the glycosylated haemoglobin level[30].

Interpreting the Result of Screening and Follow-up

If the random venous plasma glucose is below 11.1 mmol/l (200 mg/dl), it is non-diagnostic. A repeat screen is indicated a year later, provided that no high risk factors emerge in the interim. Should relevant risk factors emerge, the patient should have a fasting venous plasma glucose measured as discussed below.

If the random venous plasma glucose is equal to or greater than 11.1 mmol/l, a fasting venous plasma glucose level should be measured (see below).

ESTABLISHING THE DIAGNOSIS IN ELDERLY PATIENTS

1. who are asymptomatic of hyperglycaemia and do not have high risk factors for diabetes other than age, but have a random venous plasma glucose of 11.1 mmol/l (200 mg/dl) or greater during routine screening; or
2. who are asymptomatic of hyperglycaemia but have one or more high risk factors for diabetes other than age; or
3. who have mild symptoms of hyperglycaemia, with or without high risk factors for diabetes other than age.

Testing Procedure

A fasting venous plasma glucose level is measured.

Interpretation of the Test Result

If the fasting venous plasma glucose is below 7.8 mmol/l (140 mg/dl), an OGTT is indicated (see below).

If the fasting venous plasma glucose level is equal to or greater than 7.8 mmol/l, it should be measured again. If both readings are equal to or greater than 7.8 mmol/l, the diagnosis of diabetes mellitus is established[25,26], and an OGTT is not required. If only one reading is equal to or greater than 7.8 mmol/l, an OGTT is required to rule out the diagnosis of diabetes.

In situations of acute illness, stress or immobilization in a hospital bed, elevated fasting blood glucose levels indicate defective mechanisms to deal with glucose under stress. It is incorrect to interpret such elevated blood sugar levels as falsely positive. A provisional diagnosis of glucose intolerance or possible diabetes should be made. Blood sugar levels should be monitored and treated as indicated by the degree of hyperglycaemia. On recovery from acute illness, the diagnosis of diabetes should be ruled out by fasting plasma glucose levels or by OGTT if the former are non-diagnostic.

ORAL GLUCOSE TOLERANCE TEST

Test Procedure

The OGTT is seldom necessary unless repeated fasting glucose levels are borderline or inconsistent. It is performed in the following way[31]. Prior to the test, the patient should be ambulant and without any restriction on usual physical activity. An unrestricted diet (more than 150 g of carbohydrate per day) is taken for 3 days before the test. If possible, medications should be discontinued for 3 days before the test. The test is administered in the morning after a fast (except for water) of at least 10 but no more than 16 h. During the test, the patient should remain seated and not smoke. A loading dose of 75 g glucose solution is administered orally. Venous plasma glucose is measured immediately before the patient begins to drink the solution and every 30 min thereafter for 2 h.

Contraindications to the Test

The test should not be performed:

1. If the diagnosis of diabetes has already been established by an unequivocal elevation of plasma venous glucose level and classic symptoms of hyperglycaemia, or by two fasting venous plasma glucose levels of 7.8 mmol/l (140 mg/dl) or greater. Performance of the OGTT may cause a harmful degree of hyperglycaemia and also would not give any further information.

2. In patients who are experiencing acute medical or surgical stress as it may lead to a false-positive result. The OGTT should be delayed until several months after recovery.

3. In persons who are chronically malnourished.

4. In persons who have been confined to bed for 3 days or more.

Interpretation of the Test Result (see Table 4.3)

This method of interpretation is based on a comparison of the World Health Organisation (WHO)[26] and National Diabetes Data Group (NDDG)[25] criteria on OGTT results of two large population samples[32]. These two sets of original criteria agree on the two cut-off points relating to the 2 h value: the upper limit defining diabetes ($\geqslant$11.1 mmol/l; 200 mg/dl) and the lower limit defining normality (7.8 mmol/l; 140 mg/dl). They both define fasting hyperglycaemia as $\geqslant$7.8 mmol/l. However, they differ in that the NDDG defines a mid-test level of $\geqslant$11.1 mmol/l as abnormal and a normal fasting level as <6.4 mmol/l; 115 mg/dl, whereas the WHO does not require a mid-test level, and defines a normal fasting level as <7.8 mmol/l. Under the NDDG criteria, groups 3 and 4 in Table 4.3 are labelled as non-diagnostic, while under WHO criteria, group 3 is normal and group 4 has IGT. Modan *et al.*[32] showed that the profiles of physiological markers of IGT of subjects in groups 3–5 were similar, hence the recommendation that

Table 4.3. Classification of results of the oral glucose tolerance test

| Classification | Venous plasma glucose concentration (mmol/l) | | |
	Fasting	1 h or 'mid-test'	2 h
1. Normal	<6.4	<11.1	<7.8
2. Normal	6.4–7.7	<11.1	<7.8
3. IGT*	<7.8	⩾11.1	<7.8
4. IGT	<7.8	<11.1	7.8–11.0
5. IGT	<7.8	⩾11.1	7.8–11.0
6. Diabetic	<7.8	⩾11.1	⩾11.1

* IGT = impaired glucose tolerance.
Note: 6.4 mmol/l ≡ 115 mg/dl; 7.8 mmol/l ≡ 140 mg/dl; 11.1 mmol/l ≡ 200 mg/dl.

these three groups be labelled as IGT. Groups 1 and 2 were similar to each other for the markers examined and differed in the OGTT only by the fasting level. They are therefore classified as normal glucose tolerance.

Current Opinion on Glucose Tolerance Testing in Elderly People

The usefulness of the OGTT in the elderly has been questioned. Most patients (about 75%) diagnosed with IGT never develop diabetes. Many people diagnosed with diabetes by the OGTT never develop fasting hyperglycaemia or symptomatic diabetes[33]. Repeat OGTTs done in the same individual under standard conditions may give different results[25]. Social, employment and insurance ramifications of the label of diabetes can be economically and psychologically stressful for the elderly diabetic person. Consequently, the OGTT is rarely indicated in clinical practice[33]. It has been suggested that the diagnosis of diabetes mellitus should be limited to those with fasting hyperglycaemia in this age group[34,35].

Another reason for limiting the use of the OGTT in the clinical setting is that glucose intolerance appears to be almost physiological in the elderly. As discussed in Chapter 2, a decline in glucose tolerance starts in the third decade and continues throughout life. This is characterized by the moderate increase in 1- and 2-h postprandial plasma glucose concentrations. After a 100-g oral glucose challenge, there is a rise in arterialized venous plasma glucose concentration from 60 to 180 min of 0.7–0.8 mmol/l per decade[36]. A small increase in fasting plasma glucose concentration has also been demonstrated in some but not all studies[36]. The pathogenesis of glucose intolerance in the elderly is multifactorial, involving impaired glucose-induced insulin secretion, delayed and prolonged insulin-mediated suppression of hepatic glucose output, as well as delayed insulin-stimulated peripheral glucose uptake which appears to be the major disturbance, with skeletal muscle being the primary site of the defect[36]. The relative importance of factors such as decreased physical activity, diet changes, reduced muscle mass and obesity is not fully understood. A comparison of metabolic abnormalities in ageing, obesity and NIDDM suggested that NIDDM and glucose intolerance of ageing were distinct entities[36].

However, other lines of evidence suggest that the hyperglycaemia of ageing may indeed be pathological. The percentage of glycosylated haemoglobin increases with ageing in non-diabetic persons[37], even when no rise in fasting plasma glucose is detected[38], suggesting that at least there is increased glycosylation of haemoglobin in these persons. The findings that glucose may mediate cross-linkage of proteins and that advanced glycosylation end-products accumulate in some tissues with age and in diabetes may help explain how glucose intolerance of ageing also leads to atherosclerotic macrovascular complications of diabetes[39,40].

In conclusion, most cases of diabetes in the elderly are readily diagnosed without the OGTT. In the individual patient, when less intensive testing for diabetes is non-diagnostic, the OGTT may be the only way of obtaining a definitive diagnosis so that effective management can be commenced to improve glycaemic control and prevent complications of the disease.

The risks of an individual with IGT developing diabetes or macrovascular disease are increased, substantially unrelated to age[41]. Diagnosis of IGT in the elderly therefore demands active intervention to improve the risks. Currently, there are no generally accepted age-adjusted criteria for the diagnosis of diabetes or IGT in the elderly. The criteria described above are diagnostic for diabetes in any non-pregnant adult.

Should Annual Screening for Diabetes Mellitus in the Elderly be Limited?

Grobin's[13] study of nursing home residents reported that blood sugar levels following a 50 g oral glucose load and the percentage of subjects with abnormal screening levels did not rise after the age of 80 years. Both parameters showed a consistent drop after the age of 90 years. Age-specific prevalence of diagnosed diabetes appears to plateau at about 10% after the age of 74 years[3]. In contrast, the prevalence of diabetes diagnosed or undiagnosed in individuals over the age of 80 years has been estimated to be as high as 40%[12]. Thus, there is probably a large number of elderly persons with undiagnosed diabetes in whom the diagnosis of diabetes may reduce morbidity and probably mortality. There is no clear age above which persons with consistently normal annual screening plasma glucose levels may not benefit from further yearly screening. However, the decision should be made on an individual patient basis, taking into account coexisting diseases, general well-being and life expectancy.

EVALUATION OF THE ELDERLY PATIENT WITH DIABETES OR IGT

The vast majority of newly diagnosed diabetic persons who are 65 years of age or older have NIDDM. Some of these patients may require insulin for glycaemic control after a short trial of treatment with diet, exercise and oral hypoglycaemic agents, but they are not dependent on insulin to prevent ketoacidosis or to sustain life; they should not be classified as insulin-dependent diabetics. However, some elderly patients with long-standing NIDDM may lose the ability to secrete insulin and thus become insulin dependent and may be diagnosed at this late stage. Before starting treatment for IGT or diabetes, a comprehensive evaluation should be carried out, focusing on factors which may influence the management plan (Table 4.4).

At the time of diagnosis of IGT or diabetes, the contribution of medication and illnesses (especially infection, cancer, hyperthyroidism)

Table 4.4. Evaluation of elderly patients with impaired glucose tolerance or diabetes

---

Routine history:
  Relevant past medical history
  Risk factors for diabetes (Table 4.2)
  Family history of vascular disease, hypertension, dyslipidaemia, other endocrine
    disorders
  Eating habits
  Weight history, especially recent changes
  Level of physical activity
  Socio-economic status
  Smoking and alcohol usage
  Drug history
  Symptoms of diabetic complications
Routine physical examination:
  Including determination of body mass index and waist circumference
Laboratory tests in those with diabetes or IGT
  Urine microscopy and culture
  Fasting total cholesterol, HDL cholesterol and triglycerides
  Estimation of LDL cholesterol
  Serum uric acid
  Thyroid function tests
Other laboratory tests in those with diabetes
  Urinalysis for protein, glucose and ketones
  Glycosylated haemoglobin or fructosamine
  Liver function tests
  Serum urea and creatinine
  Electrocardiogram

---

which may affect glucose tolerance must be considered. Both patients with diabetes and IGT are at risk of macrovascular disease. Therefore, risk factors (other than diabetes or IGT) for atherosclerosis should be sought: obesity, dyslipidaemia, smoking, hypertension and lack of exercise. Elevated serum triglycerides and reduced HDL cholesterol are commonly found in patients with NIDDM. Clinical evidence of existing macrovascular disease should be sought: i.e. ischaemic heart disease, cerebrovascular disease and peripheral vascular disease. Patients with diabetes should have a baseline glycosylated haemoglobin or fructosamine measured to give an integrated measure of recent glycaemic control and monitor progress.

MANAGEMENT OF THE ELDERLY PATIENT WITH IGT

MANAGEMENT GOALS

These patients should be informed that they have an increased chance of developing diabetes and the macrovascular complications of diabetes, but it is not predictable in the individual patient. The management goals for these patients are to normalize blood glucose levels and decrease risk factors for macrovascular disease. When risk factor modifications regarding obesity, diet and exercise are undertaken, the glucose tolerance of many of these individuals often returns to normal.

MANAGEMENT STRATEGIES

The following guidelines apply to both patients with IGT or diabetes. Additional issues concerning the latter group are discussed later.

Weight, Diet and Exercise

Obese patients should aim to achieve some weight reduction by adopting a healthy life-style with a combination of correct diet and regular exercise. Weight reduction should be gradual and need not reach ideal body weight to improve glycaemic control. Patients should be encouraged to take a balanced, nutritionally correct diet and reduce their intake of simple sugars and fat. Unsaturated fat should be substituted by monounsaturated or polyunsaturated fat. Although the optimal dietary composition is unknown, a diet composed of 20% protein, 30% fat, 45–50% complex carbohydrate and less than 10% simple sugars is a generally accepted recommendation[27]. Sodium should be restricted in patients with hypertension. Alcohol restriction is recommended, especially for those with obesity, hypertriglyceridaemia or hypertension. Meal plans should be simple, flexible and adaptable to the elderly patient's ways of life and food preferences. Patients should be referred to a dietitian to facilitate successful dietary management.

Regular exercise improves body weight, plasma lipids, blood pressure, insulin sensitivity and glucose tolerance. It also maintains general fitness, balance, mobility and sense of well-being. Prior to starting regular exercise, the patient should be assessed with respect to cardiovascular, respiratory and musculoskeletal systems by the physician (see Chapter 3). A stress electrocardiogram is indicated in those with suspected ischaemic heart disease. Ideally, moderate exercise should be done for at least 20 min each time, three to four times a week, but the actual duration, frequency and progression of exercise should be individualized. Avoidance of injury during exercise should be taught.

Macrovascular Disease

Treatment of hypertension, dyslipidaemia and cessation of smoking are essential in the prevention or management of macrovascular disease. Low-dose aspirin should be considered in these patients[42] especially postmyo-cardial infarction[43] if there are no contraindications.

The severity of symptomatic peripheral vascular disease should be documented non-invasively by Doppler ultrasonography. Mild disease may improve with exercise and cessation of smoking. Patients with severe disease may benefit from referral to a vascular surgeon. Those with an asymptomatic carotid bruit should be managed conservatively, with attention to risk factors for atherosclerosis. Those with active lesions causing recurrent cerebral ischaemia will benefit from neurological referral. A baseline electro-cardiogram should be obtained in patients with suspected or known cardiovascular disease. Ischaemic heart disease should be treated vigorously as it is a major cause of death in patients with macrovascular disease. In spite of their adverse effects on lipid profiles, glycaemic control, and symptoms of hypoglycaemia, beta blockers have a definite role in reducing postinfarct mortality[43].

Hypertension

Hypertension is a risk factor for macrovascular disease. Most hypertension in patients with IGT or diabetes is essential hypertension. Treatment of essential hypertension in the elderly, including diastolic or isolated systolic hyperten-sion, has been shown to reduce stroke and cardiovascular mortality[44,45], and the benefits can be expected to extend to the elderly with IGT or diabetes. Pharmacological treatment should be considered if blood pressure remains 160/90 mmHg or higher. Maximal non-drug management, i.e. diet, exercise, weight reduction, cessation of smoking, limited alcohol intake and moderate sodium restriction should be pursued before drugs are introduced.

Elderly persons are prone to postural hypotension. No particular antihypertensive drug is contraindicated in the patient with IGT. However, side-effects of different antihypertensive drugs, e.g. hypokalaemia with diuretics, unfavourable lipid profiles with thiazides and beta blockers, postural hypotension with alpha-adrenergic blockers, central adrenergic inhibitors and vasodilators, should always be considered when choosing an antihypertensive drug.

Dyslipidaemia

Dyslipidaemia is a major risk factor for macrovascular disease. Dietary saturated fatty acid restriction and substitution with monosaturated or with polyunsaturated fatty acids under a dietitian's supervision is the first-line treatment for reduction of serum cholesterol and triglyceride levels. This can be effective even in the absence of weight reduction. Regular exercise in all patients and weight reduction for those who are overweight will also improve serum lipid levels. If non-pharmacological therapy is inadequate, lipid lowering drugs should be considered. Gemfibrozil and the 3-hydroxy-3-methylglutaryl (HMG)-coenzyme A (HMG-CoA) reductase inhibitors are useful first-line agents in patients with IGT or diabetes[46]. The former predominantly lowers fasting triglyceride and raises HDL cholesterol levels while the latter predominantly lowers low-density lipoprotein (LDL) cholesterol levels. The increased risk of drug toxicity and non-compliance with multiple drug use in the elderly must be considered before adding drugs to an elderly patient's regimen.

Diabetogenic Drugs

If the patient is taking diabetogenic drugs, they should be continued only if essential. Substitution with non-diabetogenic drugs should be tried.

MANAGEMENT OF THE ELDERLY PATIENT WITH DIABETES

MANAGEMENT GOALS

The vast majority of these patients have NIDDM. The goals of management are: to control the degree and symptoms of hyperglycaemia without precipitating large swings in glucose levels or hypoglycaemia; to prevent or delay complications; and to maintain the patient's general well-being and independence.

MANAGEMENT STRATEGIES

Target Glucose Levels

Hypoglycaemia is more frequent and can be more deleterious in older diabetic patients. The WHO criteria for ideal glycaemic control (venous plasma glucose less than 5.5 mmol/l (100 mg/dl) fasting and less than 7.8 mmol/l (140 mg/dl) 2 h postprandial) are too strict for many elderly people. Criteria for glycaemic control for older people should be adjusted as shown in Table 4.5.

Weight, Diet and Exercise

Much has been written on glycaemic control in the elderly diabetic[47]. The first line and cornerstone of treatment to control glycaemia is diet. Many elderly people with NIDDM respond well to diet and exercise alone without pharmacological intervention for glycaemic control. Gradual and moderate weight reduction is desirable in the obese diabetic. The general principles of a suitable diet are the same as described earlier for the person with glucose intolerance. In addition, attention should be directed to the distribution of carbohydrate through the day and in relation to exercise and particularly if oral hypoglycaemic agents or insulin are taken.

All patients with diabetes should follow a regular exercise programme appropriate for their mobility and fitness. Guidelines for people with glucose intolerance also apply to people diagnosed with diabetes. Any ischaemic heart disease or proliferative retinopathy must be assessed when planning an exercise programme. Glycaemic stability should be achieved prior to starting an exercise programme. Attention should be paid to the

Table 4.5. Criteria for glycaemic control for older people with diabetes (venous plasma glucose, mmol/l)

Glycaemic control	Fasting or at least 3 h since last meal	2 h postprandial
Reasonable	<7.8	<11.1
Poor	>7.8	>11.1*

* In patients taking insulin, higher post prandial levels are acceptable (e.g. up to 15 mmol/l).
Note: 7.8 mmol/l ≡140 mg/dl; 11.1 mmol/l ≡ 200 mg/dl.
(Adapted from National Health and Medical Research Council of Australia. *Diabetes in Older People*. Canberra: Australian Government Publishing Service, 1992: 6. Commonwealth of Australia copyright reproduced by permission)

presence and prevention of foot problems related to neuropathy, vasculo-pathy or skeletal deformities. Suitable footwear must be used. A podiatrist's advice can be invaluable.

Oral Hypoglycaemic Agents (See Chapter 8)

If symptomatic hyperglycaemia and high blood glucose levels persist despite adherence to diet and exercise, sulphonylureas should be considered. Short-acting sulphonylureas, e.g. tolbutamide are preferred because elderly patients are more prone to hypoglycaemia and its deleterious effects. Significant renal or hepatic impairment further increases the risk of hypoglycaemia. Only one sulphonylurea should be used at any time. It should be introduced at a low dose taken with the morning meal before gradual increase to twice a day dosage if necessary. Metformin is often useful in addition to a sulphonylurea in obese patients to assist in weight loss. However, metformin is contraindicated in the presence of cardiac, renal or hepatic impairment because of the risk of lactic acidosis.

Insulin (See Chapter 9)

If diet, exercise and maximal dosage of oral hypoglycaemic agents in combination are still inadequate in controlling hyperglycaemia and its symptoms, insulin will have to be considered instead of hypoglycaemic agents. However, insulin carries with it further risk of hypoglycaemia, and should be used only when absolutely required and at the lowest dose that is effective to keep the blood glucose levels in an acceptable range. The choice of insulin regimen depends on the individual patient's requirements and resources and will be considered elsewhere in this text. Community nursing care services are often useful in implementing and maintaining the correct insulin prescribed, and in home blood glucose monitoring.

Home Monitoring of Glycaemic Control and Ketonuria

Home blood glucose monitoring is essential in any patient who takes insulin, and is helpful in those using oral hypoglycaemic agents. This may be done using a home glucose meter or by visual colour comparison with standard charts. The frequency of monitoring depends on the stability of glycaemic control and the frequency of insulin injections. Home blood glucose monitoring can be difficult for the elderly patient with limited visual acuity, dexterity or financial resources. Community nursing services are often required for these patients.

Urine dipstick testing for glycosuria is not useful because it is affected by the renal threshold for glucose which may be elevated. Testing for ketonuria should be done when blood glucose is persistently elevated above 20 mmol/l (360 mg/dl) and during intercurrent illness.

Macrovascular Disease

Cardiovascular disease accounts for the majority of deaths in patients with diabetes. Reduction of all risk factors for atherosclerosis is a vital part of management of the diabetic patient. Principles of management of coexistent dyslipidaemia, hypertension, ischaemic heart disease, cerebral and peripheral vascular disease outlined in the previous section for patients with IGT should be applied with equal vigour to those with diabetes.

Hypertension

Hypertension is a risk factor for macrovascular disease and nephropathy in patients with diabetes. In terms of antihypertensive drug side-effects, thiazides can also worsen glycaemic control. Beta-adrenergic blockers can blunt the adrenergic symptoms of hypoglycaemia as well as delay recovery from hypoglycaemia, which is particularly dangerous in insulin-treated patients. As first-line agents, angiotensin-converting enzyme inhibitors or calcium channel blockers are often preferred to thiazides or beta blockers owing to the adverse effects of the latter on glycaemic control and lipid profiles. In patients with diabetic nephropathy, diuretics are often required for adequate antihypertensive control.

Dyslipidaemia

Dyslipidaemia in NIDDM has been extensively reviewed by others[46]. The prevalence of dyslipidaemia is increased at least twofold in persons with NIDDM, and involves all classes of lipoprotein. The most common lipid disorder seen in diabetic patients is hypertriglyceridaemia and reduced HDL cholesterol. Diet, exercise, weight reduction and improvement of glycaemic control improve but rarely correct the dyslipidaemia in patients with NIDDM completely. If after 2–3 months of such therapy, total serum cholesterol and LDL cholesterol are still above 5.2 and 3.4 mmol/l, respectively, pharmacological intervention should be considered, although are seldom used unless the total cholesterol is above 6.5 mmol/l. As with patients with IGT, HMG-CoA reductase inhibitors and gemfibrozil are the drugs of choice.

Ischaemic Heart Disease

Ischaemic heart disease is the major cause of death in persons with diabetes. Atherosclerosis progresses at a more rapid rate and is more extensive in older diabetic patients than in their non-diabetic fellows[48]. Postinfarct cardiac failure is more common and survival is lower in diabetics[15]. Thus treatment of ischaemic heart disease and risk factor modification in diabetic patients should have a high priority.

Patient Education

Education is a fundamental part of management of the elderly person with diabetes. Diabetes education programmes in elderly patients have been shown to improve knowledge, metabolic control, life-style and psychological functioning[49]. The content of diabetes education programmes needs to be adapted to elderly diabetic persons with different degrees of independence and comorbidity. Involvement of the patient's family or carer should be encouraged to maximize the benefits of education programmes.

General Management

Management of the elderly diabetic patient poses a special challenge. The elderly patient is likely to have multiple comorbid conditions which must be identified and prioritized for effective management. Financial and psychosocial resources may be limited. The elderly diabetic may have impaired cognitive dysfunction[50,51], which particularly affects memory retrieval and so can adversely affect compliance with medications. Thus directions for all medications should be in writing and education programmes may need to be repeated to be effective. The patient's drug regimen should be reviewed regularly. Polypharmacy should be minimized to prevent drug toxicity and to improve compliance. Potentially diabetogenic drugs should be used only if essential. Home care and nursing services or residential care facilities can often facilitate effective management.

SCREENING FOR DIABETIC COMPLICATIONS

Currently, many elderly people already have chronic complications of diabetes, which may be asymptomatic at diagnosis. These should be systematically screened for by history, examination and appropriate laboratory investigations. Table 4.6 presents some guidelines for initial

Table 4.6. Initial screening for chronic diabetic complications

---

Atherosclerotic disease
  Cardiovascular examination
  Electrocardiogram
  Serum total cholesterol, HDL cholesterol and triglycerides
Neuropathy
  Neurological examination, with particular attention to peripheral sensation and
    autonomic nervous system (valsalva manoeuvre, postural hypotension, sinus
    arrythmia)
Eye disease
  Visual acuity
  Fundoscopy with pupils dilated
Nephropathy
  Dipstick urinalysis for protein
  Microalbuminuria if dipstick for proteinuria is negative
  Quantification of proteinuria and creatinine clearance if dipstick for proteinuria
    is positive
  Serum creatinine and urea
  Blood pressure
Foot problems
  Vascular, neurological, musculoskeletal, cutaneous and soft tissue examination
    of the feet
  Examination and improvement of footwear

---

examination and appropriate laboratory investigations for chronic diabetic complications.

Symptoms of sensory, motor and autonomic neuropathy should be documented at the time of diagnosis of diabetes and reassessed at least every 6 months. Other neurological conditions must be ruled out before a diagnosis of diabetic neuropathy is made. The patient should be informed that symptoms of diabetic neuropathy may improve slowly with improved glycaemic control.

All elderly people with diabetes should be reviewed at least 6-monthly for refraction, and at least yearly for ophthalmoscopic examination with pupil dilatation. Detection of any retinopathy, cataract or other ocular abnormality warrants an ophthalmologist referral. Early retinopathy can be reversed by improved metabolic control or halted by laser therapy.

Renal function should be monitored at least annually by measurement of microalbuminuria and plasma creatinine. Urinalysis should be checked regularly to detect occult urinary tract infection. Strict control of hypertension is important for preventing or reversing early diabetic nephropathy.

The feet should be examined at every visit to the physician. Ulcers and infection must be treated promptly. A podiatrist should be involved in the education and management of foot care (see Chapter 7).

SUMMARY

The number of people 65 years of age or older with diabetes continues to rise as the population ages. Early diagnosis of diabetes is important to improve glycaemia, correct hyperglycaemic symptoms, prevent medical complications of diabetes as well as to maintain quality of life and independence in this age group. Routine screening for diabetes by primary physicians is recommended for all persons 65 years of age or older. Those with multiple high risk factors require definitive exclusion of the diagnosis of diabetes. The diagnostic criteria for diabetes in the elderly are identical to those for non-pregnant adults in general. Patients diagnosed with IGT are at increased risk of diabetes and macrovascular disease. Non-pharmacological measures are often successful in improving glucose tolerance in these patients and lowering their atherosclerotic risks. For those with NIDDM, diet is the cornerstone of treatment. Oral hypoglycaemic agents and insulin are valuable drugs which must be used with caution in the elderly because of the increased risk of hypoglycaemia and drug toxicity. Regular screening for diabetic complications and risk factors for atherosclerosis should be performed on all persons with diabetes. Management of diabetes in the elderly should involve education and take into account the patient's level of independent living, intercurrent illness, life expectancy and life-style.

REFERENCES

1 Wilson PWF, Anderson KM, Kannel WB. Epidemiology of diabetes mellitus in the elderly. The Framingham study. *Am J Med* 1986; **80** (Suppl. 5A): 3–9.
2 Glathaar C, Welborn TA, Stenhouse NS, Garcia-Webb P. Diabetes and impaired glucose tolerance. A prevalence estimate based on the Busselton 1981 survey. *Med J Aust* 1985; **143**: 436–40.
3 Harris MI. Epidemiology of diabetes mellitus among the elderly in the United States. *Clin Geriatr Med* 1990; **6**: 703–19.
4 King H, Rewers M, WHO Ad Hoc Diabetes Reporting Group. Global estimates for prevalence of diabetes mellitus and impaired glucose tolerance in adults. *Diabetes Care* 1993; **16**: 157–77.
5 Lipson LG. Diabetes in the elderly: diagnosis, pathogenesis, and therapy. *Am J Med* 1986; **80** (Suppl. 5A): 10–21.
6 Damsgaard EMS. Known diabetes and fasting hyperglycaemia in the elderly. Prevalence and economic impact upon health services. *Dan Med Bull* 1990; **37**: 530–46.
7 Soler NG, Fitzgerald MG, Malins JM, Summers ROC. Retinopathy at diagnosis of diabetes with special reference to patients under 40 years of age. *Br Med J* 1969; **3**: 567–9.
8 Abraira C, Emanuele N, Colwell J, *et al.* Glycemic control and complications in type II diabetes. Design of a feasibility trial. *Diabetes Care* 1992; **15**: 1560–71.

9 Nathan DM, Singer DE, Godine JE, Hodgson Harrington C, Perlmuter LC. Retinopathy in older type II diabetics: association with glucose control. *Diabetes* 1986; **35**: 797–801.

10 Ballard DJ, Humphrey LL, Melton LJ, *et al.* Epidemiology of persistent proteinuria in type II diabetes mellitus: population-based study in Rochester, Minnesota. *Diabetes* 1988; **37**: 405–12.

11 Naliboff BD, Rosenthal M. Effects of age on complications in adult onset diabetes. *J Am Geriatr Soc* 1989; **37**: 838–42.

12 Morley JE, Mooradian AD, Rosenthal MJ, Kaiser FE. Diabetes mellitus in elderly patients. Is it different? *Am J Med* 1987; **83**: 533–44.

13 Grobin W. Diabetes in the aged: underdiagnosis and overtreatment. *Can Med Assoc J* 1970; **103**: 915–23.

14 Waugh NR, Dallas JH, Jung RT, Newton RW. Mortality in a cohort of diabetic patients. Causes and relative risks. *Diabetologia* 1989; **32**: 103–4.

15 Sprafka JM, Burke GL, Folsom AR, McGovern PG, Hahn LP. Trends in prevalence of diabetes mellitus in patients with myocardial infarction and effect of diabetes on survival. The Minnesota heart survey. *Diabetes Care* 1991; **14**: 537–43.

16 Phillips PA, Rolls BJ, Ledingham JGG, *et al.* Reduced thirst after water deprivation in healthy elderly men. *N Engl J Med* 1984; **311**: 753–9.

17 Fujimoto WY. The growing prevalence of non-insulin-dependent diabetes in migrant Asian populations and its implications for Asia. *Diabetes Res Clin Pract* 1992; **15**: 167–84.

18 Centers for Disease Control. Prevalence and incidence of diabetes mellitus—United States, 1980–1987. *Morb Mortal Wkly Rep* 1990; **39**: 809–12.

19 Sparrow D, Borkon GA, Gerzof SG, Wisniewski C, Silbert CK. Relationship of fat distribution to glucose tolerance. Results of computed tomography in male participants of the Normative Aging Study. *Diabetes* 1986; **35**: 411–15.

20 Kaye SA, Folsom AR, Sprafka JM, Prineas RJ, Wallace RB. Increased incidence of diabetes mellitus in relation to abdominal adiposity in older women. *J Clin Epidemiol* 1991; **44**: 329–34.

21 Barnett AH, Eff C, Leslie RDG, Pyke DA. Diabetes in identical twins. A study of 200 pairs. *Diabetologia* 1991; **20**: 87–93.

22 Newman B, Selby JV, King M-C, Slemenda C, Fabitz R, Friedman GD. Concordance for type 2 (non-insulin-dependent) diabetes mellitus in male twins. *Diabetologia* 1987; **30**: 763–8.

23 Zimmet P, Serjeantson S, King H, Kirk R. The genetics of diabetes mellitus. *Aus NZ J Med* 1986; **16**: 419–24.

24 Krolewski AS, Warram JH. Natural history of diabetes mellitus. In: Becker KL (ed.), *Principles and Practice of Endocrinology and Metabolism*. Philadelphia: JB Lippincott, 1990: 1084–7.

25 National Diabetes Data Group. Classification and diagnosis of diabetes mellitus and other categories of glucose intolerance. *Diabetes* 1979; **28**: 1039–57.

26 WHO Expert Committee on Diabetes Mellitus, second report. *WHO Tech Rep Ser* **646**. Geneva: WHO, 1980.

27 National Health and Medical Research Council of Australia. *Diabetes in Older People*. Canberra: Australian Government Publishing Service, 1992.

28 Harris MI. Undiagnosed NIDDM: clinical and public health issues. *Diabetes Care* 1993; **16**: 642–52.

29 Mulkerrin EC, Arnold JD, Dewar R, Sykes D, Rees A, Pathy MSJ. Glycosylated haemoglobin in the diagnosis of diabetes mellitus in elderly people. *Age Ageing* 1992; **21**: 175–7.

30 Bunn HF. Evaluation of glycosylated hemoglobin in diabetic patients. *Diabetes* 1981; **30**: 613–17.

31 American Diabetes Association. *Physician's Guide to Non-insulin-Dependent (Type II) Diabetes. Diagnosis and Treatment.* Alexandria: American Diabetes Association, 1988: 7–10.

32 Modan M, Harris MI, Halkin H. Evaluation of WHO and NDDG criteria for impaired glucose tolerance. Results from two national samples. *Diabetes* 1989; **38**: 1630–5.

33 Foster DW. Diabetes Mellitus. In: Wilson JD, Braunwald E, Isselbacher KJ, *et al.* (eds), *Harrison's Principles of Internal Medicine.* New York: McGraw-Hill, 1991: 1739–59.

34 Davidson MB. The effect of aging and carbohydrate metabolism: a review of the English literature and a practical approach to the diagnosis of diabetes mellitus in the elderly. *Metabolism* 1979; **28**: 688–705.

35 Trilling JS. Screening for non-insulin-dependent diabetes mellitus in the elderly. *Clin Geriatr Med* 1990; **6**: 839–47.

36 Jackson RA, Jaspan JB. Glucose intolerance and aging. In Morley JE, Korenman SG (eds), *Endocrinology and Metabolism in the Elderly.* Boston: Blackwell Scientific, 1992: 353–72.

37 Graf RJ, Halter JB, Porte D Jr. Glycosylated hemoglobin in normal subjects and subjects with maturity-onset diabetes. Evidence for a saturable system in man. *Diabetes* 1978: **27**: 834–9.

38 Arnetz BB, Kallner A, Theorell T. The influence of aging on hemoglobin A_{1c} (HbA_{1c}). *J Gerontol* 1982; **37**: 648–50.

39 Monnier VM, Vishwanath V, Frank KE, Elmets CA, Dauchot P, Kohn PR. Relation between complications of type I diabetes mellitus and collagen-linked fluorescence. *N Engl J Med* 1986; **314**: 403–8.

40 Beisswenger PJ, Moore LL, Curphey TJ. Relationship between glycemic control and collagen-linked advanced glycosylation end products in type I diabetes. *Diabetes Care* 1993; **16**: 689–94.

41 Bennett PH. Diabetes in the elderly: diagnosis and epidemiology. *Geriatrics* 1984; **39**: 37–41.

42 ETDRS Investigators. Aspirin effects on mortality and morbidity in patients with diabetes mellitus. Early treatment diabetic retinopathy study report 14. *JAMA* 1992; **268**: 1292–300.

43 Ettinger PO. Cardiac disease in diabetes. *Postgrad Med* 1989; **85**: 229–32.

44 Dahlof B, Lindholm LH, Hansson L, Schersten B, Ekbom T, Wester P-O. Morbidity and mortality in the Swedish trial in old patients with hypertension (STOP-hypertension). *Lancet* 1991; **388**: 1281–5.

45 SHEP Cooperative Research Group. Prevention of stroke by antihypertensive drug treatment in older persons with isolated systolic hypertension. Final results of the systolic hypertension in the elderly program (SHEP). *JAMA* 1991; **265**: 3255–64.

46 Garg A, Grundy SM. Management of dyslipidemia in NIDDM. *Diabetes Care* 1990; **13**: 153–69.

47 Mooriadan AD. Management of diabetes in the elderly. In Morley JE, Korenman SG (eds), *Endocrinology and Metabolism in the Elderly.* Boston: Blackwell Scientific, 1992: 388–405.

48 Freedman DS, Gruchow HW, Bamrah VS, Anderson AJ, Barboriak JJ. Diabetes mellitus and arteriologically-documented coronary artery disease. *J Clin Epidemiol* 1988; **41**: 659–68.

49 Gilden JL, Hendryx M, Casia C, Singh SP. The effectiveness of diabetes education programs for older patients and their spouses. *J Am Geriatr Soc* 1989; **37**: 1023–30.

50 Perlmuter LC, Hakami MK, Hodgson-Harrington C, *et al.* Decreased cognitive function in aging non-insulin-dependent diabetic patients. *Am J Med* 1984; **77**: 1043–8.

51 Mooradian AD, Perryman K, Fitten J, Kavonian GD, Morley JE. Cortical function in elderly non-insulin dependent diabetic patients. Behavioral and electrophysiologic studies. *Arch Intern Med* 1988; **148**: 2369–72

5

Acute Complications of Diabetes in Elderly Patients

JEFF R. FLACK and DENNIS K. YUE*

Diabetes Centres, Bankstown-Lidcombe Hospital, Sydney, Australia and *Royal Prince Alfred Hospital, Camperdown, NSW, Australia

INTRODUCTION

The prevalence of diabetes increases with age; it is variously estimated that between 10 and 20% of persons over the age of 60 have diabetes. In some societies, this figure may be even greater given the higher prevalence of diabetes in people of certain ethnic origins. Elderly patients make up a considerable proportion of the cases referred to us for assessment, 35% of 1600 consecutive referrals being over 65 years old. Non-insulin-dependent (Type 2) diabetes predominates among these patients, but, due to better treatment and survival, an increasing number of individuals with long-standing insulin-dependent (Type 1) diabetes are represented.

Acute complications may develop over hours or days, and often resolve completely with appropriate treatment. Their recognition and prompt management are important to preserve the well-being of the individual, and in the elderly are particularly important in maintaining independence and good health.

Prevention of acute complications is naturally preferable, and in this regard patient education is of extreme importance. A multidisciplinary approach to education, clinical assessment and management of diabetes in people of all ages, preferably on an ambulatory basis, is now accepted as the best way of achieving this.

There are a number of ways of classifying the acute complications of diabetes. We have chosen a clinical one (Table 5.1). In this chapter we

Diabetes in Old Age. Edited by P. Finucane and A. J. Sinclair
© 1995 John Wiley & Sons Ltd

Table 5.1. Acute complications of diabetes

Metabolic
    Hypoglycaemia
    Persistent hyperglycaemia
    Hyperosmolar coma
    Diabetic ketoacidosis
Infections
    Urinary tract infection
    Other infections
Other
    'Self-inflicted'
    Iatrogenic: side-effects of medications, drug interactions

---

discuss each acute complication from a general perspective initially, and thence as it pertains to the elderly. We will not be considering the acute complications that may develop on the background of chronic complications, such as acute foot ulceration complicating peripheral neuropathy.

Control of the blood glucose level is a major determinant of the development and course of these complications. Therefore, self blood glucose monitoring is important. This can often be undertaken by older patients themselves, but considerations of manual dexterity and vision need to be borne in mind. However, several other factors are important in dealing with the older patient with diabetes (Table 5.2). General management principles are the same in the elderly, but may need modification in line with such factors as are present, and treatment should always be determined on an individual basis. Education of relative(s) or carer(s) is vital. Relatives may need to be taught to measure blood glucose levels as well as administer medication and supervise meals. In particular they should be aware of the general management principles for sick days and other emergencies.

Table 5.2. Factors to consider in the elderly patient

Reduced memory
Reduced vision
Reduced manual dexterity
Reduced mobility
Poor diet
High renal threshold
Intercurrent illness
Susceptibility to infection
Danger of hypoglycaemia

METABOLIC COMPLICATIONS

HYPOGLYCAEMIA

A hypoglycaemic episode (or 'hypo') is a fall of blood glucose to a level that can cause two groups of symptoms: disturbances of cerebral function and cognitive ability (neuroglycopenic symptoms), and those associated with release of counter-regulatory hormones (adrenergic symptoms). One or other symptom group may predominate, or both may be present together. Classical symptoms may include any combination of weakness, hunger, tremor, sweating, blurred vision, slurring of speech, headache or abnormal behaviour. A decreased level of consciousness leading to coma may occur. A particular cluster of symptoms tends to occur for each individual, who may or may not recognize their onset. Hypoglycaemic episodes can occur when meals are delayed, after excessive or unusual exercise, or if the wrong dose of insulin or tablet is administered. However, hypoglycaemia will often occur with no obvious precipitating cause. We now also know that the better the blood glucose control, the more likely is hypoglycaemia to occur[1].

It is important that the patient be aware of the warning symptoms of hypoglycaemia and be able to recognize them and take appropriate action. This involves carrying and consuming simple carbohydrate (sugar or orange juice) followed by some complex carbohydrate (such as a sandwich), to return the blood glucose level to normal. Education about the recognition and prompt treatment of hypoglycaemia is a vital component of management. In long-standing diabetes, when counter-regulatory hormone secretion is abnormal, and in instances where there is a rapid fall in the blood glucose level, the individual may be unable to recognize and deal with hypoglycaemia. This may result in a greater risk of serious morbidity from falls, or from neurological sequelae in the presence of prolonged hypoglycaemia. The Diabetes Control and Complications Trial[2] drew attention to the frequency of such severe hypoglycaemic episodes that required the assistance of another person for treatment.

A number of special considerations arise in relation to hypoglycaemia in elderly diabetic patients.

The Individual may be Frail

Elderly people are less able to recognize and react to impending hypoglycaemia[3] and are therefore more susceptible to physical injury, particularly since they are more likely to also have impaired balance and perhaps osteoporosis. A fractured hip or wrist, or a significant laceration, are not uncommon consequences of a fall associated with a hypoglycaemic episode. Particular care must be exercised in the management of patients who are frail or prone to falls, and in those with other (often multiple) medical problems.

The Use of Medications Needs to be Appropriate

The use of long-acting sulphonylurea agents should be discouraged due to their propensity to accumulate in older patients (who often have diminished renal function), placing the patient at risk of severe hypoglycaemia[4]. In this regard, we believe that chlorpropamide (36-h half-life) should not be used in the elderly, and that glibenclamide should be used with caution or indeed be replaced by agents less likely to cause hypoglycaemia, such as gliclazide or glipizide. Tolbutamide, a weak agent with a very short half-life, which must be given at least twice daily to be effective, is appropriate and often effective in the initial management of very elderly Type 2 patients, in whom diet alone does not give the desired blood glucose control.

It is important to advise older patients to take their medications with meals; if hypoglycaemic agents are taken at regular times but meals are delayed or missed, there is a risk of hypoglycaemia. People who rely on 'Meals on Wheels' or on meals provided by neighbours or relatives are most at risk.

Potential drug interactions should be avoided. The elderly are often on multiple medications for other medical problems such as coexistent hypertension, ischaemic heart disease, cerebrovascular disease and arthritis. Potential drug interactions, highlighted in Table 5.3, should always be remembered when one is using sulphonylurea agents. Table 5.3(a) lists agents which, when added to a patient's treatment regimen,

Table 5.3. Potential drug interactions with sulphonylureas

(a) Drugs that potentiate the hypoglycaemic action of sulphonylureas
   Other sulphonylureas
   Salicylates
   Sulphonamides
   Warfarin
   Phenytoin
(b) Drugs that antagonize the hypoglycaemic action of sulphonylureas
   Thiazides
   Frusemide
   Oestrogen
   Corticosteroids
   Propranolol

---

increase the risk of hypoglycaemia by displacing the sulphonylurea from transport proteins. The use of more than one sulphonylurea agent at a time provides no therapeutic benefit and is potentially dangerous.

Age is not a barrier to the use of insulin and many older patients can be stabilized on insulin on an ambulatory basis. Over 26% of our patients aged 65 or more are on insulin therapy, and 61% of these are on two daily injections. Care should be taken when commencing insulin therapy, however. It is prudent to start cautiously with a relatively small dose, and to build it up gradually. The use of pre-mixed insulins makes administration easier for elderly patients.

Adjustment of the dose of tablets or insulin should always be considered after a hypoglycaemic episode. One should aim for the lowest dose sufficient to achieve and maintain the desired level of control.

The Need for Good Blood Glucose Control

While care must be exercised in prescribing hypoglycaemic therapy[5], the threat of hypoglycaemia should not mean acceptance of consistently high blood glucose levels in the elderly age group. The benefit of 'tight' blood glucose control is not yet firmly established in the elderly. Nevertheless, morbidity associated with persistent hyperglycaemia must be prevented. Patients who require higher doses of tablets or insulin should receive them. The mean number of hypoglycaemic tablets in our older patients is 4.5 per day, and 23% of those on insulin are using more than 50 units per day. The general management principles detailed below can give appropriate results; most of our patients are successfully managed without adverse effects.

The Management of Hypoglycaemia

Management of the milder case is no different from that in younger age groups. In the management of the unconscious elderly patient, cerebrovascular disease is often suspected first; however, hypoglycaemia must always be considered. If possible, a low blood glucose level on a capillary sample in a reflectance meter should be confirmed on a sample measured in a laboratory. If the patient is unconscious, immediate intravenous administration of 20 ml of 50% glucose should be undertaken, followed by a further 20–30 ml over 3–5 min, and thereafter by the establishment of an intravenous infusion of 5–10% dextrose, depending on the response. Care must be taken with the fluid volume administered in those with cardiovascular impairment, common in this age group. Close assessment of urine output, respiratory status and blood pressure is mandatory. Recovery of consciousness may be slower in the elderly. Hypoglycaemia due to sulphonylurea agents is often recalcitrant to therapy until the drug is fully metabolized and excreted, which may take 24–36 h, during which time intravenous glucose supplementation will be required.

Elucidation of the cause, and management of any sequelae (stroke, fracture, lacerations, etc.), form part of the treatment plan. Future episodes must be prevented by addressing the various points above.

PERSISTENT HYPERGLYCAEMIA

Hyperglycaemia, or raised blood glucose levels, can suddenly become severe and persistent as a result of inadequate medication or excessive dietary intake. It is often brought on by physical or prolonged emotional stress, but occasionally there is no discernible cause identifiable.

Patients must understand the need to take at least their usual medication dose at times of illness, to increase the frequency of self-monitoring at such times, and to seek early medical advice during prolonged illness. Sick day diabetes management is one of the essential items of patient education frequently and correctly referred to as 'survival skills'.

Here again, special considerations arise in relation to elderly diabetic patients.

Effect of Intercurrent Illness

The older patient is less tolerant of higher blood glucose levels and is more likely to have intercurrent illness(es) which contribute to hyperglycaemia.

Nature of Symptoms

Older people with a higher renal threshold for glucose may not have polyuria. They may also be less perceptive of thirst or other 'classical' symptoms of hyperglycaemia. In the elderly, persistent hyperglycaemia can manifest itself by relatively non-specific symptoms such as lethargy, which may be inappropriately attributed to 'just ageing'. This explains the need for increased diligence in detecting hyperglycaemia by monitoring blood glucose. The lack of symptoms may lull individuals into falsely believing their diabetes is well controlled, exposing them to the risks of infection or more serious sequelae. It also explains why urine testing is often inappropriate as a means of monitoring diabetes in this age group.

Nocturia, incontinence and worsening symptoms of prostatism in men, are disturbing consequences of prolonged hyperglycaemia. Such problems often hamper the ability of older patients to manage themselves. While multiple factors often contribute to these symptoms, hyperglycaemia is a reversible problem which should be sought and corrected if present.

Secondary Failure of Oral Hypoglycaemic Agents

Weight loss and poor blood glucose control in older patients with longer standing, previously well controlled diabetes, should raise the question of secondary tablet failure. This usually occurs after several years of tablet therapy and reflects progressive failure of pancreatic beta cells, to an extent where sulphonylurea agents are no longer effective. Occasionally, changing the sulphonylurea agent is effective, with a change to glipizide claimed to be effective in 40–50% of cases[6]. Naturally, a check on dietary adherence is vital.

Metformin, a biguanide, is a useful adjunct to sulphonylurea agents and can be added with care to the treatment regimen in older individuals. Caution should be exercised in the presence of significant renal or hepatic impairment at any age, due to the possibility of inducing lactic acidosis, although this is extremely uncommon.

If, despite pushing medication to the maximum and excluding reversible causes, true secondary tablet failure persists, transfer to insulin therapy should not be withheld from the older patient. Pre-mixed insulins should be considered to avoid the need to mix insulins. Relatives or district nurses may be enlisted to supervise or administer insulin therapy, but many older patients can manage themselves.

The presence of other problems such as thyroid disorders, connective tissue disease or underlying neoplasia must always be considered.

The Need to Prevent Acute Crises

Monitoring of blood glucose levels has both motivational and therapeutic benefits. It can be carried out by older patients themselves (with patience required in educating them), or by relatives or district nursing practitioners. It is an important facet of management in preventing acute crises, and should be initiated before insulin therapy. In our view, all such patients should be so monitored.

Table 5.3(b) lists agents which, when added to a patient's treatment regimen, can aggravate hyperglycaemia by antagonizing the hypoglycaemic effect of sulphonylurea agents. The use of high-dose oral corticosteroids for conditions such as polymyalgia rheumatica or other rheumatological, respiratory, dermatological or neoplastic conditions often produces hyperglycaemia. This may not occur until a few days or even a few weeks after onset of therapy. Therefore close monitoring of the blood sugar levels is essential. It is often necessary to manage such patient's diabetes with insulin, at least for the duration of the acute episode.

Management

Reversible causes of persistent hyperglycaemia must be considered in all age groups. These include dietary indiscretions, infection and prolonged emotional stress. At such times medication levels usually need to be increased to keep blood glucose levels normal. In some patients, insulin may be necessary in patients previously managed by tablets.

There may not be a demonstrable reversible cause of sudden deterioration of blood glucose control; the event may represent true secondary tablet failure. Transfer to insulin therapy can usually be achieved in the elderly, on an ambulatory basis in most instances.

HYPEROSMOLAR COMA

Severe prolonged hyperglycaemia may culminate in this medical emergency, with high morbidity and significant mortality, that occurs predominantly in elderly individuals[7]. It is a condition where there is sufficient circulating insulin to prevent the development of diabetic ketoacidosis, yet insufficient to prevent the development of strikingly high levels of blood glucose, of the order of 45–60+ mmol/l. As patients may be unaware of the underlying diabetes, they often consume large quantities of soft drinks to quench their thirst. This contributes to the severity of the hyperglycaemia. Patients may present late, when dehydration is already severe. The condition is often complicated by cerebrovascular accidents, myocardial infarction or venous thromboses, which themselves determine the ultimate outcome.

There are four major considerations in the management of hyperosmolar coma: (i) the (often severe) dehydration; (ii) the gross hyperglycaemia; (iii) the underlying precipitant; and (iv) the sequelae.

Rehydration is important and by itself can result in lowering of the blood glucose level. We recommend the use of a low-dose insulin infusion (0.5 units/h). There is some controversy about the initial fluid of choice, whether it should be Normal Saline or Half-Normal Saline[7]. Except when hypotension is severe, replacement of fluid should be slow to avoid cardiovascular problems. It is important to note that, as in diabetic ketoacidosis, the metabolic derangements in this condition have taken days to develop, and instantaneous return to total metabolic normality should not be the aim.

Being aware of the likely precipitants of hyperosmolar coma is the key to its prevention. A high index of suspicion is required, given that hyperosmolar coma may be the initial presentation of Type 2 diabetes in an individual, or may occur in someone previously managed by diet alone or only a small dose of oral hypoglycaemic agents.

DIABETIC KETOACIDOSIS

This occurs in Type 1 diabetic individuals when there is insufficient circulating insulin to prevent the breakdown of fatty acid stores. The resultant production of ketone bodies by the liver, combined with the hyperglycaemia, induces significant metabolic derangement. Patients with typical Type 2 diabetes can also become ketoacidotic prone during times of intercurrent illness. Hyperventilation, vomiting, significant dehydration, fever (from an underlying infective cause), and reduced consciousness are common presenting features. Abdominal pain may also be present.

Elderly patients with ketoacidosis have a much worse prognosis than their younger counterparts[8]. The major problems in management are: (i) dehydration; (ii) hyperglycaemia; (iii) acidosis; (iv) low total body potassium; and (v) the underlying precipitant, which is usually infection. Elderly people are less able to tolerate hypotension associated with dehydration or the acidosis associated with this condition. Cardiovascular assessment and monitoring for arrhythmia are necessary. Careful fluid replacement is necessary to ensure adequate rehydration without inducing fluid overload[9]. Cautious use of *small* amounts of bicarbonate should only be considered when the pH approaches 7.0. It should always be remembered that as in hyperosmolar coma, the metabolic derangements in this condition have taken days to develop, and return to total metabolic normality should be gradual[10].

To prevent this complication, patient education about management of sick days is vital. The need to continue *at least* the usual treatment, and to increase the frequency of blood glucose monitoring and urinalysis for ketones at such times is fundamental. At the earliest sign of significant hyperglycaemia or sustained ketonuria, medical attention should be sought.

INFECTION

Poor blood glucose control puts the individual at increased risk of various infections, particularly of the skin and urinary tract. The development of an infection often establishes a 'vicious cycle' where the infection causes further hyperglycaemia and the increased blood glucose levels inhibit quick resolution of the infection.

As stated previously, at times of illness, 'sick day' management principles dictate that at least the usual dose of medication should be taken and, in many instances, an increase is required in order to obtain satisfactory blood glucose control to allow the infection to be cured. Patients managed on tablets may need to transfer to insulin until resolution of the acute episode. This is often necessary with severe pneumonia or significant skin infections such as carbuncles that require hospitalization and intravenous antibiotic therapy. Infections manageable in the community or with oral antibiotic therapy alone will frequently require only a small increase in tablet or insulin dose for the duration of the infection.

Elderly people are more prone to infections by virtue of a decreased immune response. The presence of poorly controlled diabetes increases the risk.

URINARY TRACT INFECTION (UTI)

UTI is often asymptomatic in the older individual and should always be sought as a cause for a deterioration in control. Microscopic haematuria, nitrites or leucocytes detected by urinary dipstick tests may be the only clues to the diagnosis in the absence of symptoms of frequency, dysuria, nocturia or incontinence. When symptoms are present, they are often mistakenly attributed to poorly controlled diabetes.

Good blood glucose control should help prevent or ameliorate infection. It is desirable to confirm the existence of infection and isolate the offending organism from a mid-stream specimen of urine. Choice of therapy will be determined by antibiotic sensitivities and consideration of prevailing renal function.

Underlying structural abnormalities of the urinary tract or other pelvic abnormalities may contribute to recurrence, and urological or gynaeco-logical assessment in such cases is mandatory. UTI is much more common in elderly males with prostatic problems and is often not diagnosed and treated.

OTHER INFECTIONS

The elderly diabetic individual may develop various other infections including cellulitis, leg or foot infections (following often minor trauma to fragile skin) and chest infections (especially in the winter months). Again it is necessary to confirm the existence of infection and to isolate and treat the offending organism.

As with UTI, poor blood glucose control can contribute to their occurrence. It is important in the elderly to diligently manage all skin trauma, cuts and abrasions to prevent the development of infection.

The use of influenza vaccines is generally recommended in this age group to lessen the chances of viral respiratory infection that may be secondarily complicated by bacterial bronchitis or pneumonia. Prophylactic antibiotic use is seldom required in the elderly diabetic individual, however, except in instances of structural respiratory abnormality or recurrent cellulitis in one site.

OTHER COMPLICATIONS

'SELF INFLICTED'

Patients with diabetes may inadvertently inflict complications upon themselves. A laceration caused by walking barefoot is not uncommon. Secondary infection and even ulceration or deep infection and osteomyelitis may occur. This is more likely in those with chronic complications of peripheral neuropathy or peripheral vascular insufficiency. Appropriate preventive education should always be given to patients.

In old people, acute foot problems leading to ulceration can develop in those who are often unable to bend over and see sufficiently well to cut their own toe-nails. Corn remedies and other attempts to self-treat foot ailments should always be discouraged. Acute burns or blisters may develop on the feet or legs from excessively hot water bottles, or from sitting too close to fires or heaters in the winter months.

Education about prevention of such serious sequelae is obviously vital. A podiatrist should be involved in the management of foot problems and the education of patients and their relatives about proper foot care. Particular care must be taken in the presence of diminished peripheral sensation and circulation.

Trauma to the feet requires specific specialist intervention to assess the extent of the problem and to determine the appropriate course of management.

'IATROGENIC'

The use of medications is associated with inherent complications that must always be borne in mind. Acute complications, such as hypoglycaemia, and various drug interactions have already been mentioned. In addition there may be problems such as nausea or diarrhoea from the introduction of metformin, or postural hypotension from antihypertensive agents.

Another area of concern is the preparation of the diabetic individual for various procedures such as colonoscopy, where dietary and medication adjustments are necessary.

Old people are far less likely to tolerate postural hypotension, and any antihypertensive agent should be introduced with due caution, commencing with a small dose. Warning the patient and relatives of all possible side-effects is mandatory, and any change in medication dosage should be written down for the patient.

Hospitalization the day before a procedure may be necessary to ensure both the success of the procedure and the appropriate management of their diabetes. The use of contrast media should also be cautious. An intravenous pyelogram in an individual with diminished renal function can induce renal failure.

SUMMARY

We have attempted to cover the common acute complications of diabetes both generally and as they pertain to the elderly. Tables 5.4 and 5.5 detail some practical points and helpful hints that we have distilled from the above discussions.

Table 5.4. Practical points

Avoid oral hypoglycaemic agents with long half-lives
Take hypoglycaemic agents with meals
Watch for drug interactions
Do not use two sulphonylurea agents together
Take care with single large insulin doses—use a twice daily dosage if necessary
Sulphonylurea-induced hypoglycaemic coma is often recalcitrant to therapy until the drug has been metabolized
Education of patients and relatives in self-care practices is vital
Good blood glucose control reduces the risk of infection
Urinary tract infection is often asymptomatic

Table 5.5. Helpful hints

Write down instructions, especially medication dosages, particularly when changing them.
Although persistent hyperglycaemia may represent secondary tablet failure, other causes must be excluded.
Anticipate hyperglycaemia when using high doses of corticosteroid.
Teach patients and relatives how to manage 'sick days'.
In hyperglycaemic emergencies, do not attempt to achieve instantaneous, total metabolic normality.
Warn patients about all important side-effects of medications.
Introduce antihypertensive agents gradually.
Be aware that preparation for various procedures may render the patient at risk of hypoglycaemia—plan ahead, establish and use appropriate protocols.

Appropriate management of the increasing numbers of elderly diabetic individuals in our society should reduce the frequency of acute complications and ensure a good quality of life.

REFERENCES

1 Amiel S. Reversal of unawareness of hypoglycaemia. *N Engl J Med* 1993; **329**: 876–7.
2 Diabetes Control and Complications Trial Research Group. The effect of intensive treatment of diabetes on the development and progression of long-term complications in insulin-dependent diabetes mellitus. *N Engl J Med* 1993; **329**: 977–86.
3 Meneilly GS, Cheung E, Tuokko H. Counterregulatory hormone responses to hypoglycaemia in the elderly patient with diabetes. *Diabetes* 1994; **43**: 403–10.
4 Peters AL, Davidson MB. Use of sulphonylurea agents in older diabetic patients. *Clin Geriatr Med* 1990; **6**: 903–21.
5 Stepka M, Rogala H, Czyzyk A. Hypoglycaemia: a major problem in the management of diabetes in the elderly. *Aging Milano* 1993; **5**: 117–21.
6 Shuman CR. Glipizide: an overview. *Am J Med* 1983; **75** (Suppl. 5B): 55–9.
7 Marshall SM, Alberti KGMM. Hyperosmolar non-ketotic diabetic coma. In: Alberti KGMM, Krall LP (eds), *The Diabetes Annual* Vol. 4. Amsterdam: Elsevier Science Publishers, 1988: 235.
8 Malone ML, Gennis V, Goodwin JS. Characteristics of diabetic ketoacidosis in older versus younger adults. *J Am Geriatr Soc* 1992; **40**: 1100–4.
9 Jolobe O. Characteristics of diabetic ketoacidosis in older patients. *J Am Geriatr Soc* 1993; **41**: 888.
10 Alberti KG. Diabetic emergencies. *Br Med Bull* 1989; **45**: 242.

6

Chronic Complications of Diabetes

PETER J. WATKINS

Diabetic Department, King's College Hospital, London, UK

The chronic complications of diabetes affect many organs and tissues, as diverse as the eyes and feet. Large vessel disease also progressively takes its toll, so that ischaemic heart disease, cerebrovascular disease and peripheral vascular disease may come to dominate the lives of elderly diabetic patients. Neuropathy and renal disease are also important.

Differentiating between problems which are a consequence of diabetes and those which result from age-related degenerative processes can present a diagnostic challenge to the clinician. In the clinical situation, however, this distinction may be unimportant, particularly if the problem is not remediable. The need to assess elderly diabetic patients accurately, to separate those problems which are best left alone from those which require treatment and then to select the best management strategies all points to a need for skilled clinicians who are well trained in diabetes care.

CLASSIFICATION OF COMPLICATIONS

Problems in elderly diabetic patients arise chiefly from the increased frequency of common disorders occurring in the diabetic state, namely major arterial disease and cataract. The specific complications are well known and are the result of microangiopathy (retinopathy, nephropathy) or neuropathy.

Diabetes in Old Age. Edited by P. Finucane and A. J. Sinclair
© 1995 John Wiley & Sons Ltd

PATHOGENESIS OF COMPLICATIONS

Protracted and persistent hyperglycaemia over many years (decades) in genetically susceptible tissues seems the most likely cause of specific diabetic complications. This very general statement takes account of volumes of clinical and scientific observations. The facts are:

1. Specific diabetic complications increase with duration of diabetes.

2. Many diabetic patients are spared complications even after many years of diabetes, for example 70% of long-standing early-onset insulin-dependent diabetes mellitus (IDDM) patients never develop proteinuria, and about 10% never develop any retinopathy.

3. Complications though often occurring together do not necessarily do so: thus blind patients are often free from renal disease or neuropathy and patients with severe neuropathy can be free from other complications. Patients with advanced nephropathy, however, tend to have multiple complications in association with their renal disease.

Specific causes of complications are not well understood. Fundamental metabolic and vascular changes are likely to be responsible; they are not exclusive and metabolic changes can alter vascularity. The importance of basement membrane thickening (the original basis of the 'microvascular disease'), which occurs with both ageing and increasing duration of diabetes, is becoming progressively blurred.

Glycation of many proteins results from persistent hyperglycaemia. Glucose binds proteins mainly linking lysine residues. Glycation can alter protein structure (e.g. collagen) and function (some enzymes). Pharmacological deglycation using aminoguanidine has proved beneficial in animal diabetic renal damage but its effects in humans are unknown. The value of glycated haemoglobin in assessing diabetic control is discussed elsewhere.

The enzyme aldose reductase is present in many tissues. It converts glucose to the sugar alcohol sorbitol, which is in turn metabolized to fructose. Activation of this pathway in the presence of hyperglycaemia leads to tissue depletion of myoinositol and reduction of $Na^+/K^+/ATPase$ activity. The effects of the aldose reductase inhibitor drugs are discussed below in the neuropathy section.

The importance of genetic factors in the development of complications is becoming clearer, although so far no specific genetic markers for any complication have been identified, making it impossible to predict which patients will develop problems. The familial clustering of families with or without nephropathy in US patients attending for renal replacement treatment in Minneapolis, or among the Pima Indians of Arizona presents the best evidence for a genetic basis for diabetic renal disease.

DIABETIC CONTROL AND DIABETIC COMPLICATIONS

The value of controlling diabetes to eliminate symptoms of the disease is beyond question. The value of *tight* metabolic control of diabetes must, however, be seen as a conflict between the major hazard which results, namely hypoglycaemia, and its potential advantages in terms of preventing complications. This conflict becomes acute in the elderly where the problems of hypoglycaemia are added to other potential causes of blackouts, and in whom there must be diminishing returns in terms of preventing complications, chiefly because of the reduced time-scale. Individual patients with long-standing diabetes trained over decades regarding the importance of tight control may adapt with difficulty to decreasing standards of control needed to diminish the disastrous effects of hypoglycaemia.

BENEFITS OF GOOD (BUT NOT TIGHT) CONTROL

1. Elimination of symptoms especially nocturia, sometimes nocturnal incontinence, pruritus vulvae and balantis; and in particular improvement of well-being and energy, with restoration of lost weight.

2. Elimination of glycosuria, which is important in the presence of urinary tract infections to accelerate recovery.

3. Possible reduction of pain in patients suffering painful forms of neuropathy.

TIGHT CONTROL OF DIABETES

Many studies, most notably the recently reported Diabetes Control and Complications Trial (DCCT) from the USA have shown that very good metabolic control of diabetes at an early stage in young-onset IDDM patients delays the onset and slows the progression of retinopathy, neuropathy and nephropathy. The price is a substantial increase in the risk of severe hypoglycaemia. Unfortunately, its effects on non-insulin-dependent diabetes mellitus (NIDDM) patients in older age groups is not known, nor is there any demonstration of advantages which might arise from the use of insulin rather than oral hypoglycaemic agents. The results of the United Kingdom Prospective Diabetes Survey (UKPDS) of more than 5000 NIDDM patients are keenly awaited, and may throw light on this important question. In the most elderly patients, however, whose life expectancy is brief, there is almost no chance that improving control will affect complications of diabetes, but then, in a short time-scale they may not advance much in any case.

With regard to major arterial disease, there is no evidence that controlling diabetes can alter the course of this disease. Other factors then become much more important especially control of blood pressure and elimination of smoking.

PREVENTING THE SEQUELAE OF DIABETIC COMPLICATIONS

Primary prevention of diabetic complications in the elderly may not be possible, but secondary prevention of their sequelae is often feasible and effective. Preventing foot problems is one of the most rewarding aspects of good diabetes practice and highly dependent on good and effective advice. Eye screening is also of great value and leads to useful treatments to preserve or restore vision. Detection of hypertension and its proper treatment is of great value in prevention of strokes and possibly retards the progression of renal disease as well, although published studies have only reported results in younger IDDM patients.

Even where serious complications do arise, for example foot ulceration and sepsis, immediate reporting of the problem combined with emergency treatment can save limbs, and proper counselling then can serve to prevent further problems.

Detailed descriptions of appropriate screening procedures and the action to be taken are described below in the relevant sections.

WHO ARE 'ELDERLY' DIABETIC PATIENTS?

Different elderly diabetic patients may have entirely different requirements with regard to the development and management of diabetic complications. Their clinical care can be considered under the following categories.

Newly Diagnosed NIDDM Patients

Presentation as a consequence of established diabetic complications becomes increasingly common as age increases. Diabetes is often discovered in patients presenting with foot ulceration, sepsis or gangrene; in those attending optometrists with declining vision; or in patients who develop painful neuropathy syndromes described below. Thus, of 27 of our own patients presenting with painful proximal motor neuropathy (femoral neuropathy or amyotrophy), eight NIDDM were not previously known to have diabetes.

Furthermore, newly diagnosed elderly diabetic patients who present in a more conventional way (by symptoms or screening) are often found to have specific complications at the time of diagnosis, indicating the undetected presence of diabetes over many years. Studies by retinal photography show that approximately one-fifth of all new NIDDM patients have retinopathy at diagnosis, and proteinuria can also be found when they are first examined. These well known findings indicate the importance of a full examination at the time of discovery and diagnosis of diabetes, even when the diabetes itself appears in every other way easy to manage, possibly even by diet alone.

Among hospital in-patients, inclusion of blood glucose measurement in the biochemical screening tests now performed almost routinely commonly yields a diagnosis of diabetes among patients with a wide range of disorders and may sometimes explain the nature of the problem in cardiac, orthopaedic, ophthalmological, neurological, gynaecological or urological patients and many others.

Patients with Long-established Diabetes

Patients with long-established diabetes reach old age with or without complications of their condition. Some remain unscathed even after more than 60 years of diabetes; even after 30 years, the annual incidence of new cases of nephropathy declines sharply making the prognosis for those spared up to 30 years relatively good. Some patients, unfortunately reach old age with established complications which may be single or multiple; thus some patients are blind and can be so for many years without other problems; others may have foot problems but are otherwise in good health. Those less fortunate may be overwhelmed with problems especially those who are crippled with extensive arterial disease.

Modification of diabetes treatment may be needed at this stage, and should be reviewed in the light of problems experienced by individual patients. Emphasis is given to minimizing hypoglycaemia, especially when cerebrovascular disease becomes a problem. There is a potential need for insulin especially in some forms of neuropathy associated with pain; and patients should avoid the use of inappropriately long-acting renally metabolized oral hypoglycaemic agents especially in the presence of renal impairment, using instead such drugs as gliclazide or tolbutamide.

NEUROPATHY

Peripheral nerve damage in diabetes is common and increasingly so in old age. It takes three forms:

1. Progressive diffuse polyneuropathy, i.e. symmetrical sensory neuropathy associated with autonomic neuropathy.

2. Reversible mononeuropathies and radiculopathies including proximal motor (femoral) neuropathy, cranial nerve palsies and acute painful neuropathies.

3. Pressure palsies, notably carpal tunnel syndrome, ulnar nerve compression and rarely foot drop.

These different forms of nerve damage must have different aetiologies with different impacts from vascular and metabolic factors. Most striking is the difference in behaviour of these main groups; namely, that the common symmetrical sensory neuropathy (with autonomic neuropathy) is a slowly progressive disorder, while those with radiculopathies and pain are expected to recover. Identification and management of these problems is therefore quite distinct and extremely important. Pressure palsies are commoner in patients with diabetes than in controls, but not specific: carpal tunnel syndrome occurs the most frequently, is the chief cause of painful fingers, and always important to diagnose because it is so easy to treat by simple surgery under local anaesthetic.

SYMMETRICAL SENSORY NEUROPATHY

Nerve function gradually declines with age; this decline is accelerated in some, but by no means all, diabetic patients leading to the development of symmetrical sensory neuropathy. It is not known why some patients are prone to and others spared from this disease. Tight control of diabetes over many years retards the decline of nerve function in younger IDDM patients. It is not known whether the same applies to older NIDDM patients and the results of the large British study (UKPDS) are awaited. Aldose reductase inhibitor drugs which improve the metabolic redox status in the nerve can slow the decline of nerve function in diabetic patients, but the long-term clinical value is still being assessed and they are only available in a few countries. Administration of gamma linolenic acid (evening primrose oil) may have a similar protective effect, but further studies are still needed.

Symmetrical sensory neuropathy is a very common condition affecting a high proportion of both newly diagnosed and long-standing elderly patients. It is normally symptomless, and this can be particularly serious when selective small fibre involvement leads to loss of thermal and pain sensation, leaving other modalities relatively intact. The lack of symptoms represents a lurking hazard because of the potential for unsuspected foot injuries, which are the commonest manifestation of sensory neuropathy.

Some patients are aware of their neuropathy: symptoms include grumbling paraesthesiae in the toes of both feet which may resolve with improved diabetes control or sometimes persist for many years. Numbness (and sometimes a sensation of coldness) can be severe and patients feel they are walking on cotton wool, but that is relatively uncommon.

Diagnosis

Clinical neurological examination is the chief basis for a diagnosis of neuropathy. Testing for sensory modalities (cotton wool, pinprick) can reveal a 'stocking' loss, but pain and temperature deficits from small fibre damage are commoner and less easy to detect. Absence of ankle reflexes is confirmatory but their loss in old age is so common that the diagnostic information is limited. Appraisal of foot deformities is vital in the prevention and management of major foot problems (see Chapter 7).

The only simple quantitative test for neuropathy is measurement of vibration perception threshold (VPT) and even this is of relatively limited value in the elderly in whom thresholds are normally higher than in younger people. Nevertheless, the Biothesiometer (Newbury, Ohio) is simple to use. Readings exceeded 35 V are associated with a considerably increased risk of foot ulceration, and above 50 V indicate severe neuropathy. The graduated tuning fork (Reidell-Seiffer graduated tuning fork, Firma Martin, Tuttlingen, Germany) is also a useful tool, very simple, cheap and relatively reproducible; a score above five indicates neuropathy. Electromyography is not normally needed unless for research purposes. Symptoms correlate poorly with all measurements of neuropathy.

AUTONOMIC NEUROPATHY (AN)

Autonomic function declines with age in the same way that peripheral nerve conduction progressively slows through life. Deterioration of neurological function is accelerated in diabetes, though this decline is not uniform. Thus, in some patients it is scarcely different from normal, while in others it is accelerated to the point of severe symptomatic AN, which is associated with an increased mortality. Symptomatic AN is surprisingly uncommon compared with the extremely common finding of abnormal autonomic function tests, which can be demonstrated in any diabetic population; furthermore, symptomatic AN is particularly rare in the elderly population, and in most instances other explanations need to be sought for the various features attributed to AN (Table 6.1). For detailed descriptions of symptomatic AN, further reading elsewhere is suggested, while the following paragraphs are directed specifically to the elderly population.

Table 6.1. Clinical features of autonomic neuropathy

	Clinical syndromes	Other abnormalities
Cardiovascular:	Postural hypotension Tachycardia	
Sweating:	Gustatory sweating	
Genitourinary:	Impotence Neurogenic bladder	
Gastrointestinal:	Diarrhoea Gastroparesis	Oesophageal mobility Gall-bladder emptying
Respiratory:	Arrests ?Sudden death	?Sleep apnoea Cough reflex
Eye:		Pupillary responses Pupillary size
Neuroendocrine responses:		Catecholamines Glucagon Pancreatic polypeptide

(Cough reflex, Pupillary responses, Pupillary size, Catecholamines, Glucagon, Pancreatic polypeptide) all reduced

Postural Hypotension

A fall in systolic blood pressure (BP) of more than 30 mmHg is not rare in the diabetic population. It is increasingly likely to occur in elderly patients where complex factors are involved, and it is not always due to AN. Its chief symptom is giddiness on standing (for which there are other causes) which is most commonly transient and rarely leads to complete incapacity with an inability to stand at all. The diagnosis must be confirmed by actual measurement of the lying and standing blood pressure: readings should be taken for at least 3 min during standing since the BP fall is often gradual.

Treatment is only needed if symptoms are troublesome. Attention must be given foremost to causes other than diabetes (notably cardiovascular disease, cerebrovascular disease, parkinsonism, Addison's disease), and to elimination of the many drugs which exacerbate hypotension: these include most hypotensives, diuretics, tranquillizers, antidepressives and hypnotics. Supine hypertension may have to be accepted in order to prevent upright hypotension. Postural hypotension is always worse after long periods in bed, so that ambulation should be encouraged. In difficult cases many measures can be tried, best summarized as follows: elevation of the head of the bed; full length elastic stockings; increased salt intake; fludrocortisone administration slowly increasing the dose from 100 to 400 µg daily. Other measures are generally less satisfactory.

Gastrointestinal Symptoms

Diarrhoea or vomiting in elderly patients are scarcely ever attributable to AN. Other causes and treatments must always be sought.

Genitourinary Symptoms

Impairment of bladder emptying can be described as a common feature of diabetic neuropathy, but it is rarely symptomatic and bladder emptying problems normally have another cause especially in elderly men where prostatism is the only common problem. Even if there is significant neurogenic bladder impairment, improvement of the outlet almost always alleviates the symptoms. Occasionally intermittent self-catheterization or (less ideally) permanent indwelling catheterization provides the only solution.

Impotence

Impotence is a common symptom especially in diabetic men with about one-half of those over 55 years of age being affected. Younger patients, even in their third and fourth decades sometimes have this problem. While neuropathy plays an important role, vascular mechanisms are also relevant, while psychogenic impotence is probably the commonest cause overall.

The onset of neuropathic impotence is usually gradual, progressing slowly over months, but complete erectile failure is usually present within 2 years of the onset of symptoms. Ejaculation can be retained in the earlier stages. Retrograde ejaculation sometimes occurs. This history contrasts with psychogenic impotence, which begins suddenly and in which nocturnal erections may persist.

Impotence may also be due to vascular occlusion of the branches of the internal pudendal artery. Furthermore, in rare cases, erectile failure may be caused by thrombosis of the bifurcation of the aorta (Leriche's syndrome).

The diagnosis of neuropathic impotence in diabetes is difficult. The use of an intracavernosal injection of the muscle relaxant, papaverine, is to some extent useful in distinguishing neurogenic from vasculogenic impotence; it causes an erection in the former but not in the latter. This is helpful both in terms of diagnosis and giving guidance in the choice of treatment. Autonomic function tests give some clue as to the presence of AN, but they do not establish conclusively in an individual whether it is the cause of impotence.

The rational treatment of diabetic impotence depends on a careful history, in particular to evaluate any psychological component. If such a factor is present, then the patient and his partner may be helped by appropriate discussion and advice. Intracavernous injection of papaverine causes an erection in patients not suffering from severe vascular disease, and offers a treatment which some men and their partners find satisfactory. However, infection and penile fibrosis are potential complications. The use of a vacuum pump applied to a condom is less invasive, and is satisfactory for some patients, particularly if they are properly instructed in its use.

A rigid penile implant is often successful, especially in younger patients when ejaculation is retained. Inflatable prostheses are also available but are expensive and more often prone to failure. Elderly patients are not usually suitable candidates for surgery and are more likely to accept the situation if it is carefully explained.

Diagnosis

The diagnosis of AN is often difficult. Standard bedside autonomic function tests decline with age and after 70 years discrimination between normal and abnormal is nearly impossible. Of course normal tests (Table 6.2) eliminate the diagnosis of AN.

Loss of heart rate variability during deep breathing is the most reliable and simplest test of AN. It is best assessed using a cardiotachograph during deep respirations (6 breaths/min) taking average readings during six breaths. It can be performed using an ordinary electrocardiograph during a single deep breath (5 s inspiration, 5 s expiration). The heart rate difference (maximum rate during inspiration minus minimum rate during expiration) in people aged less than 55 is normally greater than 10. The heart rate increase on standing up should be greater than 12 at 15 s, and normally there is also an overshoot. The Valsalva manoeuvre can be included among the tests; a mercury sphygmomanometer is used, the patient blowing hard through the empty barrel of a 20 ml syringe to maintain the mercury column at 40 mm for 10 s. Maximum heart rate during blowing, followed by minimum heart rate after cessation, are recorded. There should be a bradycardia after cessation of blowing. The ratio of maximum to minimum heart rate is normally greater than 1.21 and clearly abnormal when less than 1.10. Many other sophisticated tests need special equipment.

Guidelines are as follows: peripheral neuropathy, should be present in cases of AN; lying and standing BP should always be measured; heart rate

Table 6.2. Normal values for autonomic function tests*

	Normal	Abnormal
Heart rate variation (deep breathing)	>15	<10
Heart rate on standing (at 15 s)	>15	<12
Heart rate on standing 30:15 ratio	>1.04	<1.00
Valsalva ratio	>1.21	<1.20
Postural systolic pressure fall at 2 min	<10 mmHg	>30 mmHg

*These tests decline with age. The figures given here apply generally in those less than 60 years old.

variability and heart rate changes on standing can be measured but as explained above, interpretation may be difficult.

MONONEUROPATHIES, RADICULOPATHIES AND ACUTELY PAINFUL NEUROPATHIES

The rapid onset, severity and eventual resolution of these syndromes contrast sharply with the slow progression of sensory neuropathy and AN. They are sometimes precipitated within a few weeks of starting insulin. These conditions can occur at any age, become commoner in older patients (though none of them is common), and sometimes mark the presentation of the diabetes itself. They rarely recur in later years. They are not associated with other classical diabetic complications.

Pain

This is sometimes of considerable severity and has highly characteristic features: it is protracted and unremitting. Constant burning sensations, paraesthesiae, or shooting pains occur, but the most characteristic symptom

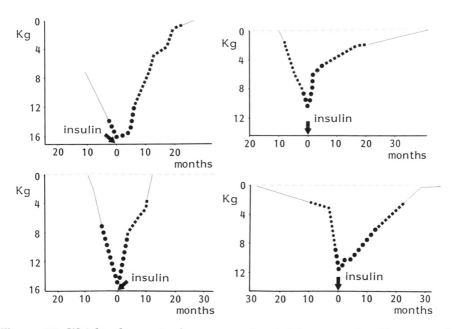

Figure 6.1. Weight change in four cases of painful neuropathy. Documented weight loss without painful symptoms (—); moderate symptoms (···); severe symptoms (●●●); residual symptoms (■■■)

is a cutaneous hypersensitivity leading to acute discomfort on contact with clothing and bedclothes. The pain leads to insomnia, depression and weight loss (Figure 6.1). Patients are so distressed that they may seek several opinions on their condition. The weight loss can be so striking that malignancy is often considered in the differential diagnosis, and the condition itself has been described as neuropathic cachexia.

The distribution of the pain is either in a stocking distribution involving feet and legs to a variable level, occasionally to the groins; or in a radicular distribution affecting two or three adjacent roots generally over the lower trunk. The thighs are affected in cases of femoral neuropathy.

Femoral Neuropathy (Proximal Motor Neuropathy: Amyotrophy)

Pain with or without wasting of one or both thighs is the cardinal feature of this disagreeable condition. It normally begins in one thigh and if the opposite side is affected, symptoms usually develop within a few weeks of the first. The wasting can be so severe that climbing stairs is nearly impossible and the leg may buckle causing falls. The knee jerk is absent, while ankle jerk may be intact. Patients are often first referred to a rheumatologist for treatment of 'arthritis'. Other neurological conditions notably spinal compressive disorders must be excluded. Full recovery is the rule in 6–12 months (Figure 6.2). Recurrence is rare.

Cranial Nerve Palsies

Third and sixth nerve palsies presenting with diplopia of sudden onset are characteristic. Pain behind the eye occurs sometimes in third nerve palsies; the pupil is usually spared, and ptosis does not normally occur. Full examination and careful follow-up are needed, but extensive investigation is not normally required. Complete recovery occurs spontaneously in about 3 months.

Management of Pain

The promise that symptoms always eventually remit may sustain patients during the wretched months of their illness. Diabetic control should be optimal, and insulin should be given if any doubt exists. Regular analgesics are essential, although drugs of addiction should be avoided. Tricyclic antidepressants are helpful: a useful combination is a preparation containing a phenothiazine (fluphenazine) with nortriptyline. Carbamazepine can be tried; mexiletine is of doubtful value, as is capsaicin cream. Application of Opsite (a thin adhesive film) can help to alleviate contact discomfort. Vitamins, antiplatelet drugs, aldose reductase inhibitors, and

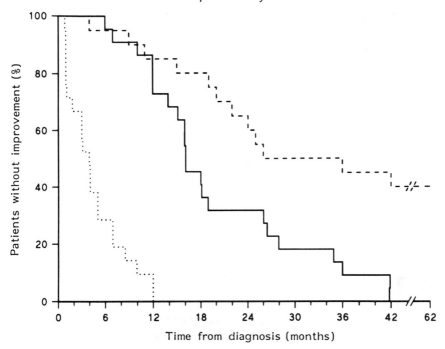

Figure 6.2. Rates of recovery of symptoms and signs of femoral neuropathy in 27 diabetic patients. The 'improvement of pain' (.....) is the time until the first report of improvement in sensory symptoms, from 22 patients. The 'disappearance of discomfort' (—) is the time until complete resolution of sensory symptoms, in 23 patients. The 'recovery of knee jerks' (– – – –) is time course of return to normal of the abnormalities of patella tendon reflexes in 20 patients. No recovery was observed later than 42 months after diagnosis, follow up was for a median of 62 months

sympathetic blockade are of no value. Electrical nerve stimulators applied to the site of pain may help and patients can take an active part in their treatment.

THE EYE

Declining vision is always of concern to the elderly and represents an extremely common problem. The chief causes of deteriorating eyesight in the elderly are either specific for diabetes, or those which occur in any ageing population regardless of the presence of diabetes. They are:

1. cataract;

2. diabetic retinopathy, including macular oedema;

3. macular degeneration;

4. glaucoma;

5. central vein thrombosis.

DIABETIC RETINOPATHY

Retinopathy is quite often present when diabetes is diagnosed in older patients, and occasionally is so severe that visual deterioration is the presenting symptom. Estimates show that up to 20% of newly diagnosed NIDDM patients have established retinopathy (Figure 6.3) and that the proportion affected at diagnosis increases with age. Methods of investigation influence these findings, with careful analysis of retinal photography yielding the greatest numbers. Prevalence of retinopathy increases with duration of diabetes, with a tendency for those taking insulin to develop more retinopathy than those on other treatments. Retinopathy after 15 years of known diabetes is less common than in young-onset (under 30 years old) IDDM patients. The difference is especially striking for proliferative retinopathy, with a prevalence in older patients which is approximately one-half that for younger IDDM patients. Conversely, maculopathy is predominantly a problem of older NIDDM patients although not all authors confirm this observation.

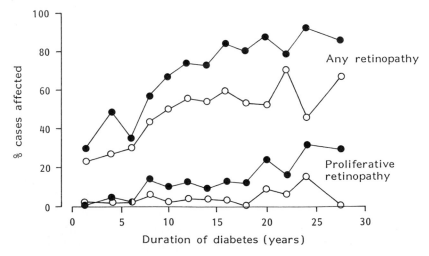

Figure 6.3. Frequency of retinopathy (any degree) or proliferative retinopathy by duration of diabetes (in years) in persons receiving or not receiving insulin who were diagnosed to have diabetes at or after 30 years of age. ●—●, taking insulin; o—o, not taking insulin. (From Klein R. *et al*. 1984[7]. Reproduced by permission of the American Medical Association)

Pathophysiology

Capillary abnormalities are the earliest changes to occur in diabetes; small areas of capillary closure with associated retinal non-perfusion can be seen using fluorescein angiography with retinal photography. The areas of non-perfusion increase in size until visible lesions appear. Subsequently, arteriolar and arterial occlusion may develop as areas of non-perfusion increase still further.

The cause of these early abnormalities is not well understood. Endothelial cell proliferation and then degeneration occur; capillary closure is associated with disappearance of the endothelial cells. The underlying abnormalities are numerous. There may be an early increase of retinal blood flow and there are numerous coagulation and biochemical abnormalities.

Capillary closure and retinal ischemia result in excessive leakage from diseased capillaries, well seen using fluorescein angiography. When this is severe, maculopathy and macular oedema can occur. Ischaemic areas may be seen as cotton wool spots, and provide the stimulus for growth of new vessels. The nature of the 'angiogenic' factor is still uncertain.

Early Changes

There are unconfirmed observations suggesting an early breakdown of the blood–retinal barrier with leakage of fluorescein into the vitreous. Increased retinal blood flow may also be an early feature of diabetes.

Background Retinopathy

Microaneurysms, hard exudates, and haemorrhages constitute the chief lesions of background retinopathy. Unless they occur at or near the macula, they alone are unlikely to cause blindness. Progression of these lesions to the more serious preproliferative or proliferative retinopathies occurs at a very variable rate: in some, it is imperceptibly slow with almost no development over several decades; in others it occurs at a much faster rate. It is not possible to predict the rate of progression in individual patients. Poor diabetic control and hypertension may both contribute to the faster progression of retinopathy.

Background retinopathy eventually affects 80–90% of all older NIDDM patients after 20–25 years of diabetes.

Microaneurysms

These are the earliest recognizable abnormalities of diabetic retinopathy. They represent minute bulges or dilatations of retinal capillaries. They appear as tiny red dots; more of them are seen using fluorescein angiography. They are abnormally permeable but by themselves not harmful.

Hard Exudates

These are yellow-white discrete patches of lipid, which often occur in rings around leaking capillaries. They may coalesce to form extensive sheets of exudate. They cause blindness only when they develop on the macula.

Haemorrhages

These appear as small (dot) and large (blot) red spots on the retina. They harm vision when they appear on the macula.

Maculopathy

Disease at the macula is one of the causes of blindness in diabetes. This is defined as background retinopathy with macular oedema. It is usually insidious in its development and visual acuity can be shown to decline over months or even years. The appearance of hard exudates often in rings, close to the macula (exudatative maculopathy) gives warning that the disease may spread on to the macula; when it does so visual acuity falls, usually irreversibly. It is probably commoner in NIDDM patients than in those with IDDM; thus, in the British Multicentre Study on Photocoagulation, 56 of 99 maculopathy patients were in the 30–59 year old group at diagnosis while only nine were under 30 years of age at diagnosis of diabetes.

Macular Oedema

This is a thickening or swelling of the macular portion of the retina. It occurs both in the presence of hard exudates and less commonly in their absence. It is very difficult to visualize by direct ophthalmoscopy; the macular region appears indistinct and has a subtle grey discoloration. Fluorescein angiography reveals extensive capillary leakage. It may progress rapidly so that early recognition and treatment (laser photocoagulation) are required, even then vision is threatened.

Ischaemic Maculopathy

Peripheral capillaries are destroyed and the prognosis for vision is very poor especially in the elderly. There is sometimes little to be seen on retinal examination and fluorescein angiography may be needed to establish the diagnosis.

Preproliferative Lesions

Ischaemia of the retina probably predisposes to the development of dangerous formation of new vessels, perhaps in response to an 'angiogenic factor'. Lesions indicating an ischaemic and therefore 'preproliferative' retina are:

1. Multiple dot and blot haemorrhages.

2. Cotton wool spots (previously 'soft exudates'); these are small zones of intracellular oedema in the retinal nerve fibre layer developing in an area of ischaemia from capillary closure. They are indistinct, large (disc size) and pale.

3. Venous beading, loops, reduplication.

4. Arterial streaking manifested by parallel white streaks on either side of the arteries.

5. IRMA (intraretinal microvascular abnormality) are fine vascular loops lying within the retina, probably representing true intraretinal neovascularization.

6. Atrophic-looking retina.

Proliferative Retinopathy

New vessel formation occurs either on the optic disc (new vessels on the disc, NVD) or in the periphery of the retina (new vessel elsewhere, NVE). Disc new vessels may grow forward into the vitreous and the risk of vitreous haemorrhage is very great, resulting in blindness in about 30% of cases after 3 years if untreated. The hazard is less for NVE, although they often precede the development of NVD.

Large preretinal haemorrhages may occur, not always affecting vision, but vitreous haemorrhages are more serious causing blindness rapidly, painlessly and without warning. The vitreous usually clears after some weeks with some recovery of vision, but with repeated haemorrhages vision deteriorates permanently.

Proliferative retinopathy affects up to 15% NIDDM patients treated with diet or tablets after 25 years, 30% of NIDDM patients on insulin, compared with 56% of IDDM patients diagnosed under 30 years of age.

Advanced Diabetic Eye Disease

The development of fibroglial proliferation usually following new vessel formation and haemorrhage leads to the appearance of white fibrous strands, which contract and cause severe retinal detachment and tears.

When new vessel formation occurs in the anterior chamber and on the iris (rubeosis iridis) a particularly painful and intractable form of glaucoma develops (rubeotic glaucoma). When conservative management for this condition fails, enucleation is sometimes needed for the relief of pain.

Indications for Referral to an Ophthalmologist

These include:

1. decline of corrected visual acuity from any cause;

2. the presence of preproliferative lesions;

3. proliferative retinopathy with or without vitreous haemorrhage; and

4. lesions which herald the development of maculopathy, especially the appearance of exudates near the macula.

Treatment by Laser Photocoagulation

The prevention of blindness requires treatment of appropriate lesions by photocoagulation before vision has deteriorated and before vitreous haemorrhage has occurred. The indications are:

1. NVD;

2. NVE, less urgent than NVD;

3. Exudative retinopathy: this is treated by photocoagulation when vision begins to decline or when exudates encroach on the macula.

Relatively few elderly patients require photocoagulation and further information on photocoagulation is to be found elsewhere. Patients who have lost vision from vitreous opacification can benefit from vitrectomy.

SCREENING AND PREVENTION

Primary prevention of retinopathy in the elderly is probably impossible, but identification of the causes of visual decline lead to useful treatment for restoring vision most frequently by cataract extraction, or sometimes preservation of vision by photocoagulation (see above) or glaucoma treatment. Otherwise, many visual aids are available for those in whom visual loss is properly identified.

Visual Acuity

Regular testing of visual acuity is the key to proper care of the eyes in diabetes. Using a Snellen chart, the best corrected vision should be recorded using either the patient's own glasses or a 'pin-hole' held in front of the eye. Both declining vision and poor vision are indications for careful retinal examination and referral to an ophthalmologist. Visual acuity should be tested at diagnosis and then regularly, normally annually or thereabouts, or more frequently if pathology is detected.

The simplicity of testing visual acuity means that it can be performed by practice or hospital nurses or by optometrists. The results can be recorded in the cooperation card carried by the patient and is then available for all those attending the patient.

Fundus Examination

This should be undertaken in a darkened room after the pupils have been dilated with Tropicamide 1% eye drops. The examination can be performed by any trained physician, hospital diabetic physicians having the greatest experience of detecting retinopathy (other than ophthalmologists whose sophisticated skill should not be used for screening). Optometrists in some areas have developed well organized schemes for examining diabetic patients, supported by suitable quality safeguards and training programmes. Regular fundus examination is desirable, perhaps annually, but it becomes mandatory if visual acuity begins to deteriorate.

Retinal Photography

Screening by retinal photography is gaining popularity. It may be undertaken either by cameras yielding polaroid prints, or by standard retinal photography always through dilated pupils. Several studies have indicated that some lesions, especially fine peripheral new vessels, may be missed by these techniques. Perhaps the best use for retinal photography will be to demonstrate the absence of any retinal lesions; once present specialized examination is needed. Retinal photography cannot replace the need for visual acuity testing or in general the need for proper fundus examination.

Fluorescein Angiography

This is useful in detecting exudation from intraretinal vascular abnormalities and areas of ischaemia, and will confirm the presence of new vessels if that is required. It is a specialized technique used only by ophthalmologists.

THE LENS: REFRACTIVE CHANGES AND CATARACT

Refractive Changes

The development of myopia (2–3 dioptres) is common in uncontrolled diabetes; it is occasionally the presenting symptom and may be diagnosed as such by an astute optician. This refractive shift is due to osmotic changes in the lens. The refractive change is reversed after starting insulin (and much more rarely after starting tablets) and patients become hyper-metropic for a time, perhaps 2 or 3 weeks, during which they may experience difficulty with reading and with their insulin injection technique. They are sometimes alarmed unless warned. The use of temporary glasses at this time is helpful.

The onset of cataract formation is sometimes accompanied by the development of myopia while blurred vision and diplopia are common symptoms during hypoglycaemia.

Cataract

Cataract formation in diabetics is one of the most frequently observed problems and is commoner than in non-diabetics. Cataracts have an increased prevalence in adult diabetics with a three- to fourfold increased risk in the age range 50–64 years, this excess risk decreasing in later years so that after 69 years there is little increased risk.

Cataract takes various forms. It can appear as the dots, flakes, spokes or subcapsular opacities ('snowstorm') of cortical cataract, or with nuclear sclerosis in which opacities are dense, central and may have yellow–brown discoloration. The rate of progress of lens opacities is difficult to predict. It is usually slow and, as interference with vision is usually late and treatment often effective, it is justifiable to be reasonably optimistic to the patient. The word 'cataract' may be frightening and is better avoided in describing the minor lens opacities, which are so often seen in elderly diabetics.

Treatment for mature cataract is by surgical extraction followed by lens implant, contact lens application or the provision of spectacles. A high success rate is expected, although occasional disappointments occur if extensive retinopathy has been hidden by the presence of the lens opacities.

GLAUCOMA

Glaucoma occurs in diabetic patients as in others; evidence of an increased prevalence is weak and a reported association with AN has not been confirmed. The association of proliferative retinopathy with rubeosis iridis and intractable glaucoma is particularly disagreeable. The presence of glaucoma usually means that the eyes should not be dilated for retinal examinations.

DIABETES AND THE KIDNEY

Detection of proteinuria is crucial for good management of all diabetic patients and the appropriate urine test should be performed at every consultation. When proteinuria is discovered, the physician is alerted to a range of diagnoses, many of which can be simply and effectively treated. These include hypertension, renal disease from diabetes or from any other cause, cardiac failure or just a severe urinary tract infection. Associated with proteinuria from diabetic nephropathy is the substantially increased risk of generalized arterial disease, which is often the chief problem and cause of death in older patients in whom demise from renal failure is relatively rare. The patient with newly diagnosed proteinuria therefore needs a full clinical examination, above all a blood pressure check and assessment of renal function and a decision regarding the extent of renal investigation appropriate to the individual patient.

PROTEINURIA IN DIABETIC PATIENTS

Most diabetic patients with proteinuria have diabetic nephropathy, especially if its onset is gradual and retinopathy is also present (see below). However, other renal diseases are more likely to be discovered among older NIDDM than younger IDDM patients: thus, among our patients presenting in end-stage renal failure, one-third of NIDDM patients had non-diabetic renal diseases compared with only 10% among IDDM patients. The range of conditions included hypertensive renal disease and pyelonephritis (the commonest causes), glomerulonephritis and other less common disorders.

The overall prevalence of proteinuria in NIDDM patients is approximately 15% though estimates vary considerably. Proteinuria is commonly present at diagnosis of NIDDM (but never in IDDM), and progresses to affect approximately one-third of all patients whose diabetes is of longer duration. The annual incidence of proteinuria for NIDDM patients has not been established.

No racial group is known to escape diabetic nephropathy, but it is especially common among Asian patients. In the UK as many as one-half of the NIDDM patients reaching diabetic end-stage failure are from ethnic minorities.

Investigation of Proteinuria

Detection of proteinuria should be performed using Albustix. If more than a trace positive is recorded, 24-h urine protein excretion should be measured and serum creatinine determined. A mid-stream urine is assessed for the presence of infection; however, a urinary tract infection is unlikely to be the cause of heavy proteinuria. If the proteinuria is substantial (more than 0.5 g/24 h) it may be appropriate to perform further investigations.

If the proteinuria has evolved slowly over several years, is associated with retinopathy, and if there is no haematuria, it is most likely to be due to diabetic nephropathy. Extensive investigation is not then needed, although a renal ultrasound examination is generally performed mainly to exclude obstructive lesions in the lower urinary tract. The kidneys are generally of normal size in patients with diabetic nephropathy.

When the clinical features are atypical for diabetic, nephropathy, other renal diagnoses need to be considered, though a firm diagnosis does not always lead to useful specific treatment. Special situations include the presence of haematuria or the sudden onset of proteinuria with or without nephrotic features when, as well as evaluation by blood count, erythrocyte sedimentation rate, antinuclear factor and serum complement measurement, a renal biopsy may be considered if the general condition of the patient allows. Unequal kidney size leads to a consideration of renal artery stenosis, although the hazards of arteriography and the relatively limited benefits of angioplasty may not be warranted in the very old. Small shrunken kidneys indicate end-stage renal disease and further investigation is not normally fruitful.

Microalbuminuria

It is now possible to detect tiny amounts of albuminuria indicating the earliest stages of renal damage. Microalbuminuria is defined as an albumin excretion of 30–300 µg/min. It can be detected using semiquantitative reagent strips, but these readily produce false-positive results so that it is necessary to check the result by more sophisticated laboratory tests on a timed overnight urine sample. Microalbuminuria may indicate the very earliest stages of diabetic nephropathy, but in the elderly especially, its presence often reflects other forms of renal damage, most commonly from hypertension. Many patients with microalbuminuria never develop definite renal disease, but there is a substantially increased mortality from coronary artery disease in this group.

Testing for microalbuminuria is not a recommended procedure in elderly patients, mainly because it is relatively non-specific (e.g. hypertensive renal damage causes microalbuminuria) and relatively expensive. Apart from indicating to the physician to check the blood pressure, it does not lead to any other useful investigation or treatment.

COURSE OF DIABETIC NEPHROPATHY

1. Hyperfiltration (a raised glomerular filtration rate, GFR) occurs early in the cause of IDDM but is much less likely to be present at the known onset of NIDDM.

2. Incipient nephropathy (microalbuminuria 30–300 µg/min) is the stage of microalbuminuria when renal function is still normal. It may persist for several years or indefinitely. The progression of microalbuminuria in the elderly has not been examined in detail, but in IDDM at least 20% of these patients do not progress to overt proteinuria.

3. Persistent proteinuria (albuminuria >300 µg/min) represents established renal disease. At this stage the serum creatinine may persist for some years in the normal range, but the GFR will slowly decline, while hypertension gradually develops and increases.

The rate of decline of GFR is linear in relation to time (Figure 6.4) and in the clinic can be usefully plotted using the inverse creatinine value: it varies considerably from one patient to another, and in some of the older patients may be so slow as to be almost imperceptible. Indeed, with good hypotensive treatment, decline of renal function can be halted so that even raised serum creatinine levels may not change over several years. Slowing the progression of renal impairment in this way represents a major advance in understanding the disease and its management, and emphasizes the importance of detecting and treating hypertension.

Protein restriction has a very limited place in reducing the rate of decline of GFR, and it normally suffices to ensure that patients avoid an excessive protein intake (defined as more than 1 g/kg per day). There is at present no convincing evidence to suggest that giving hypotensive treatment to normotensive elderly nephropathic patients is advantageous, and even in the young it remains controversial.

4. Clinical renal impairment (serum creatinine 120–400 µmol/l). By this stage renal impairment is manifest, although patients are not necessarily symptomatic. The development of oedema is one of the earliest clinical features of renal impairment, often associated with anaemia and a rather non-specific decline of health.

5. End-stage renal disease (serum creatinine >400 µmol/l). Patients are normally ill at this time and will eventually develop classical uraemic symptoms notably from fluid retention and subsequently nausea and

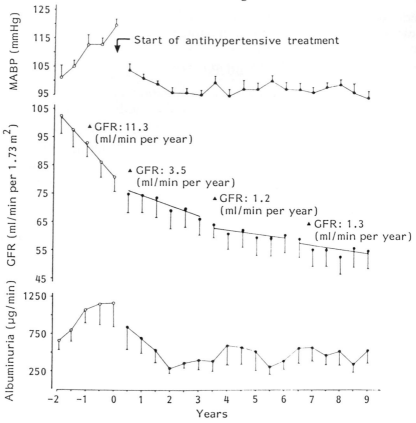

Figure 6.4. Average course of mean arterial blood pressure (MABP), glomerular filtration rate (GFR) and albuminuria before (o) and during (●) long-term effective antihypertensive treatment of nine insulin-dependent diabetic patients with diabetic nephropathy. (Reprinted by permission from Parving H.-H., Smidt, U. M., Hommel, E., *et al.* Effective antihypertensive treatment postpones renal insufficiency in diabetic nephropathy. *Am J Kidney Dis* 1993; **22**: 188–95)

vomiting, which can be alleviated to some extent by moderate protein restriction. They are best seen in conjunction with a renal physician so that a proper treatment plan is developed. This will be influenced by the presence of vascular disease, which will almost certainly be extensive especially in elderly patients.

MANAGEMENT OF RENAL FAILURE

Peripheral and later pulmonary oedema are the earliest and commonest clinical manifestations of renal failure in the diabetic patient. It is important at this point to distinguish true cardiac failure from fluid retention resulting from renal failure, though often both are present. If oedema cannot readily be controlled by diuretic treatment, and especially if the patient's general health is declining, renal dialysis must be considered. Uraemic symptoms can to some extent be controlled by a protein-restricted diet, although by this stage most patients will need renal support anyway. This is usually needed earlier in diabetic than non-diabetic patients and very likely when the serum creatinine is in the range 450–550 µmol/l. About one-quarter to one-third of renal unit patients are diabetic, as more older patients are accepted for treatment the proportion of NIDDM patients is increasing and already exceeds half of all the diabetic patients. Continuous ambulatory peritoneal dialysis (CAPD) is the treatment of first choice to alleviate renal failure in the elderly, and now quite feasible in patients in their 70s, leading to a good quality of life. In 1992, of all patients admitted to the Renal Unit for renal support treatment at King's College Hospital, 38% were over 65 and 20% over 75 years of age (B. Hendry, personal communication). CAPD is the commonest mode of treatment, since very few diabetics over 65 years old are suitable for transplantation. Mortality is 10–20% higher than among non-diabetic patients, chiefly because of the extensive cardiovascular disease.

Management of the diabetes during CAPD is not normally a major problem, except when high concentration glucose bags are used when hyperglycaemia can rapidly develop. NIDDM patients either remain on their normal treatment, though many require conversion to insulin, when a fixed insulin mixture twice daily will usually suffice. Peritoneal insulin is very effective, but unless patients are very skilful with aseptic techniques, the peritonitis rate is unacceptably high.

Contraindications to starting CAPD must be carefully considered. Dementia from cerebrovascular disease and strokes, and carcinomatosis are clear contraindications. Patients with gross cardiac disease and cardio-megaly have a very poor prognosis, though the alleviation of symptoms in those with cardiac failure can be very impressive. Social circumstances, vision and ability to cope all need to be taken into consideration.

MANAGEMENT OF DIABETES IN RENAL FAILURE

Short-acting sulphonylureas which are metabolized and not renally excreted should be used. Gliclazide or tolbutamide are best suited for these patients. Glibenclamide which is still very popular may cause profound hypoglycaemia and should not be used in these patients. Biguanides should never be given to renal failure patients both because of side-effects and the potential hazard of lactic acidosis.

As renal failure progresses, some patients need less oral hypoglycaemic treatment and may revert to diet alone. Some, however, deteriorate especially when intercurrent illness supervenes and still need insulin treatment. The diabetes management thus needs constant review as the disease progresses.

MANAGEMENT OF HYPERTENSION

Regular measurement of blood pressure in the elderly nephropathic diabetic patient is crucial and leads directly to treatment, which effectively reduces morbidity and progression of renal damage. The gains from adequate hypotensive treatment are substantial, namely reduction of progression of renal impairment, sometimes halting it (but not reversing it), together with prevention of strokes and heart failure.

The level of blood pressure which requires treatment is not easily determined. For patients in the age range 65–75 years levels persistently greater than 160/100 mmHg probably merit treatment, though argument remains about the value of treating diastolic pressures less than 105 mmHg. Nevertheless, if nephropathy is clearly established, even in this age group, it is probably wise to keep the blood pressure below 160/95 mmHg. Above 75 years of age, decisions to treat hypertension become very difficult, since both cerebrovascular and renal problems may be exacerbated.

Treatment of hypertension should include general measures, such as weight reduction and avoidance of excessive alcohol and salt. First choice of drug treatment lies between angiotensin-converting enzyme (ACE) inhibitors, calcium channel antagonists, or possibly selective beta blockers. ACE inhibitors may give added renal protection in patients with nephropathy because they specifically reduce intraglomerular pressures; on the other hand, the principal hazard of their use is in precipitating acute renal failure in patients with renal artery stenosis, so that careful monitoring during the first month of treatment is important. Loop diuretics (e.g. frusemide, bumetanide) are often needed as well, especially when oedema develops in association with vasodilatation. Specific considerations are required in some groups, namely the relative contraindication to the use of beta blockers in patients with peripheral vascular disease, cardiac failure or asthma; and avoidance of thiazide diuretics which exacerbate hyperglycaemia and hyperlipaemia especially in NIDDM. Hypertension in Afro-Caribbean patients is exceptionally common and often resistant to treatment, and in these patients verapamil can be more effective than other agents.

URINARY TRACT INFECTIONS

Urinary tract infections occur in diabetic people with the same frequency as in non-diabetic people, but they are sometimes exceptionally severe and may cause the renal papillae to slough—necrotizing papillitis. Infection is particularly troublesome in the rare patient with urinary retention from neurogenic bladder. Diabetic control is easily disturbed by urinary infection, as with any infection, and must be regained quickly, with insulin if necessary, while the infection is treated with antibiotics.

Pyelonephritis with septicaemia is not uncommon in diabetes, with occasional formation of perinephric abscesses. The source of the infection may not be immediately apparent and sometimes patients present in profound shock without an obvious site of infection.

OTHER DIABETIC COMPLICATIONS

Almost all patients with diabetic nephropathy also have retinopathy and when the renal disease is advanced so is the eye disease. Thus, in NIDDM as in IDDM renal failure patients, three-quarters have proliferative retinopathy and nearly one-third are blind. There is a constant need for monitoring retinopathy and ensuring that photocoagulation treatment is appropriately applied.

Diabetic foot problems are common in nephropathy patients, both from neuropathy and peripheral vascular disease. About one-third of our NIDDM renal failure patients had at some stage had a neuropathic foot ulcer, while amputations for severe peripheral vascular disease are not rare. The presence of a podiatrist in a diabetic renal clinic has a major impact in reducing foot morbidity and may halve the amputation rate.

MACROVASCULAR DISEASE

Major arterial disease affecting the coronary circulation, cerebral arteries and causing peripheral vascular disease of feet and legs may represent the most serious of the problems affecting elderly diabetic patients. The prevalence is higher in a diabetic than a non-diabetic population, but it is much greater in those patients who develop proteinuria from diabetic nephropathy. Three-quarters of diabetic patients diagnosed over 60 years of age die from cardiovascular disease, chiefly from myocardial infarction. The proportion is even higher among those with nephropathy. Other risk factors are well known, namely smoking, hypertension, hyperlipidaemia and obesity.

The clinical features of major arterial disease are very similar to those in non-diabetic patients, but there are a number of differences which are described below.

1. Atheromatous arterial disease has a tendency to a more peripheral distribution in diabetes, especially in the legs, but probably in the coronary

vessels as well. Distal lesions are not always amenable to manipulation by angioplasty or arterial surgery, but none the less, proximal lesions are still common and often treatable. Diabetic patients should be offered these treatments using exactly the same criteria as those used for non-diabetics.

2. Medial arterial calcification (Monckeberg's sclerosis) of distal arteries is a feature of diabetes, and becomes much commoner in those with severe neuropathy. This may result from a medial degeneration in sympathetically denervated vessels. Calcification is further increased and more distal in its distribution in nephropathy patients. Calcified vessels become more rigid than normal, though the effects on blood flow are uncertain.

3. Symptomless myocardial infarction is commoner in a diabetic population. The presence of AN is thought to be responsible for the absence of chest pain, but the evidence is conflicting.

Mortality in acute myocardial infarction is doubled in diabetic patients. Autonomic abnormalities, high non-esterified fatty acid levels, and the dubious entity of 'diabetic cardiomyopathy' have all been blamed.

SKIN AND JOINTS

CHEIROARTHROPATHY

Patients with very long-standing diabetes may develop a mild curvature of the fingers, which makes it impossible to place the hand and fingers flat on a smooth surface. This defect is accompanied by some tightening of the skin over the fingers and is thought to be due to a collagen defect. There is no disability.

CHONDROCALCINOSIS

This can occur in association with haemochromatosis affecting especially the knees. Acute arthritis sometimes results. There is no other specific joint disease affecting the diabetic apart from the rare Charcot or neuroarthropathic foot problems, which are described elsewhere.

NECROBIOSIS LIPOIDICA DIABETICORUM

This lesion is specific to diabetes. It is rare, affecting chiefly younger diabetic women; it is exceptionally rare in the elderly. The shin is the commonest site of involvement with obviously dilated capillaries (telangiectasis), an atrophic base, and a slightly raised pinkish rim; ulceration can occur. The lesions are normally permanent.

GRANULOMA ANNULARE

This is a raised pinkish lesion sometimes circular in configuration occurring especially on the limb, with a rather dubious relationship to diabetes.

VITILIGO

This is an autoimmune disorder causing patchy depigmentation, which may have an association with IDDM.

XANTHOMAS

These are discrete yellow eruptions, which appear in crops and are associated with severe hyperlipidaemia.

ACANTHOSIS NIGRICANS

Pigmentation affecting axillae and groin with a velvety skin. This is associated with insulin resistance resulting from an absence of insulin receptors.

LIPOHYPERTROPHY

This is represented by fatty lumps occurring at the sites of insulin injection especially if injections are given repeatedly into the same place.

LIPOATROPHY

This was formerly seen at the sites of insulin injections before the introduction of purified insulins. Lipatrophic diabetes (absence of subcutaneous fat, lipaemia and hepatomegaly) is very rare.

CONCLUSIONS

Specific diabetic complications need to be identified and managed in elderly diabetic patients just as they are in younger groups. Primary prevention is probably not possible by this stage of life, but the consequences can often be averted, notably in the case of the feet. Many older patients are beset with major problems from arterial disease which may dominate their health problems, and management then may become much more complex. Great skill and co-ordination of services is needed in the care of elderly diabetic patients.

FURTHER READING

1 Dyck PJ, Thomas PK, Asbury AK, Winegrad AI, Porte D (eds), *Diabetic Neuropathy*. Philadelphia: WB Saunders Company, 1987.
2 Bannister R, Mathias CJ (eds), *Autonomic Failure*. Oxford University Press, 1992.
3 Watkins PJ. Clinical observations and experiments in diabetic neuropathy. *Diabetologia* 1992; **35**: 2–11.
4 The Diabetes Control and Complications Trial Research Group. Effect of intensive treatment of diabetes on the development and progression of long term complications in insulin dependent diabetes mellitus. *N Engl J Med* 1993; **329**: 977–986.
5 Brenner BM, Stein JH (eds), *The Kidney in Diabetes Mellitus*. New York: Churchill Livingstone, 1989.
6 Drury PL, Watkins PJ. Diabetic renal disease and its prevention. *Clin Endocrinol* 1993; **38**: 445–450.
7 Coppack SW, Watkins PJ. The natural history of diabetic femoral neuropathy. *QJ Med* 1991; **79**: 307–313.
8 Klein R, Klein BEK, Moss SE, *et al.* Wisconsin epidemiologic study of diabetic retinopathy: III. Prevalence and risk of diabetic retinopathy when age at diagnosis is 30 or more years. *Arch Ophthalmol* 1984; **102**: 527–532.

7

The Diabetic Foot

MATTHEW J. YOUNG* and ANDREW J. M. BOULTON
University Department of Medicine, Manchester Royal Infirmary, Manchester, UK

INTRODUCTION

The earliest descriptions of foot ulceration associated with diabetes date from the nineteenth century. In 1934 Joslin reported that gangrene was a menace to diabetic patients[1]. Sixty years later foot problems remain one of the commonest reasons for hospital admission among diabetic patients. The rate of lower limb amputation is 15 times higher in diabetic patients compared with non-diabetic patients[2]. More than 50% of diabetic amputees need an amputation in the contralateral limb during the first 4 years after the loss of the first leg[3]. It has been estimated that 20% of all hospital admissions among diabetic patients in the USA are for foot problems and hospital costs alone have been estimated at $200 million in 1980[4,5]. In the UK the total annual cost of major leg amputations in diabetic patients has been estimated at £13.4m during the financial year 1985–86[6]. Conversely, diabetic foot problems are potentially the most preventable long-term complications of diabetes. It is now the stated aim of the WHO/IDF to reduce the number of amputations for diabetes in Europe by 50% within 3 years, as set out in the St Vincent Declaration[7]. Education of the patient together with a multidisciplinary team approach to the management of foot problems in specially organized diabetic foot clinics has been shown to reduce the incidence of major leg amputation, and the duration of in-patient admission for the treatment of foot ulceration, in diabetic patients[8,9].

---

* Present address: Department of Diabetes, The Royal Infirmary, Edinburgh, UK

Diabetes in Old Age. Edited by P. Finucane and A. J. Sinclair
© 1995 John Wiley & Sons Ltd

The average age of patients with diabetic foot problems is over 60 years[9]. Peripheral neuropathy and peripheral vascular disease, the main antecedents of foot ulceration, are more prevalent with increasing age[10], which makes diabetic foot problems an increased component of diabetes care in the elderly.

Foot ulceration is not the only complication of the diabetic foot syndrome and, in addition to a discussion about the aetiology and management of diabetic foot ulceration, this chapter will also discuss the diagnosis and management of Charcot neuroarthropathy.

RISK FACTORS FOR FOOT ULCERATION IN DIABETES

Foot problems in diabetes can develop from a number of component causes. The main contributing factors include sensorimotor and autonomic neuropathy, peripheral vascular disease, limited joint mobility and high foot pressures. The existence of other long-term complications of diabetes also influences the development of foot ulceration. In addition, these factors are compounded by increasing age, particularly in those patients who live alone.

PERIPHERAL SENSORIMOTOR NEUROPATHY

Peripheral sensorimotor neuropathy is the primary cause or contributory cause in 90% of diabetic foot ulceration[8,9]. The incidence of diabetic peripheral sensorimotor neuropathy increases with the duration of diabetes but, as the prevalence depends on the diagnostic criteria that are used, the prevalence rates which have been reported from different epidemiological studies vary considerably[11]. In a prospective study of a large cohort of diabetic patients followed over 25 years, 50% exhibited objective signs of neuropathy[10], while in a recent multicentre study which screened a large hospital-treated diabetic population it was found that the overall prevalence of neuropathy was 28.5%[12]. In the same study, more than one-half of all the patients with Type 2 diabetes, aged over 60, were found to have neuropathy.

The most common symptoms of sensory neuropathy are numbness, lancinating pain, 'pins and needles', burning pain and hyperaesthesiae typically with nocturnal exacerbation. The clinical signs are usually sensory loss in a glove and stocking distribution. While loss of pain, fine touch and temperature sensation are related to small (often unmyelinated) fibre involvement, loss of vibration perception and proprioception is believed to be related to large (usually myelinated) fibre damage. Usually both small and large fibres are affected but occasionally there is disproportionate involvement of one or other fibre type (most commonly small fibres)[13]. It must be remembered that in some patients the presenting feature of peripheral neuropathy, and indeed of diabetes itself, may be foot ulceration, as the progression to an insensitive foot may occur without any positive symptoms. Thus, the absence of symptoms must never be equated with absence of risk of ulceration.

The diagnosis of diabetic peripheral neuropathy for clinical trials purposes is a complex issue, which usually involves the use of clinical examination, nerve conduction measurements, and quantitative sensory tests[14]. For routine screening purposes clinical examination using a 128 Hz tuning fork will suffice. The vibration perception threshold (VPT) can be measured quantitatively using a Biothesiometer (Biomedical, Newbury, Ohio, USA). Such measurements have shown to be increased in association with other measurements of diabetic peripheral neuropathy and increase with normal ageing; therefore, the use of age-related normal values are generally recommended. Other authors have claimed that the increased coefficient of variation in older patients makes the measurement of VPT unreliable and that it should be supplemented by other tests of neuropathy[15]. For screening purposes, however, this may not be necessary. A VPT of greater than 25 V has been shown in a cross-sectional survey to be associated with foot ulceration, and, in a recent prospective study, was strongly predictive of subsequent foot ulceration over a 4-year period[16]. In the latter study patients with a VPT >25 V were seven times more likely to develop a foot ulcer than a patient with a VPT <25 V over a 4-year period. This increased to 11 times when recurrent ulceration was considered, as no patient with a VPT <25 V developed a second ulcer. This study also revealed a relationship between foot ulceration and increasing age but, even after correcting for this, VPT remained a strong predictor of foot ulceration risk.

Motor fibre loss is another significant result of peripheral neuropathy leading to small muscle atrophy in the foot. As a consequence, there is an imbalance between flexor and extensor muscle function resulting in clawing of the toes, prominent metatarsal heads and anterior displacement of the metatarsal footpads[17,18] (Figure 7.1). Abnormally high foot pressures usually develop under these areas and, as discussed below, can lead to foot ulceration in the susceptible foot.

In addition the gait pattern is significantly altered in patients with diabetic neuropathy[19] and this may alter the foot pressure distribution making the foot more prone to the effects of high pressure. Gait problems, with increasing falls, and the risks of injury to the feet, are increased in neuropathic diabetic patients. Such problems are more pronounced in elderly neuropathic patients, and worse in those with visual handicap, increasing the risk of foot ulceration in these patients[20].

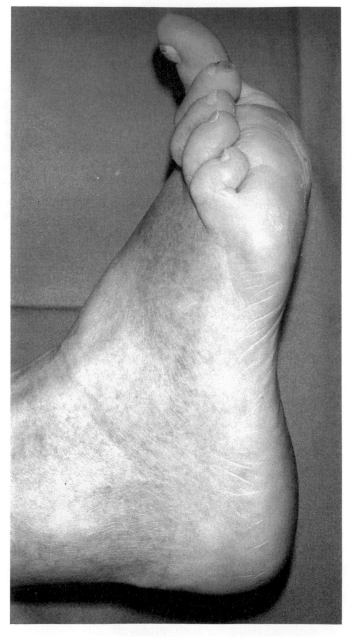

Figure 7.1. At-risk foot showing prominent metatarsal heads and clawed toes

AUTONOMIC NEUROPATHY

Autonomic neuropathy encompasses a wide spectrum of problems in the cardiovascular, gastrointestinal and genitourinary systems and is known to be associated with the development of foot ulceration in diabetic patients[21]. In the foot, denervation of the sweat glands[22] leads to dry, atrophic skin and callus formation. Severe cracking of the skin often occurs under these circumstances and facilitates microbial infections.

Loss of sympathetic tone in small vessels also leads to reduced resistance and increased arteriovenous shunting[23]. Venous PO_2 is raised in the neuropathic limb to a level approaching that of arterial blood, and has been measured at higher levels than in the endoneurium[24]. Thus in a diabetic patient with autonomic neuropathy, but without coexisting major vessel occlusive vascular disease the blood flow is increased at rest and distended dorsal foot veins can be seen[25]. Initially, the overall increase in blood flow is reflected by an increase in capillary pressure; however, this leads to microvascular sclerosis, and when taken in conjunction with the increased shunting in the diabetic neuropathic foot may lead to inadequate nutritional flow and subsequent tissue ischaemia, greatly increasing the risk of ulceration[26]. The coexistence of autonomic neuropathy and macrovascular disease may cause a further deterioration in the level of tissue oxygenation.

PERIPHERAL VASCULAR DISEASE

Both the micro- and macrocirculation in the lower extremities are affected by diabetes. In the microcirculation the skin capillary pressure is increased in patients with Type 1 diabetes, either of recent onset or of long duration, and this abnormality reverses when the diabetes control improves[27]. This increase in the capillary pressure is probably responsible for the loss of the blood flow autoregulation, increased arteriovenous shunting, impaired hyperaemic response, changes in capillary blood flow and basement membrane thickening[28]. However, in diabetic patients with sensory neuropathy, gangrene can develop in the absence of pain. These changes are independent of the existence of autonomic neuropathy, although these two abnormalities are usually found together. Acute improvement of the glycaemic control in patients with autonomic neuropathy results in redistribution of skin blood flow with increased capillary and reduced arteriovenous shunt flow[29].

Macrovascular disease is also more common in diabetic patients. Peripheral vascular disease is estimated to occur 20 times more often in diabetic patients than in non-diabetic patients[30]. Lipid disorders[31], platelet dysfunction[32], increased coagulation[33] and endothelial cell dysfunction[34] have been implicated in the pathogenesis of the atherosclerosis[35]. Peripheral vascular disease usually has the same clinical presentation as that seen in non-diabetic patients with intermittent claudication, rest pain, ulceration and gangrene being the main clinical features[36], but the symptoms may be masked by coexisting peripheral neuropathy. Although, as in non-diabetic patients, the femoropopliteal segments are most often affected, smaller vessels below the knee, such as the tibial and peroneal arteries are more severely affected in diabetic than in non-diabetic patients[37].

Medial arterial calcification is another common finding in diabetic patients and can be recognized on X-ray films by its 'pipe-stem' appearance[38]. Medial arterial calcification is reported to be associated with diabetic peripheral somatosensory and autonomic neuropathy[38-40]; however, few previous studies have examined the distribution of medial arterial calcification quantitatively within the diabetic foot. Medial arterial calcification is significantly associated with an increased prevalence of cardiovascular mortality[41-43], although this may also be related to the increase in medial arterial calcification associated with diabetic nephropathy[38], an independent marker of increased mortality in diabetes[44]. In a recent study[45], we demonstrated that diabetes alone does not increase the prevalence of medial arterial calcification in matched groups of controls and non-neuropathic subjects; however, there was significantly heavier arterial calcification in the feet of neuropathic diabetic patients. A linear regression model revealed that VPT, duration of diabetes and serum creatinine were all independent predictors of the degree of medial arterial calcification. Medial arterial calcification, when present, is known to alter the pulse waveform and falsely elevate ankle pressures in diabetic patients[46-48]. For this reason it has been suggested that toe systolic pressure measurements might replace ankle-pressure measurements as an index of arterial inflow to the diabetic foot[48] as the ankle pressure index, measured by Doppler ultrasound, may be misleadingly high, despite the presence of occlusive peripheral vascular disease[46-48]. A recent study which demonstrated that toe systolic pressures are reduced in diabetic patients with peripheral neuropathy, despite normal or increased ankle systolic pressures would support this view[49]. If ankle pressures are to be used appropriately then all cases where the ankle systolic pressure is low can be accepted as indicative of occlusive vascular disease, but where the ankle systolic pressure, or ankle brachial pressure index, is normal or elevated then this should be interpreted with caution, particularly in elderly and neuropathic diabetic patients.

LIMITED JOINT MOBILITY

Diffuse collagen abnormalities are common in diabetic patients[50]. The main pathogenic mechanism for these abnormalities is glycation of collagen, which results in thickening and increased cross-linking of collagen bundles[51]. One of the clinical manifestations of this change is thick, tight and waxy skin, leading to restriction of joint movements. Patients with limited joint mobility are unable to oppose the palms of their hands (the prayer sign, Figure 7.2)[52]. The term cheiroarthropathy was used to describe this condition. As other joints, including those in the foot, can also be affected, a more appropriate term is limited joint mobility, and this is now in general use[53,54]. Limited joint mobility in the foot mainly involves the subtalar joint, which provides the foot with shock-absorbing capacity during walking[55]. This results in increased plantar foot pressures, and, in the neuropathic foot, may be a contributory factor to the development of foot ulceration[56]. Limited extension of the great toe, 'hallux rigidus', can also predispose to ulceration by limiting the adaptive extension of the toe during the final 'toe-off' phase of walking, thus increasing the vertical and shear forces on the toe.

FOOT PRESSURE ABNORMALITIES

The two main factors responsible for the development of high foot pressures, motor neuropathy and limited joint mobility, have already been discussed. Callus formation, which itself is a result of high foot pressures and dry skin, may also act as a foreign body and results in further increases of these pressures[57]. In contrast, the age and body weight of a patient do not significantly influence the foot pressure[58,59].

Intermittent moderate stress on healthy tissue for an excessive time, as in the case of abnormal pressures applied on the plantar surface of the foot during excessive walking, can lead to tissue inflammation and, finally, to ulceration[60]. At the microscopic level, it is believed that pressure overcomes the nutritive flow of the skin and this leads to localized tissue necrosis and breakdown[61]. The demonstration of increased arteriovenous shunting[62-64] in the diabetic foot, and the impaired hyperaemic injury response[65,66] in neuropathic patients may also contribute to the increased risk of ulceration. Studies in dogs have shown that repetitive moderate trauma leads to the eventual breakdown of the skin and ulceration[67]. Thermography of the feet of patients with diabetic neuropathy has shown hot spots of inflammation in areas of high foot pressures and repetitive trauma[68]. Sensory dysfunction is crucial for the development of neuropathic ulceration: in non-neuropathic subjects, the pain which accompanies the inflammation will usually force them to rest the foot before it progresses to ulceration, whereas patients with loss of pain awareness will continue to walk long after an ulcer has developed. Therefore, high foot pressures alone, in the absence of sensory neuropathy, do not result in foot ulceration. This can be illustrated in patients with rheumatoid arthritis, in whom joint involvement in the feet

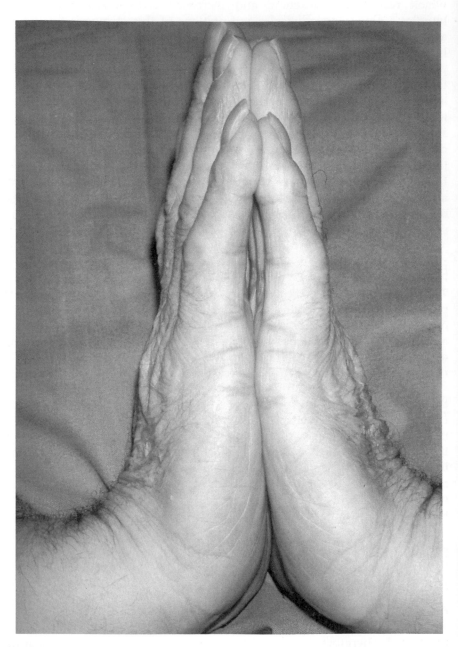

Figure 7.2. The prayer sign

results in high foot pressures comparable with those found in diabetic patients, but not ulceration[69].

Different methods have been designed for the measurement of high foot pressures. The first method, developed by Harris and Beath in 1947[70], was semiquantitative and consisted of a multilayer inked rubber mat which makes contact with a piece of paper. When pressure is applied on the mat, ink marks the paper with the density of the impression in proportion to the applied pressure. Measurements in diabetic patients using this method showed high loading under the feet, particularly the metatarsal heads[71].

The first studies which provided quantitative measurements of foot pressures were conducted using a strain gauge system[72,73]. The main findings of these studies were that loads under the diabetic feet were higher than in non-diabetic subjects and that plantar ulcers usually occurred at sites of maximum load.

The optical pedobarograph, which was based on the original system of Chodera[74], and developed at Sheffield University, is another apparatus which has been extensively used for studying foot pressures in diabetic patients[75]. In comparison with other systems using capacitance or resistance element matrices[76,77], the optical pedobarograph provides better spatial resolution and reliability. Cross-sectional studies have shown that foot pressures in neuropathic diabetic patients are higher compared with non-neuropathic patients and that foot ulcers develop in areas with high pressures[78].

In the first prospective study to examine the relationship between high foot pressures and ulceration, 86 diabetic patients, with a mean age of 56 years, including those with and without high foot pressures, were followed up for a mean period of 30 months[79]. All the plantar ulcers which developed during this study (17% of all feet) occurred in patients with high foot pressures at baseline, while in the group of patients with neuropathy and high pressures at baseline the ulceration rate during the study was 18% per year. Therefore, high foot pressures, especially in neuropathic patients, are highly predictive of subsequent foot ulceration and may be useful in identifying the at-risk patient.

OTHER RISK FACTORS

History of Previous Foot Problems

A history of previous foot problems in diabetic patients strongly suggests that the patient is at high risk for future problems, especially in the case of lower limb amputation[2,3]. Studies in patients with traumatic or diabetic amputations, have shown that amputation alone does not cause an increase in the loads under the remaining foot. However, in a neuropathic diabetic patient amputation is associated with high pressure under the remaining foot, probably related to neuropathy and limited joint mobility in the remaining foot[80].

In the prospective study of the prediction of foot ulceration using VPTs recurrent ulceration was common, affecting over 50% of the patients. In addition, in a recent audit of dressing policy at the Manchester Foot Hospital the median number of ulcers per patient was 2 (range 1–12)[81], again suggesting that over one-half of the patients reulcerated, despite preventative care and advice. The likely causes for this are as yet unknown but it appears that those patients who do not wear their recommended shoes (which are usually supplied), or do not follow the appropriate advice are those who subsequently reulcerate.

Reduced Resistance to Infection

There are many reasons for impaired resistance to infection in a diabetic ulcer. Diabetes is associated with impaired neutrophil function, particularly in the presence of a high blood glucose[82] and macro- and microcirculatory abnormalities lead to relative hypoxia in the wound[83]. Multiple microbes, often a mixture of aerobic and anaerobic bacteria are usually found in cultures from foot ulcers. The commonest pathogenic organisms in diabetic foot ulcers are staphylococci and streptococci, usually faecal in origin, although the clinical relevance of organisms grown from superficial swabs is variable, as other organisms may colonize the wound surface and the quality of the sample and the method of transport and culture markedly influence the reliability of the result[84]. The treatment of infections associated with foot ulceration is detailed further in the management of foot ulceration.

Smoking and Alcohol

Smoking is known to be associated with foot ulceration, probably by increasing the prevalence of vascular disease[85]. Recurrent neuropathic foot ulceration has been reported as being more common in diabetic patients with a high alcohol consumption[86].

Other Complications of Diabetes

Foot pressures in patients with nephropathy are higher than in diabetic patients without renal impairment, and in combination with neuropathy, which is also more common in such patients, impose a serious risk for foot ulceration[87].

THE EFFECTS OF AGEING ON THE DIABETIC FOOT

Lower limb amputation is more common in older, usually Type 2, diabetic patients[2]. The average age of diabetic foot clinic attenders is over 60 years of age[9]; therefore, the elderly must be at particular risk of foot ulceration. Reduced mobility, particularly at the hip, in patients over 60 impairs their ability to inspect the feet and leads to the continued progression of foot lesions, often beyond a point of repair, before they are discovered[88]. In addition, patients with severely impaired vision depend on other people for foot inspection, and when they are not easily available, such as an elderly person living alone, this may make foot care very difficult to perform adequately.

Diabetes alone probably does not add to the prevalence of bunions, clawed toes and medial arterial calcification that is seen in the elderly[45,89]. Neuropathy, however, is more prevalent in the elderly, increasing with both age and duration of diabetes. Once this is superimposed on the normal ageing process, skeletal abnormalities including spontaneous fractures are significantly more common[89]. Add the increased prevalence of peripheral vascular disease in the older Type 2 diabetic patient to the increase in neuropathy and difficulties with foot care and it fully explains the particular predilection for foot abnormalities that exists in older diabetic patients.

THE PATHWAY TO FOOT ULCERATION

A model of the pathways to amputation was developed by Pecoraro *et al.*[83]. A similar model can be applied to foot ulceration, where foot ulceration develops as the result of a number of component causes acting together, but which singularly may not have resulted in the development of a foot ulcer.

Peripheral neuropathy is the first of these component causes. When peripheral neuropathy is present, patients rarely complain of the presence of an ulcer. They rarely limp and may not even be aware that the ulcer has formed. In such cases the first warning signs of the existence of an ulcer will probably be visual, such as the bleeding when the footwear is removed or, in most serious situations, the development of gangrene. It is not uncommon for neuropathic diabetic patients to present because of the smell caused by purulent discharge. They may also have a curious indifference to the condition of their feet, which can be likened to sensory inattention. This can make the importance of education about foot care difficult to impress upon them[91].

However, peripheral neuropathy is not the only component cause, because, as explained above, without trauma, the foot would not ulcerate spontaneously merely because of neuropathy. Thus the two must act synergistically. This trauma may take the form of an acute event, for example a penetrating injury due to a nail or glass on the floor, or more commonly repetitive minor trauma from walking or tight shoes. In its turn, the pressure from walking is increased by limited joint mobility and callus, which as outlined above are increased in patients with peripheral neuropathy. Thus the circle is closed and the components interact to make the patient at risk of foot ulceration.

Peripheral vascular insufficiency may be added as an additional component, to make the skin less viable and reduce the pressure at which ischaemia and tissue breakdown develop. Impaired wound healing follows to continue the cycle of tissue destruction when an ulcer has formed.

MANAGEMENT OF THE DIABETIC FOOT SYNDROME

The prevention and management of diabetic foot problems must address each of these component causes and associated risk profiles outlined above. The success of such strategies should be gauged by their effect on ulceration and amputation rates. As mentioned in the introduction, the care of the diabetic patient with foot problems is improved significantly by the formation of a diabetic foot care team, preferably in a foot clinic setting[9,92]. The diabetic foot care team should include a doctor, nurse and chiropodist, all with an interest in diabetes. The team should have access to hospital facilities with a good relationship between themselves and the local vascular and/or orthopaedic surgeon, orthotist and limb fitting centre. A visiting orthotist to supply and fit the shoes is ideal. The full integration of, and cooperation between, team members is essential. Inconsistent or inappropriate advice and care from different members of the team can often lead to all such advice being ignored with potentially serious consequences.

While others have tried to update it, or have introduced more descriptive systems, the most widely used system of diabetic foot ulcer classification is still the Wagner classification of foot ulceration[93]. The first grade in the Wagner classification is actually grade 0, which refers to the high risk diabetic foot without actual ulceration. This is also termed the 'at-risk' foot.

THE 'AT-RISK' FOOT

It is important to stress once again that the feet of patients with diabetes do not ulcerate spontaneously. Foot ulceration is usually due to the combination of the factors outlined above. When these factors and the other known associations with diabetic foot ulceration are present, but the foot is intact, the foot, and the patient, are said to be 'at risk'. The main 'at-risk' groups are listed in Table 7.1.

IDENTIFICATION AND MANAGEMENT OF THE 'AT-RISK' FOOT

The identification of 'at-risk' patients who might benefit from foot care education and treatment is of paramount importance. Patients who are not previously known to be 'at risk' should be assessed at all new clinic appointments and at least annually thereafter. Once the patient has been identified as being 'at risk' then the feet should be examined at every clinic visit. This simple method of risk reduction is frequently overlooked[94,95], and yet it is the basis of foot ulcer prevention.

It is also important to stress that standard clinical examination will identify most of the 'at-risk' patients without the need for pedobarography or other expensive screening systems, although these can be used where they are available. When screening patients for the risks of foot ulceration the following categories should be assessed.

Peripheral Neuropathy

Despite the potential problems of age-related changes in neurological function, routine clinical examination, including reflexes and vibration perception using a 128 Hz tuning fork will readily identify the neuropathic patient at risk of foot ulceration. Semmes-weinstein monofilaments are a quick method for assessing the at-risk foot in leprosy and have been used by some diabetes units in the UK[96]. Peripheral neuropathy can be detected by use of the neuropathy disability score (NDS)[12]: This is derived from

Table 7.1. 'At-risk' groups for diabetic foot ulceration

Patients with:
    a history of previous ulceration
    peripheral neuropathy
    peripheral vascular disease
    limited joint mobility
    bony deformities
    diabetic nephropathy
    visual impairment
    a history of alcohol excess
Patients who live alone
Elderly patients

---

examination of the ankle reflex, vibration sensation using a 128 Hz tuning fork, pinprick sensation, and temperature (cold tuning fork) sensation at the great toe. Each sensory modality is scored as either normal = 0 or reduced/absent = 1 for each side and the ankle reflexes as normal = 0, present with reinforcement = 1 or absent = 2 per side. Thus the total maximum abnormal score is 10. A score of 6 or over can be regarded as indicative of significant peripheral neuropathy. Such a score correlates well with VPT measurements[12], which, as described above, have recently been shown to predict foot ulceration in diabetic patients[16]. If a Biothesiometer is available then a VPT of greater than 25 in both feet will predict up to 84% of those patients who will develop foot ulceration over the next 4 years[16].

Autonomic neuropathy can be recognized clinically by the absence of sweating in the feet and distended dorsal foot veins while the foot is level with the heart or by more sophisticated cardiovascular tests[97].

As yet there are no licensed specific treatments for diabetic peripheral neuropathy in the UK although Tolrestat (Alredase, Wyeth Pharmaceuticals, Radnor, PA, USA)[98-100] is now licensed in many countries around the world. Gamma-linoleic acid (Efamol, Scotia Pharmaceuticals, Guildford, UK) has also now been shown to improve mild neuropathy in a multicentre study[101], but this does not have a licence for the treatment of neuropathy at present. The mainstay of risk reduction must therefore lie with foot care education and the amelioration of other risk factors if present.

Foot care education should be concise and repeated regularly in order to have the maximum effect on patients' behaviour[102]. Video presentations have been shown to be effective at imparting knowledge about foot care[103], but they should not supplant one-to-one or small group education. The main aspects of foot care education are detailed in Table 7.2, but should include the need for regular, at least once daily, inspection of the feet for new lesions and the need to have shoes measured each time they are acquired; these are two aspects which appear, from experience, to be regularly overlooked in the majority of patients with ulcers. Although education is the potential saviour of the diabetic foot, there is a considerable body of evidence to suggest that while knowledge about diabetic foot problems may increase, attitudes to, and compliance with, the necessary care may remain unchanged. The limitations of current education and preventative methods are highlighted by the number of patients, even in specialist clinics, who have recurrent ulceration. The lack of perceived vulnerability has been highlighted as one reason for this[104,105]. Until this is addressed effectively education programmes may be limited in their success.

As mentioned repeatedly in this text the elderly pose particular problems when trying to impart effective foot care advice and strategies. Many are

Table 7.2. General principles of foot care education

1. Target the level of information to the needs of the patient. Those not at risk may require only general advice about foot hygiene and shoes.
2. Assess the ability of the patient to understand and perform the necessary components of foot care. If this is limited then the spouse or carer should be involved at the beginning of the process.
3. Suggest a positive approach to foot care with 'do's' rather than 'don'ts' as the principle of active rather than passive foot care is more likely to be successful and acceptable to the patient:
   - inspect the feet daily;
   - report any problems immediately;
   - have your feet measured every time new shoes are bought;
   - buy shoes with a square toe box and laces;
   - inspect the inside of shoes for foreign objects every day before putting them on;
   - attend a fully trained chiropodist regularly;
   - cut your nails straight across and not rounded;
   - keep your feet away from heat (fires, radiators and hot water bottles) and check the bath water before stepping into it;
   - always wear something on your feet to protect them and never walk barefoot.
4. Repeat the advice at regular intervals and check that it is being followed.
5. Disseminate advice to other family members and other health care professionals involved in the care of a patient.

unable to perform routine foot care because of poor eyesight and reduced mobility which make it difficult to inspect the foot[88], and so a spouse or carer should be taught how to provide foot care. There is a particular problem when the patient lives alone, especially if they are partially sighted, and this may be insoluble despite home support services.

Peripheral Vascular Disease

The foot pulses are the best guide to the presence of peripheral vascular disease in diabetes. Any areas of cyanosis or peripheral necrosis also indicate arterial insufficiency. Ankle systolic pressures are commonly used to assess the arterial inflow to the diabetic foot but may be falsely elevated in diabetic patients with peripheral neuropathy due to medial arterial calcification in the vessels around the ankle[45]. Toe systolic pressures may be more reliable but are more difficult to measure[48]. If the ankle systolic is more than 75 mmHg above the brachial systolic then this is highly indicative of medial arterial calcification and the poor reliability of the ankle pressure to indicate lower extremity arterial disease[106]. However, it is also possible that medial arterial calcification is falsely elevating the ankle pressure into the normal range in some neuropathic patients. Therefore absent pulses and a normal ankle pressure should be interpreted with caution, and perhaps with a plain radiograph of the foot. A low ankle pressure, and an ankle pressure index of <0.9, suggests arterial occlusive disease and the need for further investigation[106].

Diabetic patients with neuropathy may have significant ischaemia with no pain because of the loss of pain sensation. The absence of foot pulses indicates vascular disease even if the popliteal pulse is present and there is no complaint of claudication or rest pain.

Diabetic patients with evidence of peripheral vascular disease should be referred for vascular assessment with arterial reconstruction or angioplasty where appropriate[107]. Peripheral autonomic neuropathy is usually present in patients with foot ulceration, who can therefore be said to have performed autosympathectomy. Surgical sympathectomy is still attempted in a number of diabetic patients but, because of this autosympathectomy, and associated medial arterial calcification, it is unlikely to produce any substantial benefit.

Limited Joint Mobility

The prayer sign (Figure 7.2), in which the ulnar border of the hands do not meet when holding the hands together as though at pray is a simple screening test for limited joint mobility[53]. Measurement of the metatarsophalangeal and subtalar joints is more accurate but time-consuming[54-56].

There is no specific treatment for limited joint mobility. General pressure reducing management, as outlined below, should be applied. A rocker bottom shoe may help in cases of hallux rigidus as this replaces the normal angulation of the metatarsophalangeal joints at toe off in the gait cycle with a fixed curve in a rigid sole shoe and so reduces the loading at the great toe.

Elevated Plantar Foot Pressures

Not every clinic needs a pedobarograph to detect high plantar foot pressures. It should be remembered that high plantar pressures are only a predictor of ulceration in patients with peripheral neuropathy and non-neuropathic patients with high pressures do not seem to be at the same degree of risk.

Clinical examination of the feet, noting prominent metatarsal heads (Figure 7.1) or rocker bottom deformity, as seen in Charcot feet (Figure 7.3), will predict most high pressure areas without the need for measurement. If plantar pressures are to be measured in a routine clinic setting at all, then a Harris Beath Mat will give a qualitative assessment which will suffice for most purposes[70], and it is possible that ultrasound measurements

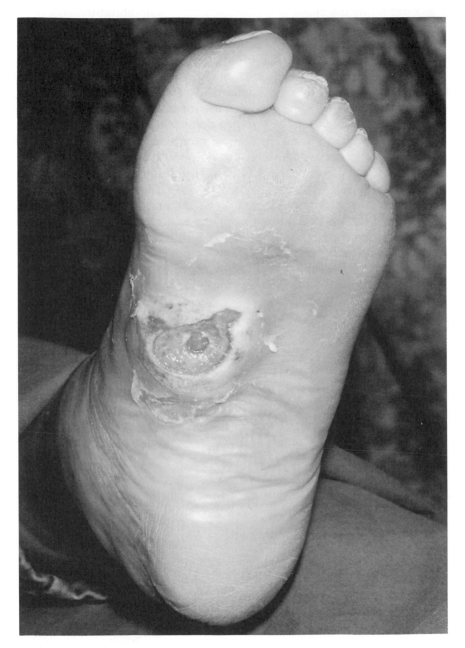

Figure 7.3. Anteroposterior view of sole of a Charcot foot showing plantar prominence, which has ulcerated

of plantar tissue thickness will provide information about the risk of foot ulceration in the future[108].

Extra-depth shoes with cushioned insoles should be provided. These shoes should be deep enough at the toe box to allow room for clawed toes without any rubbing, which is a frequent cause of ulceration in standard shoes. The shoes for diabetic patients with neuropathy should be laced, or made with a strap, as 'slip-on' shoes are unable to grip the mid-foot and prevent forward migration of the foot within the shoe[109,110]. Custom-made shoes are not necessary for most diabetic neuropathic patients. They should be reserved for those with major foot deformity. Most of the extra-depth shoes supplied in our clinic are from an 'off-the-shelf' range of lengths and widths[9] (Figure 7.4).

Padded hosiery may also help to relieve pressure. This has the advantage of being able to protect the dorsum of the foot from over-tightened laces. With care, and regular rotation, these socks have been shown to reduce pressure for at least 6 months[111,112]. It is important to measure for shoes with the socks on as they have a considerable bulk and could cause a pressure problem if the shoes are not supplied to accommodate.

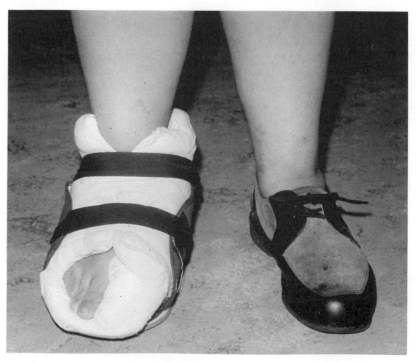

Figure 7.4. 'Scotch-Cast' Boot (right foot) and extra depth shoe (left foot) used in the prevention and treatment of diabetic foot ulceration

The surgical removal of prominent metatarsal heads may also be considered for diabetic patients with good blood supply[113].

Bony Deformity

Any bony prominence that can increase plantar pressure or pressure within shoes is a potential source of foot ulceration. For this reason, prominent metatarsal heads, Charcot feet, usually with mid-foot collapse, bunions and clawed toes all predispose to foot ulceration.

Extra-depth and extra-wide shoes will accommodate clawed toes and bunions. Although surgical correction of a bunion may be considered, this should only be performed in the presence of a good blood supply. It should also be remembered that the resultant rigid hallux may actually increase pressure in certain cases. The surgical removal of prominent metatarsal heads may also be considered for diabetic patients with good blood supply[113].

Charcot feet should be accommodated in custom shoes. Surgical removal of any plantar bony prominence is a successful way to reduce plantar pressure once the Charcot process has finally settled.

Callosities

Excessive callus increases plantar pressure and can lead to tissue break-down in the underlying skin. The presence of haemorrhage into a callus is a sign of early ulcer formation with at least a 50% chance of finding an ulcer when it is removed[114,115]. There is evidence that shows that callus is a more reliable predictor of foot ulceration risk than high foot pressures in neuropathic patients and can be detected by simple clinical rather than expensive technical methods[116]. Therefore, the regular removal of excess callus, preferably by a state-registered (qualified) chiropodist, should be a routine part of foot care for diabetic patients, particularly those with peripheral neuropathy[57].

Previous Ulceration

Patients with previous ulceration should have a review of their risk factors and the cause of the previous ulcer in order to try and prevent recurrence. There should be regular follow-up with chiropody and assessment of the feet at every clinic visit. Reinforcement of foot care education at frequent intervals should also be given as patients with foot ulceration have usually failed to heed the advice they have been given[117].

Other Diabetes Complications

Patients with nephropathy and retinopathy may also benefit from intensive follow-up and review, particularly in specialist clinics such as diabetes–renal clinics where the expertise of diabetologist, renal physician and foot care team can be focused in one place[118].

Referral to a Chiropodist

Once a patient has been identified as being at increased risk of foot ulceration, for whatever reason, that patient should see a chiropodist regularly. The interval between treatments will depend on the rate of nail growth and callus formation but is usually about six weekly. As elderly patients are already at increased risk of foot ulceration the majority should be referred for chiropody. Unless otherwise at risk the average follow-up interval may not need to be as frequent as this. An additional benefit from regular chiropody is that it ensures that the patient's feet are examined regularly and gives increased opportunities for the reinforcement of diabetic foot care advice.

THE MANAGEMENT OF DIABETIC FOOT ULCERATION

WAGNER CLASSIFICATION—GRADES 1–3

Site

Diabetic foot ulcers are predominantly neuropathic in origin, and therefore form at sites of pressure. The commonest sites of ulceration are the metatarsal heads and the tops of clawed toes in shoes that are too shallow at the toe-box (Figure 7.5), but any pressure point can ulcerate. Superficial ulcers form when pressure leads to a reduction in skin blood flow, to autolysis and to a breakdown in the dermal layer which leads to an ulcer. Neuropathic diabetic patients, who are unable to feel these changes, continue to stress the skin, by walking or keeping the same tight shoes on, even after it has broken down.

Deep ulcers are superficial ulcers that have continued to be walked on by a neuropathic patient. This continues the cycle of tissue destruction and enlarges the ulcer cavity. If this process continues it may lead to the involvement of underlying tendons (Wagner grade 2) and eventually to bone, causing osteomyelitis (Wagner grade 3). Occasionally penetrating injuries will cause the primary formation of a deep abscess.

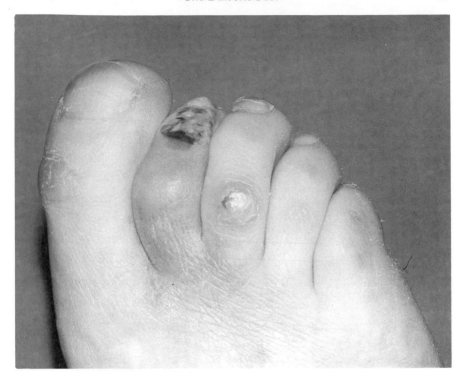

Figure 7.5. Shoe induced ulceration of clawed toes in a neuropathic diabetic patient

A particularly serious problem is the ulceration of unprotected heels (Figure 7.6) in neuropathic patients while in hospital, this may occur during bed rest or during operations while resting on an operating table, even for a short period of time. It is particularly tragic as it is easily preventable with leg troughs yet prolongs in-patient stay and may lead to the loss of a limb. Trauma, including the heat of hot water bottles, gas fires (Figure 7.7) or inappropriate self-'chiropody' is an occasional cause of ulceration[119].

Assessment

The risk factors that led to the ulcer must be identified to prevent recurrence. A neuropathic and vascular assessment should be performed in each patient with a foot ulcer using the methods outlined above. The differential diagnosis between purely neuropathic, neuroischaemic and predominantly ischaemic ulceration can usually be made on clinical grounds using the examination techniques outlined above. The precipitating factor, which may be unknown to the patient, may be deduced from the site or nature of

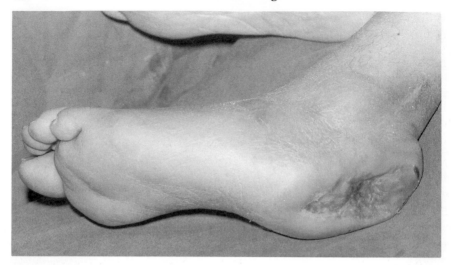

Figure 7.6. Heel ulcer due to pressure from resting on unprotected heels in a neuropathic patient

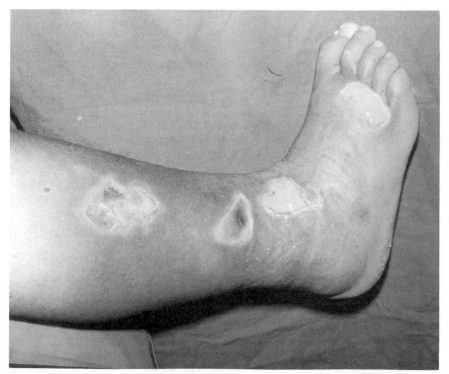

Figure 7.7. Extensive burns on the leg of a neuropathic diabetic patient who had fallen asleep in front of the gas fire to be woken by the smell of burning

the ulcer. Inappropriate footwear is probably the commonest cause of foot ulceration, even in patients who have been supplied with appropriate shoes, as the lure of high heels and pointed toes is often too tempting to resist. Any assessment of the 'at-risk' patient or patient with a foot ulcer should therefore pay particular attention to their shoes.

Management

As increased pressure caused the ulcer, the relief of pressure must be the main way to treat it. Metatarsal head ulceration can be unloaded in a variety of ways. Bed rest is perhaps the most effective, but is difficult to enforce, carries its own risks, principally venous thrombosis, heel ulceration, and pneumonia in the elderly, and, especially if in hospital, is expensive. If the person lives on their own or has an infirm spouse then bed rest at home is, of course, impossible. For this reason a number of ambulatory methods of off-loading ulcer sites have been devised. The majority of these comprise of some form of cast which distributes the pressure of walking across the whole of the sole of the foot[120]. Removable casts, such as the 'Scotch-Cast Boot' (Figure 7.4)[121] may be abused by patients not wearing them, but this is perhaps preferable to the problems of iatrogenic injury from a non-removable (by the patient) total contact cast[122]. The use of total contact casts is, however, contraindicated in patients with oedema secondary to deep infection. The patient may need admission for investigation and treatment of osteomyelitis, surgical debridement or intravenous antibiotics, but once the initial infection is controlled then out-patient care, using off-loading casts or similar, can often be restarted.

Shoe-induced ulcers can be easily unloaded by the provision of, or recommencement of wearing, appropriately fitting wide and extra-depth shoes[109,110].

Callus should be debrided at every clinic visit. The formation of excessive callus is a sign that the patient is still walking.

Evidence of vascular insufficiency should prompt referral to a vascular surgeon, particularly if the ulcer is slow to heal. Previous concerns about the long-term patency of arterial grafts in diabetic patients should be discounted. There is evidence to show that a successful arterial bypass operation has the same graft survival rate in diabetic patients as patients without diabetes[123], and restoration of impaired blood flow may remove the need for amputation, or at least markedly reduce its scope.

Infection is difficult to assess in the diabetic foot ulcer. Necrosis, slough and erythema are not universal and systemic features are rare. Culture from the ulcer surface is likely to produce a mixed growth of dubious significance[124] as the average isolate from a wound swab is over three organisms[125]. The deeper the tissue, or isolation from the bloodstream increases the reliability of the pathogenicity of the isolate. Culture from ulcer scrapings during debridement, or better, deep surgical debridement, may provide a more reliable guide to the principal organism which is responsible for the infection; however, this too may be misleading and the broad-spectrum antibiotics are the first choice in the treatment of infected ulcers. The provision of 'prophylactic' antibiotics has its advocates. If prophylactic antibiotics are not instituted then they should be started with the minimum of clinical suspicion. These should be broad spectrum and Co-amoxiclav is regularly used in this unit, as is clindamycin, which is also a useful antibiotic for foot infections. Combination therapy for initial blind treatment of deep infection might be ampicillin, flucloxacillin and metronidazole, or ciprofloxacin and metronidazole although this is often based on personal choice rather than hard scientific evidence.

X-rays of the foot are recommended to detect osteomyelitis in the majority of patients and should be routinely performed in patients with deep ulcers. If osteomyelitis is suspected then further investigations, with Tc[99]m radioisotope bone and labelled white cell scanning, should be performed[126]. A number of case studies have suggested that magnetic resonance (MRI) scanning can detect the difference between Charcot feet and infection[127,128]. The controlled trial evidence for this claim is still quite limited, given the effectiveness of the current methods, and the limited availability of MRI scan time in most hospitals within the UK, an isotope bone scan followed by a white cell scan is still the preferred method of diagnosing osteomyelitis in most units. Levin has suggested that if the ulcer can be probed to bone then this is likely to be complicated by osteomyelitis in 100% of cases and therefore advocates empirical treatment[129]. If the patient is systemically well and there is no evidence of spreading infection then even the patient with osteomyelitis, particularly of toes alone, can often be managed as an out-patient. Hospitalization is usually required where osteomyelitis of the metatarsals or mid-foot is suspected, when there is severe cellulitis, when the patient is unable to comply with the advice to rest, or where there is vascular insufficiency.

When indicated, for example with spreading infection, or deep-seated infection within the foot, surgical debridement should aim to remove all the infected tissue, preferably in one operation. This may necessitate partial amputation, commonly of a metatarsal and associated toe, the 'ray amputation', which should then heal well if the blood supply is adequate[130] (Figure 7.8). The removal of all the infected and/or necrotic tissue should produce an improvement in the patients' metabolic state and, in neuro-pathic patients with adequate blood supply, even extensive tissue loss will heal.

It is important to measure the size of the ulcer in order to gauge progress. The minimum should be a measure of the diameter of the ulcer in two planes at right angles, tracing the perimeter and/or photographs are also

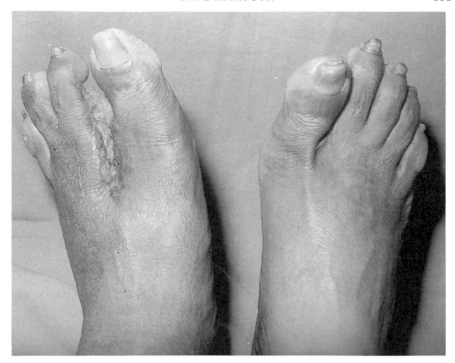

Figure 7.8. Ray amputation of second toe and associated metatarsal

useful to measure progress. An accurate system for assessment of the depth or volume of an ulcer has still to be achieved.

Dressings are the subject of much debate. Dressings alone will not heal an ulcer, pressure relief is the main component of ulcer management. If an ulcer is off-loaded it should heal and for this reason the dressing has long been considered as merely a cover for the surface to reduce bacterial contamination. 'Active' dressings have been advocated in the treatment of chronic venous ulcers but have not been widely adopted in diabetes. The dry dressing is still in common use, but recent wound care theory suggests that a moist wound environment encourages granulation tissue[131]. Hydrocolloid dressings, and alginates under an occlusive dressing, can be recommended, based on a recent audit of their use in the Manchester Foot Hospital from 1990 to 1992, which, despite isolated case reports suggesting that infection might be a problem[132], found no increase in infection rate in those patients treated with Granuflex compared with other dressings[81]. However, macerated wound edges are sometimes a problem with hydrocolloids, and these dressings are not in universal favour[133]. A recent review of the antibacterial effects of honey in superficial wounds[134] has renewed interest in this ancient remedy[135].

In higher grade ulcers the dressings should conform to the ulcer cavity. Hydrocolloid pastes and dressings (e.g. Granuflex paste and Granuflex dressing, Squibb Convatec, Uxbridge, UK)[136], and iodine based dressings (e.g. Iodosorb, Perstop Pharma, Basingstoke, UK) are regularly used in such circumstances, once the wound has started to heal and the slough has gone. As a general rule, deep ulcers often have tendons at their bases and they should not be allowed to get too dry.

Chemical debridement with desloughing agents such as topical streptokinase (Varidase topical, Lederle Laboratories, Gosport, UK) may be required in the early stages of the treatment of foot ulceration if there is an adherent slough. Necrotic eschar is, however, probably best removed mechanically.

The use of wound healing factors is in its infancy but may hold great promise for the future. Autologous, blood derived, wound healing factor has been used for many years, particularly in the United States, but adequate controlled studies in patients are uncommon[137,138]. Small placebo-controlled trials of recombinant biosynthetic platelet-derived growth factor in venous ulceration[139] and a recent trial in diabetic neuropathic foot ulceration[140] showed that it might speed ulcer healing and larger trials are now under way.

Diabetes control should be optimized if possible, as there is evidence to suggest that healing is impaired with poor blood glucose control, although this does not necessarily mean a need for insulin in a non-insulin-dependent patient.

After-care

Once an ulcer is healed that patient is left in the highest risk category of all for a further ulcer. Education, foot care, chiropody, footwear and careful follow-up are all necessary to try and prevent a recurrence[141], although, as outlined above, recurrent ulceration is still a significant problem, even in 'centres of excellence'.

LOCALIZED GANGRENE: WAGNER—GRADE 4

Site

Localized gangrene is commonly found at the ends of toes (Figure 7.9), but may also occur at the apex of the heel. These are regions where there are endarteries with little or no collateral circulation if a branch fails. As well as being a sign of global arterial insufficiency in the foot, digital gangrene can occur as a result of infection leading to an infective vasculitis[142].

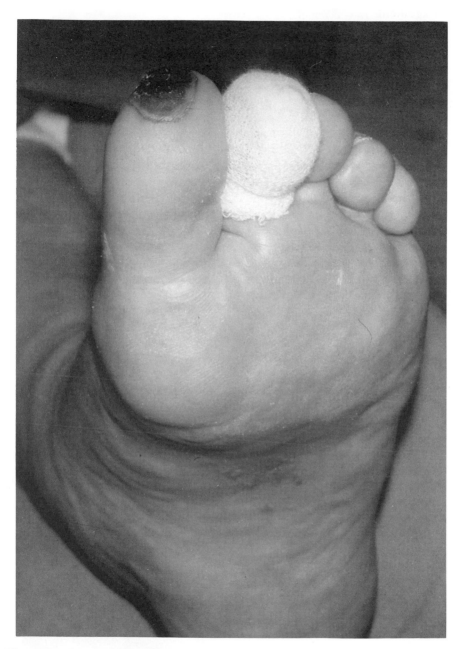

Figure 7.9. Localized gangrene at the end of the great toe

Management

Vascular assessment is mandatory for these patients. If treatable occlusive arterial insufficiency is found then angioplasty and proximal reconstructive surgery is useful and may significantly reduce the amount of tissue loss. However, the vascular disease of diabetic patients is often below the trifurcation of the popliteal artery. Reconstructive surgery, particularly with *in-situ*, or reversed, saphenous vein as a conduit, can now be performed at the level of the dorsalis pedis artery to restore pulsitile flow below the tibial arteries[107].

Infection should be treated promptly to prevent gangrene and rapidly spreading infection leading to a severely ill and toxic patient.

Well circumscribed localized necrosis with viable tissue borders can often be left to separate undisturbed, 'auto-amputation'. The wound left behind should then be treated as a superficial ulcer in the usual way, and often heals well (Figure 7.10).

More extensive or spreading necrosis in a toxic patient, particularly if there is no reversible arterial lesion, may require primary amputation. This decision should only be taken after review by a vascular surgeon, as

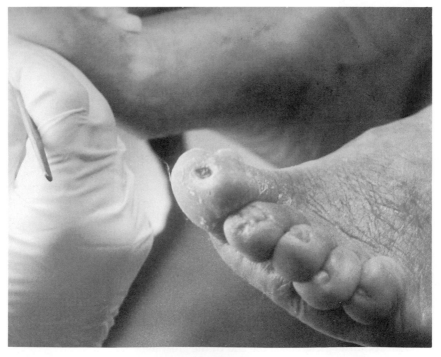

Figure 7.10. Gangrene has separated to leave a clean ulcer, which subsequently healed well

arterial reconstruction or angioplasty can markedly improve the level at which amputation stump is viable.

After-care

The remaining foot of an amputee is at an exceedingly high risk of ulceration and further surgery[143]. General after-care should be as for other ulcers but with particular attention to the intact foot. The foot with a partial amputation is often mechanically very different and this may produce new pressure points at risk of ulceration. In addition, amputation, at whatever level, has special orthotic needs, which must be addressed. Insoles, shoe infills and prostheses all require careful and regular review to ensure that they are functioning correctly.

EXTENSIVE GANGRENE: WAGNER—GRADE 5

Site and Causation

Wagner grade 5 lesions are described as extensive necrosis of the foot and are due to arterial occlusion and failure of arterial inflow.

Management

Primary amputation is the usual treatment for extensive gangrene. However, the extent of amputation can be reduced in some patients by pre-amputation arterial reconstructive surgery. There is little likelihood of walking after an above-knee amputation in an elderly patient. For this reason, a vascular assessment should be performed in all patients prior to amputation, as a femoropopliteal or similar bypass operation might improve the viability of a distal stump. Again this may not always be possible in diabetic patients, because the arterial disease is often below the popliteal trifurcation. In addition, if the necrosis extends beyond the dorsalis pedis artery it will preclude distal bypass surgery. Angioplasty is possible in a number of diabetic patients and probably has a similar prognosis to that of non-diabetic patients. Unfortunately, although the techniques are constantly improving, angioplasty is only suitable for more proximal, and relatively short, segments of occlusion or luminal narrowing, and the diffuse ragged atheroma which is frequently found in diabetic patients means that this technique is often technically impossible. However, this cannot usually be determined by clinical means and angiography should not be withheld even if the patient might not be fit for bypass surgery.

It is also important to point out that not every amputation is a destructive event. If it is likely that the patient would otherwise spend a considerable period of time in hospital then a successful amputation can lead to the patient being discharged earlier, and if the adjustment to an artificial limb is made, earlier mobilization, with a consequent increase in the sense of well-being compared to patients with indolent ulceration[144].

Diabetes and infection control should be attended to as a priority, as these patients are often very ill due to the toxic effects of the necrotic tissue burden. Triple antibiotic therapy (e.g. ampicillin, flucloxacillin and metronidazole) is the first-line choice. Rehydration and blood glucose control may require the use of intravenous insulin infusions in the seriously ill or hyperglycaemic patient.

Coexistent coronary and cerebral vascular disease in these patients often makes the anaesthetic choice difficult and regional anaesthesia is a common choice.

After-care

The mortality rate in patients following major amputation is high and the care of the remaining foot is particularly important. The patient is likely to die from other major vessel problems, particularly coronary artery disease and treatment for these conditions should be addressed in the follow-up period.

THE DIABETIC CHARCOT FOOT

The original text of Jean Marie Charcot's descriptions of patients with tabes dorsalis who developed a destructive arthropathy which starts 'rather suddenly, without precipitating cause' was published in 1868, and was recently translated into English[145]. The first case report of neuroarthropathy in a diabetic patient was described in 1936[146]. Since that time the devastating effects of Charcot neuroarthropathy in the diabetic foot have been well described in the literature[147-149]. Diabetes is now believed to be the leading cause of Charcot neuroarthropathy in the developed world[150], but it is the firmly held belief of those who regularly treat patients with Charcot feet that such changes are 'frequently overlooked'[151]. The prevalence of Charcot change among 68 000 diabetic patients attending the Joslin Clinic was estimated at 0.15%[147] but prevalence rates as high as 7% in other clinic populations[152], and 16% in a selected group of 54 neuropathic diabetic patients with previous foot ulceration[89], have also been reported.

Eighty per cent of the patients who develop Charcot neuroarthropathy have a known duration of diabetes of over 10 years and the modal age is about 60 years[151]. The duration of diabetes appears to be more important than age alone, but this is compounded in Type 2 diabetes, which frequently undergoes a long disease duration prior to diagnosis. The long duration of diabetes prior to the initiation of the Charcot process probably reflects the degree of neuropathy that is usually present in these patients. Recently, it has been suggested that a specific small fibre neuropathy of cool perception is present in diabetic patients with Charcot neuroarthropathy[153], although this would seem unlikely given the wide range of conditions, including leprosy and syphilis, in which Charcot neuroarthropathy occurs, and the density of neuropathy at the time of the initiating event. Recent work has not confirmed this pattern of neuropathy and it would seem that Charcot patients have a more severe neuropathy and not a qualitatively different pattern of nerve damage; autonomic neuropathy does, however, appear to be a universal finding in diabetic Charcot patients[154].

The initiating event of the Charcot process is often a seemingly trivial injury[151], which may result in a minor periarticular fracture[155] or in a major fracture[156,157], despite the inability of the patient to recall the injury in many cases. The reasons why such trivial injuries should lead to such major catastrophic destruction in the foot have not yet been fully explained. It has been reported that both Types 1 and 2 diabetic patients have a decreased bone mass when compared with age- and sex-matched control subjects[158]. Although renal failure secondary to diabetic nephropathy may contribute to this problem[159], there are suggestions that bone mass is reduced in diabetic patients with normal renal function. Edmonds *et al.*[160] have shown that radionuclide uptake is increased in the feet of neuropathic diabetic patients and suggested that increased bone blood flow and arteriovenous shunting led to increased osteoclastic activity and a reduced bone mineral density in the feet of diabetic patients. If present, a reduction in bone mineral density would lead to a direct reduction in bone strength, as over 90% of the variance in bone strength is due to differences in bone mineral density[161]. Decreased bone mineral density, the increased repetitive trauma from higher foot pressures in neuropathic patients[79], and the increased risk of tripping and falling in elderly diabetic patients[19,20], might then predispose to Charcot neuroarthropathy in diabetic patients. A recent radiographic survey of patients with diabetic neuropathy has demonstrated a high incidence of unperceived traumatic foot fractures in these patients, and may represent a less destructive outcome of the same processes[89]. It is possible that prevention of minor trauma, and the prompt treatment of reported injuries might reduce the incidence of Charcot neuroarthropathy, but this remains to be proven.

Following the initiating injury there is a rapid onset of swelling, an increase in temperature in the foot, and often an ache or discomfort. The patient may have noticed a change in the shape of the foot and others describe the sensation, or the sound, of the bones crunching as they walk. The blood supply to the Charcot foot is always good[147], indeed there are case reports of the Charcot process starting in patients following arterial bypass surgery[162]. It is assumed that autonomic neuropathy plays a part in the increased vascularity of bone, possibly by increased arterio-venous shunting[159], and this increases osteoclastic activity, resulting in the destruction, fragmentation, and remodelling of bone (Figure 7.11). It is these processes which, if left untreated, lead to the characteristic patterns of deformity in the Charcot foot[151], including the collapse of the longitudinal and transverse arches leading to a rocker bottom foot.

The natural history of Charcot neuroarthropathy passes from this acute phase of development through a stage of coalescence, in which the bone fragments are reabsorbed, the odema lessens and the foot cools, into the stage of reconstruction, in which the final repair and regenerative modelling of bone takes place to leave a stable, chronic Charcot foot[163]. The time course of these events is variable but intervention must be made in the earliest phase to prevent subsequent deformity.

Radiographs of the foot should be performed to make the initial diag-nosis. The characteristic appearances of bone destruction, fragmentation,

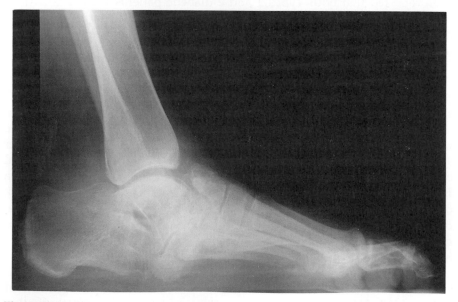

Figure 7.11. Charcot neuroarthropathy. Lateral X-ray showing destruction of talus and mid-foot

loss of joint architecture and new bone formation should be determined[148]. Confirmation of Charcot neuroarthropathy should be obtained by three phase Tc^{99} m isotope bone scans, which demonstrate the intense vascularity of the rapid bone turnover that accompanies the Charcot process in its active phase. Labelled white cell scans, or one of the other alternatives outlined in the management of foot ulceration above, may be performed where there is a suspicion of osteomyelitis as this cannot always be ruled out on the basis of history and radiographs alone[164]. The current vogue for computerized tomography and MR scanning of Charcot feet can often produce small details of the pattern of Charcot involvement but are difficult to interpret and often have little to add to well taken standardized radiographs of the foot (Figure 7.12)[165].

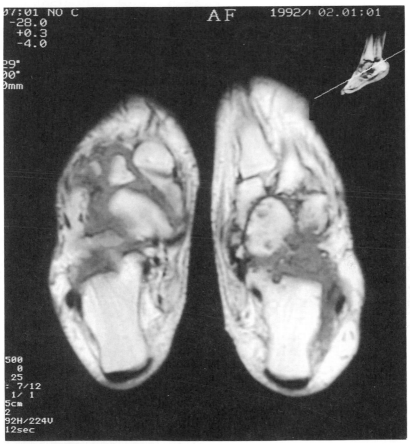

Figure 7.12. Magnetic resonance image of the talus and mid-foot of the patient in Figure 7.11. Note the bilateral Charcot changes. Such images are often difficult to interpret, even for experienced radiologists

The management of the Charcot foot has always been difficult and varies from the expectant to the markedly interventional[166]. The first principles of management are rest and freedom from weight-bearing. Non-weight-bearing is useful to reduce the activity but this frequently restarts when walking is recommended. In the United States in particular, the practice of prolonged, 1 year or more, immobilization in a plaster of Paris cast is the usual treatment[151]. The total-contact cast is usually the method employed, but this requires frequent changes as the oedema reduces. Plaster casting will stabilize the foot, but again, while casting reduces activity initially, when the plaster is finally removed after 6–12 months the acute destructive process may restart. Surgical fusion of the joints of the foot in their anatomical positions has met with little success[151]. The American vogue for surgical stabilization in the acute phase of Charcot neuroarthropathy has now largely been abandoned because if often accelerated the destruction of bone and joint alignment; but surgery may still be used, for example to remove a plantar prominence once the process has finally settled[167,168], which can be assessed by following skin temperature and radiographic change[169]. In the UK total contact casting or bed rest are still the mainstays of treatment. The Scotch-Cast Boot[121] can also be used to rest the active Charcot foot, and is particularly useful to provide pressure redistribution of a rocker bottom foot with an ulcer at its apex (Figure 7.4).

As yet there is no definitive treatment aimed at the underlying over-activity of osteoclasts in the active destructive phase of Charcot neuroarthropathy. Reflex sympathetic dystrophy (Sudeck's atrophy) is thought to be a similar process to Charcot neuroarthropathy, precipitated by an injury and associated with swelling, increased skin temperature, pain, and bone destruction. A successful clinical trial of the use of intravenous pamidronate (Aredia, Ciba-Geigy), which is believed to inhibit osteoclast activity, in patients with reflex sympathetic dystrophy[170], and which has been used for the treatment of osteoporosis, led to the suggestion that this drug might prove useful in acute Charcot neuroarthropathy. In patients with Charcot neuroarthropathy, treatment with intravenous bisphosphonate has resulted in a rapid resolution of symptoms and signs, including increased foot temperature and swelling, and a marked improvement in the biochemical markers of bone turnover, particularly alkaline phosphatase concentrations[171]. Follow-up of up to 2 years has seen no recurrence of the Charcot process in a series of 10 patients (unpublished observation).

CONCLUSIONS

The diabetic foot syndrome is a significant cause of morbidity and mortality in elderly diabetic patients. However, by recognizing the known risk associations, and taking steps to reduce their effect, the incidence of foot ulceration can be significantly reduced. If in turn, foot ulceration is managed in a systematic and appropriate manner the incidence of amputations due to ulceration can be significantly reduced, and may even exceed that required in the St Vincent Declaration. This must be the ultimate goal in treating diabetic foot problems and, as attainable, should be attained.

REFERENCES

1 Joslin EP. The menace of diabetic gangrene. *N Engl J Med* 1934; **211**: 16–20.
2 Most RS, Sinnock P. The epidemiology of lower extremity amputations in diabetic individuals. *Diabetes Care* 1983; **6**: 87–91.
3 Ebskov B, Josephsen P. Incidence of reamputation and death after gangrene of the lower extremity. *Prosthet Orthotics Int* 1980; **4**: 77–80.
4 Bessman AN. Foot problems in diabetes. *Compr Ther* 1982; **8**: 32–7.
5 Kozak GP, Rowbotham JL. Diabetic foot disease: A major problem. In: Kozak GP, Hoar CS, Rowbotham JL (eds), *Management of Diabetic Foot Problems*. Philadelphia: WB Saunders, 1984: 1–8.
6 Connor H. The economic impact of diabetic foot disease. In: Connor H, Boulton AJM, Ward JD (eds), *The Foot in Diabetes*. Chichester: John Wiley & Sons, 1986: 150–9.
7 WHO/IDF. Diabetes care and research in Europe. The St Vincent Declaration. *Diabetic Med* 1990; **7**: 360.
8 Assal JP, Gfeller R, Ekoe JM. Patient education in diabetes. In: *Recent Trends in Diabetic Research*. Stockholm: Almqvist and Wiksell, 1982: 276–89.
9 Thomson FJ, Veves A, Ashe H, *et al.* A team approach to diabetic foot care—the Manchester experience. *Foot* 1991; **1**: 75–82.
10 Pirart J. Diabetes mellitus and its degenerative complications: A prospective study of 4400 patients observed between 1947 and 1973. *Diabetes Care*, 1978; **1**: 168–88.
11 Melton LJ, Dyck PJ. Clinical features of the diabetic neuropathies: Epidemiology. In: Dyck PJ, Thomas PK, Lambert EH, *et al.* (eds), *Diabetic Neuropathy*. Philadelphia: WB Saunders, 1987: 27–35.
12 Young MJ, Boulton AJM, Macleod AF, Williams DRR, Sonksen PH. A multicentre study of the prevalence of diabetic peripheral neuropathy in the United Kingdom hospital clinic population. *Diabetologia* 1993; **36**: 150–4.
13 Thomas PK, Brown MJ: Diabetic polyneuropathy. In: Dyck PJ, Thomas PK, Lambert EH, *et al.* (eds), *Diabetic Neuropathy*. Philadelphia: WB Saunders, 1987: 56–65.
14 Consensus Statement: report and recommendations of the San Antonio Conference on Diabetic Neuropathy. *Diabetes* 1988; **37**: 1000–4.
15 Thomson FJ, Masson EA, Boulton AJM. Quantitative vibration perception testing in elderly people: an assessment of variability. *Age Ageing* 1992; **21**: 171–4.
16 Young MJ, Breddy JL, Veves A, Boulton AJM. The use of vibration perception to predict diabetic neuropathic foot ulceration: A prospective study. *Diabetes Care* 1994 ; **17**: 557–60.

17 Cavanagh PR, Young MJ, Adams JE, Vickers KL, Boulton AJM. Correlates of structure and function in the diabetic foot. *Diabetologia* 1991; **34** (Suppl. 2): A39.

18 Boulton AJM. The diabetic foot. *Med Clin North Am* 1988; **72**: 1513–30.

19 Cavanagh PR, Derr JA, Ulbrecht JS, Maser RE, OrchardTJ. Problems with gait and posture in neuropathic patients with insulin dependent diabetes mellitus. *Diabetic Med* 1992; **9**: 469–74.

20 Cavanagh PR, Simoneau GG, Ulbrecht JS. Ulceration, unsteadiness, and uncertainty: the biomechanical consequences of diabetes mellitus. *J Biomech* 1993: **26** (Suppl. 1): 23–40.

21 Gilmore JE, Allen JA, Hayes JR. Autonomic function in neuropathic diabetic patients with foot ulceration. *Diabetes Care* 1993; **16**: 61–7.

22 Ryder REJ, Marshall R, Johnson K, Ryder AP, Owens DR, Hayes TM. Acetylcholine sweat spot test for autonomic denervation. *Lancet* 1988; i: 1303–5.

23 Edmonds ME, Roberts VC, Watkins PJ. Blood flow in the diabetic neuropathic foot. *Diabetologia* 1982; **22**: 9–15.

24 Boulton AJM, Scarpello JHB, Ward JD. Venous oxygenation in the diabetic neuropathic foot: evidence for arteriovenous shunting? *Diabetologia* 1982; **22**: 6–8.

25 Ward JD. The diabetic leg. *Diabetologia* 1982; **22**: 141–7.

26 Flynn MD, Tooke JE. Aetiology of diabetic foot ulceration: a role for the microcirculation? *Diabetic Med* 1992; **9**: 320–9.

27 Sandeman DD, Shore AC, Tooke JE. Relation of skin capillary pressure in patients with insulin-dependent diabetes mellitus to complications and metabolic control. *N Engl J Med* 1992; **327**: 760–4.

28 Newrick PG, Cochrane T, Betts RP, Wards JD, Boulton AJM. Reduced hyperaemic response under the diabetic neuropathic foot. *Diabetic Med* 1988; **5**: 570–3.

29 Flynn MD, Boolell M, Tooke J, Watkins PJ. The effect of insulin infusion on capillary blood flow in the diabetic neuropathic foot. *Diabetic Med* 1992; **9**: 630–4.

30 Ganda OP. Pathogenesis of accelerated atherosclerosis in diabetes. In: Kozak GP, Hoar CS, Rowbotham JL (eds), *Management of Diabetic Foot Problems*. Philadelphia: WB Saunders, 1984: 17–26.

31 Uusitupa MIJ. Five year incidence of atherosclerotic vascular disease in relation to general risk factors, insulin level, and abnormalities of lipoprotein composition in non-insulin-dependent and non-diabetic subjects. *Circulation* 1990; **82**: 27–36.

32 Colwell JA, Halushka PV. Platelet function in diabetes mellitus. *Br J. Haematol* 1980; **44**: 521–6.

33 Juhan-Vague I, Alessi MC, Vague P. Increased plasma plasminogen activator inhibitor 1 levels. A possible link between insulin resistance and atherosclerosis. *Diabetologia* 1991; **34**: 457–62.

34 Bossaler C. Impaired muscarinic endothelium dependent relaxation and cyclic guanosine 5′-monophosphate formation in atherosclerotic human coronary artery and rabbit aorta. *J Clin Invest* 1987; **79**: 170.

35 Colwell JA, Lopes-Virella M, Halushka PV. Pathogenesis of atherosclerosis in diabetes mellitus. *Diabetes Care* 1981; **4**: 121–33.

36 Levin ME. The Diabetic Foot: Pathophysiology, evaluation and treatment. In: Levin ME, O'Neal LW (eds), *The Diabetic Foot*. St Louis: CV Mosby, 1988: 1–50.

37 LoGerfo FW, Coffman JD. Vascular and microvascular disease of the foot in diabetes. *N Engl J Med* 1984; **311**: 1615–19.

38 Edmonds ME, Morrison N, Laws JW, Watkins PJ. Medial arterial calcification and diabetic neuropathy. *Br Med J* 1982; **284**: 928–30.
39 Goebel F-D, Fuessi HS. Mönckeberg's sclerosis after sympathetic denervation in diabetic and non-diabetic subjects. *Diabetologia* 1983; **24**: 348–50.
40 Everhart JE, Pettitt DJ, Knowler WC, Rose FA, Bennett PH. Medial arterial calcification and its association with mortality and complications of diabetes. *Diabetologia* 1988; **31**: 16–23.
41 Lachman AS, Spray TL, Kerwin DM, Shugoll GI, Roberts WC. Medial calcinosis of Mönckeberg. A review of the problem and a description of a patient with involvement of peripheral, visceral and coronary arteries. *Am J Med* 1977; **63**: 615–22.
42 Nillson SE, Lindholm H, Bülow S, Frostberg N, Emilsson T, Stenkula G. The Kristianstad survey 63–64 (Calcifications in arteries of lower limbs). *Acta Med Scand* 1967; **428** (Suppl.): 1–46.
43 Janka HU, Stadl E, Mehnert H. Peripheral vascular disease in diabetes mellitus and its relation to cardiovascular risk factors: screening with Doppler ultrasonic technique. *Diabetes Care* 1980; **3**: 207–13.
44 Jensen T, Borch-Johnsen K, Kofoed-Enevoldsen A, Deckert T. Coronary heart disease in young type 1 (insulin-dependent) diabetic patients with and without diabetic nephropathy: incidence and risk factors. *Diabetologia* 1987; **30**: 144–8.
45 Young MJ, Adams JE, Anderson GF, Boulton AJM, Cavanagh PR. Medial arterial calcification in the feet of diabetic patients and matched non-diabetic control subjects. *Diabetologia* 1993; **36**: 615–21.
46 Cutajar CL, Marston A, Newcombe JF. Value of cuff occlusion pressures in assessment of peripheral vascular disease. *Br Med J* 1973; **2**: 392–5.
47 Emanuele MA, Buchanan BJ, Abraira C. Elevated leg systolic pressures and arterial calcification in diabetic occlusive vascular disease. *Diabetes Care* 1981; **4**: 289–92.
48 Dormandy J (ed.), *European Consensus Document on Critical Limb Ischaemia*. Berlin: Springer-Verlag, 1989.
49 Stevens MJ, Goss DE, Foster AVM, Pitei D, Edmonds ME, Watkins PJ. Abnormal digital pressure measurements in diabetic neuropathic foot ulceration. *Diabetic Med* 1993; **10**: 909–15.
50 Larkin JG, Frier BM. Limited joint mobility and Dupuytrens contracture in diabetic, hypertensive and normal populations. *Br Med J* 1986; **292**: 1494.
51 Goodfield MJB, Millard LG. The skin in diabetes mellitus. *Diabetologia* 1988; **31**: 567–75.
52 Lundbaek K. Stiff hands in long term diabetes. *Acta Med Scand* 1957; **158**: 447–51.
53 Rosenbloom AL, Silverstein JM, Lezotte DC, Richardson K, McCallum M. Limited joint mobility in childhood diabetes indicates increased risk for microvascular disease. *N Engl J Med* 1981; **305**: 191–4.
54 Campbell RR, Hawkins SJ, Maddison PJ, Reckless JPD. Limited joint mobility in the diabetes mellitus. *Ann Rheum Dis* 1985; **44**: 93–7.
55 Delbridge L, Perry P, Marr S, Arnold N, Yue DK, Turtle JR, Reeve TS. Limited joint mobility in the diabetic foot: Relationship to neuropathic ulceration. *Diabetic Med* 1988; **5**: 333–7.
56 Fernando DJS, Masson EA, Veves A, Boulton AJM. Relationship of limited joint mobility to abnormal foot pressures and diabetic foot ulceration. *Diabetes Care* 1991; **14**: 8–11.

57 Young MJ, Cavanagh PR, Thomas G, Johnson MM, Murray H, Boulton AJM. The effect of callus removal on dynamic plantar foot pressures in diabetic patients. *Diabetic Med* 1992; **9**: 55–7.

58 Veves A, Fernando DJS, Walewski P, Boulton AJM. A study of plantar pressures in a diabetic clinic population. *Foot* 1991; **1**: 89–92.

59 Cavanagh PR, Sims DS Jr, Sanders LJ. Body mass is a poor predictor of peak plantar pressure in diabetic men. *Diabetes Care* 1991; **14**: 750–5.

60 Brand PW. Repetitive stress in the development of diabetic foot ulcers. In: Levin ME, O'Neal LW (eds), *The Diabetic Foot*. St Louis: CV Mosby, 1988: 83–90.

61 Boulton AJM. The diabetic foot. Neuropathic in origin? *Diabetic Med* 1990; **7**: 852–8.

62 Partsch H. Gestyorte Gefassregulation bei ulzero-multierenden. Neuropathien der unteren Extremitaten. *Vasa* 1978; **7**: 119–25.

63 Boulton AJM, Scarpello JHB, Ward JD. Venous oxygenation in the diabetic neuropathic foot: evidence for arteriovenous shunting? *Diabetologia* 1982; **22**: 6–8.

64 Edmonds ME, Roberts VC, Watkins PJ. Blood flow in the diabetic neuropathic foot. *Diabetologia* 1982; **22**: 9–15.

65 Rayman G, Williams SA, Spencer PD, Smaje LH, Wise PH, Tooke JE. Impaired microvascular response to minor skin trauma in Type 1 diabetes. *Br Med J* 1986; **292**: 1295–8.

66 Walmsley D, Wales JK, Wiles PG. Reduced hyperaemia following skin trauma; evidence for an impaired microvascular response to injury in the diabetic foot. *Diabetologia* 1989; **32**: 736–9.

67 Koziak M. Etiology and pathology of ischaemic ulcers. *Arch Phys Med Rehab* 1959; **40**: 62–9.

68 MacFarlane IA, Benbow SJ, Chan AW, Bowsher D, Williams G. Diabetic peripheral neuropathy: the significance of plantar foot temperatures as demonstrated by liquid crystal contact thermography. *Diabetic Med* 1993; **10** (Suppl. 1): P104.

69 Masson EA, Hay EM, Stockley I, Veves A, Betts RP, Boulton AJM. Abnormal foot pressures alone may not cause ulceration. *Diabetic Med* 1989; **6**: 426–8.

70 Silvino N, Evanski PM, Waugh TR. The Harris and Beath footprinting mat: Diagnostic validity and clinical use. *Clin Orthop Related Res* 1980; **151**: 265–9.

71 Barrett JP, Mooney V. Neuropathy and diabetic pressure lesions. *Orthop Clin N Am* 1973; **4**: 43–7.

72 Stokes IAF, Furis IB, Hutton WC. The neuropathic ulcer and loads on the foot in diabetic patients. *Acta Orthop Scand* 1976; **46**: 839–47.

73 Ctercteko GC, Dhanendran M, Hutton WC, LeQuesne LP. Vertical forces acting on the feet of diabetic patients with neuropathic ulceration. *Br J Surg* 1981; **68**: 608–14.

74 Chodera J. *Examination Methods of Standing in Man*. Vols 1–3. FU Czech Academy of Science 1957.

75 Betts RP, Franks CI, Duckworth T. Analysis of pressures and loans under the foot. 1. Quantification of the static distribution using the PET computer. 2. Quantification of the dynamic distribution. *Clin Phys Physiol Meas* 1980; **1**: 101–24.

76 Cavanagh PR, Ulbrecht JS. The diabetic foot: A quantitative approach to the assessment of neuropathy, deformity, and plantar pressure. In: Jahss M (ed.), *Disorders of the Foot*, 2nd edn. New York: WB Saunders, 1991: 1864–907.

77 Young MJ, Murray HJ, Veves A, Boulton AJM. A comparison of the Musgrave and optical pedobarograph systems for measuring foot pressures in diabetic patients. *Foot* 1993; **3**: 62–4.

78 Boulton AJM, Hardisty CA, Betts RP, Franks CI, Worth RC, Ward JD, Duckworth T. Dynamic foot pressure and other studies as diagnostic and management aids in diabetic neuropathy. *Diabetes Care* 1983; **6**: 26–33.

79 Veves A, Murray HJ, Young MJ, Boulton AJM. The risk of foot ulceration in diabetic patients with high foot pressure: A prospective study. *Diabetologia* 1992; **35**: 660–3.

80 Veves A, Van Ross ERE, Boulton AJM. Foot pressure measurements in diabetic and non-diabetic amputees. *Diabetes Care* 1992; **15**: 905–7.

81 Knowles A, Westwood B, Young MJ, Boulton AJM. A retrospective study to assess the outcome of diabetic ulcers that have been dressed with Granuflex and other dressings. *Proceedings of the Joint Meeting of the Wound Healing Society and the European Tissue Repair Society*, Amsterdam, August, 1993: P68.

82 Wilson RM. Neutrophil function in diabetes. *Diabetic Med* 1986; **6**: 509–12.

83 Pecoraro RE, Ahroni JH, Boyko EJ, Stensel VL. Chronology and determinants of tissue repair in diabetic lower-extremity ulcers. *Diabetes* 1991; **40**: 1305–13.

84 Louie TJ, Gartlett JG, Tally FP. Aerobic and anaerobic bacteria in diabetic foot ulcers. *Ann Intern Med* 1976; **85**: 461–3.

85 Delbridge L, Appleberg M, Reeves TS. Factors associated with the development of foot lesions in the diabetic. *Surgery* 1983; **93**: 78–82.

86 Young RJ, Zhou YQ, Rodriguez E, Prescott RJ, Ewing DJ, Clark BF. Variable relationship between peripheral somatic and autonomic neuropathy in patients with different syndromes of diabetic polyneuropathy. *Diabetes* 1986; **35**: 192–7.

87 Fernando DJS, Hutchison A, Veves A, Gokal R, Boulton AJM. Risk factors for non-ischaemic foot ulceration in diabetic nephropathy. *Diabetic Med* 1991; **8**: 223–5.

88 Thomson FJ, Masson EA. Can elderly diabetic patients co-operate with routine foot care? *Age Ageing* 1992; **21**: 333–7.

89 Cavanagh PR, Young MJ, Adams JE, Vickers KL, Boulton AJM. Radiographic abnormalities in the feet of neuropathic diabetic patients. *Diabetes Care* 1994; **17**: 201–9.

90 Pecoraro RE, Reiber GE, Burgess EM. Pathways to diabetic limb amputation: basis for prevention. *Diabetes Care* 1990; **13**: 513–21.

91 Walsh CH, Soler NG, Fitzgerald MG, Malins JM. Association of foot lesions with retinopathy in patients with newly diagnosed diabetes. *Lancet* 1975; i: 878–80.

92 Edmonds ME, Blundell MP, Morris HE, Maelor-Thomas E, Cotton LT, Watkins PJ. Improved survival of the diabetic foot: the role of the specialist foot clinic. *QJ Med* 1986; **232**: 763–71.

93 Wagner FW. The dysvascular foot: a system for diagnosis and treatment. *Foot Ankle* 1981; **2**: 64.

94 Cohen SJ. Potential barriers to diabetes care. *Diabetes Care* 1983; **6**: 499–500.

95 Bailey TS, Yu HM, Rayfield EJ. Patterns of foot examination in a diabetes clinic. *Am J Med* 1985; **78**: 371–4.

96 Kumar S, Fernando DJS, Veves A, Knowles A, Young MJ, Boulton AJM. Semmes-weinstein monofilaments: a simple, effective and inexpensive screening device for identifying diabetic patients at risk of foot ulceration. *Diabetes Res Clin Pract* 1991; **13**: 63–7.

97 Ewing DJ, Martyn CN, Young RJ, Clarke BF. The value of cardiovascular autonomic function tests: 10 years experience in diabetes. *Diabetes Care* 1985; **8**: 491–8.

98 Masson EA, Boulton AJM. Aldose reductase inhibitor in the treatment of diabetic neuropathy. A review of the rationale and clinical evidence. *Drugs* 1990; **39**: 190–202.

99 Boulton AJM, Levin S, Comstock J. A multicentre trial of the aldose reductase inhibitor, tolrestat, in patients with symptomatic diabetic neuropathy. *Diabetologia* 1990; **33**: 431–7.

100 Giugliano D, Marfella R, Quatraro A, *et al.* Tolrestat for mild diabetic neuropathy. *Ann Intern Med* 1993; **118**: 7–11.

101 The gamma-linoleic acid multicentre trial group. Treatment of diabetic neuropathy with gamma-linoleic acid. *Diabetes Care* 1993; **16**: 8–15.

102 Barth R, Campbell LV, Allen S, Jupp JJ, Chisholm DJ. Intensive education improves knowledge, compliance, and foot problems in Type 2 diabetes. *Diabetic Med* 1991; **8**:111–17.

103 Knowles EA, Kumar S, Veves A, Young MJ, Fernando DJS, Boulton AJM. Essential elements of footcare education are retained for at least a year. *Diabetic Med* 1992; **9** (Suppl. 2): S6.

104 Stuart L, Wiles PJ. Knowledge and beliefs towards footcare among diabetic patients: a comparison of qualitative and quantitative methodologies. *Diabetic Med* 1992; **9** (Suppl. 2): S3.

105 Stuart L, Wiles PJ. The influence of a learning contract on levels of footcare. *Diabetic Med* 1993; **10** (Suppl. 3): S3.

106 Orchard TJ, Strandness DE. Assessment of peripheral vascular disease in diabetes. *Diabetes Care* 1993; **16**: 1199–209.

107 Gibbons GW, Freeman D. Vascular evaluation and treatment of the diabetic. *Clin Podiatr Med Surg* 1987; **4**: 377–81.

108 Young MJ, Coffey J, Taylor PM, Boulton AJM. Plantar ultrasound: a new, non-invasive technique to predict foot ulcer risk. *Diabetic Med* 1993; **10** (Suppl. 3): S39.

109 Tovey FE. The manufacture of diabetic footwear. *Diabetic Med* 1984; **1**: 69–71.

110 Tovey FE, Moss MJ. Specialist shoes for the diabetic foot. In: Connor H, Boulton AJM, Ward JE (eds), *The Foot in Diabetes*. Chichester: John Wiley & Sons, 1987: 97–108.

111 Veves A, Masson EA, Fernando DJS, Boulton AJM. Use of experimental padded hosiery to reduce foot pressures in diabetic neuropathy. *Diabetes Care* 1989; **12**: 653–5.

112 Veves A, Masson EA, Fernando DJS, Boulton AJM. Studies of experimental hosiery in diabetic neuropathic patients with high foot pressures. *Diabetic Med* 1990; **7**: 324–6.

113 Gudas CJ. Prophylactic surgery in the diabetic foot. *Clin Podiatr Med Surg* 1987; **4**: 445–8.

114 Rosen RC, Davids MS, Bohanske LM. Hemorrhage into plantar callus and diabetes mellitus. *Cutis* 1985; **35**: 339–41.

115 Harkless LB. You see what you look for and recognise what you know. *Clin Podiatr Med Surg* 1987; **4**: 331–9.

116 Murray HJ, Young MJ, Boulton AJM. The relationship between callus formation, high pressures and neuropathy in diabetic foot ulceration. *Diabetic Med* 1994; **11** (Suppl. 2); A19.

117 Masson EA, Angle S, Roseman P, Soper C, Wilson I, Cotton M, Boulton AJM. Diabetic foot ulcers—do patients know how to protect themselves? *Practical Diabetes* 1989; **6**: 22–3.

118 Boulton AJM, Gokal R, Masson EA. The formation of a combined diabetic nephropathy clinic. *Postgrad Med J* 1988; **64** (Suppl. 3): 84.

119 Boulton AJM. The diabetic foot. *Med Clin North Am* 1988; **72**: 1513–30.

120 Pollard JP, Le Quesne LP. Method of healing diabetic forefoot ulcers. *Br Med J* 1983; **286**: 436–7.

121 Burden AC, Jones GR, Jones R, Blandford RL. Use of the 'Scotchcast boot' in treating diabetic foot ulcers. *Br Med J* 1983; **286**: 1555–7.

122 Mueller MJ, Diamond JE, Sinacore DR. Total contact casting in treatment of diabetic plantar ulcers. *Diabetes Care* 1989; **12**: 384–8.

123 Stipa S, Wheelcock FC. A comparison of femoral artery grafts in diabetic and non-diabetic patients. *Am J Surg* 1971; **121**: 223–8.

124 Joseph WS, Axler DA. Microbiology and antimicrobial therapy of diabetic foot infections. *Clin Podiatr Med Surg* 1990; **7**: 467–81.

125 Hunt JA. Foot infections are rarely due to a single microorganism. *Diabetic Med* 1992; **9**: 749–52.

126 Hetherington VJ. Technectium and combined Gallium and Technectium scans in the neurotrophic foot. *J Am Podiatr Assoc* 1982; **72**: 458–63.

127 Durham JR, Lukens ML, Campanini DS, Wright JG, Smead WL. Impact of magnetic resonance imaging on the management of diabetic foot infections. *Am J Surg* 1991; **162**: 150–3.

128 Wang A, Weinstein D, Greenfield L, et al. MRI and diabetic foot infections. *Magn Reson Imaging* 1990; **8**: 805–9.

129 Levin S. Digest of current literature. *Infect Dis Clin Pract* 1992; **1**: 49–50.

130 McKeown KC. The history of the diabetic foot. In: Boulton AJM, Connor H, Cavanagh PR (eds), *The Foot in Diabetes*, 2nd edn. Chichester: John Wiley, 1994: 5–13.

131 Porter M. Making sense of dressings. *Wound Management* 1992; **2**: 10–12.

132 Lithner F. Adverse effects on diabetic foot ulcers of highly adhesive hydrocolloid occlusive dressings. *Diabetes Care* 1990; **13**: 814–15.

133 Tovey FE. Diabetic foot ulceration. *Wound Manage* 1993; **3**: 12–14.

134 Greenwood D. Honey for superficial wounds and ulcers. *Lancet* 1993; **341**: 90–1.

135 Zumla A, Lulat A. Honey: a remedy rediscovered. *J R Soc Med London* 1989; **82**: 374–5.

136 Turner TD. Hydrogels and hydrocolloids—an overview of the products and their properties. In: Turner TD, Schmidt RJ, Harding KG (eds), *Advances in Wound Management*. Chichester: John Wiley & Sons, 1985: 89–95.

137 Knighton DR, Ciresi K, Fiegel VD, Schumerth S, Butler E, Cerra F. Stimulation of repair in chronic, non-healing cutaneous ulcers using platelet derived wound healing formula. *Surg Gynecol Obstet* 1990; **170**: 56–60.

138 Krupski WC, Reilly LM, Perez S, Moss KM, Crombleholme PA, Rapp JH. A prospective randomized trial of autologous platelet derived wound healing factors for the treatment of chronic non-healing wounds: A preliminary report. *J Vasc Surg* 1991; **14**: 526–36.

139 Robson MC, Phillips LG, Thomasen A, Robson LE, Pierce GF. Platelet derived growth factor BB for the treatment of chronic pressure ulcers. *Lancet* 1992; **339**: 23–5.

140 Young MJ, Larsen J, Knowles A, Parnell L, Ward JD, Boulton AJM. The treatment of diabetic neuropathic foot ulcers with biosynthetic platelet derived growth factor. *Diabetic Med* 1992; **9** (Suppl. 2): 76.

141 Day JL. Patient education—how may recurrence be prevented? In: Connor H, Boulton AJM (eds), *The Foot in Diabetes*. Chichester: John Wiley, 1987: 135–43.
142 Edmonds M, Foster A, Greenhill M, Sinha J, Philpott-Howard J, Salisbury J. Acute septic vasculitis not diabetic microangiopathy leads to digital necrosis in the neuropathic foot. *Diabetic Med* 1992; **9** (Suppl. 1): P85.
143 Goldner MG. The fate of the second leg in the diabetic amputee. *Diabetes* 1960; **9**: 100–3.
144 Mawdsley SK, Carrington AL, Morley M, Kincey J, Boulton AJM. A comparison of the quality of life between diabetic foot ulcer patients and diabetic lower limb amputees. *Diabetic Med* 1994; **11** (Suppl. 1): 32.
145 Charcot JM. On some neuropathies apparently related to a lesion of the brain or spinal cord. Translated by Hoche G, Sanders LJ. *J Hist Neurosci* 1992; **1**: 75–87.
146 Jordan WR. Neuritic manifestations in diabetes mellitus. *Arch Intern Med* 1936; **57**: 307–10.
147 Sinha S, Munichoodappa CS, Kozak GP. Neuroarthropathy (Charcot joints) in diabetes mellitus. *Medicine* 1972; **51**: 191–210.
148 Cofield RH, Morrison MJ, Beabout JW. Diabetic neuroarthropathy in the foot: patient characteristics and patterns of radiographic change. *Foot Ankle* 1983; **4**: 15–22.
149 Sammarco GJ. Diabetic arthropathy. In: Sammarco GJ (ed), *The Foot in Diabetes*. Philadelphia: Lea & Febiger, 1991.
150 Frykberg RG. Osteoarthropathy. *Clin Podiatr Med Surg* 1987; **4**: 351–76.
151 Sanders LJ. Frykberg RG. Charcot Foot. In: Levin ME, O'Neal LW, Bowker JH (eds), *The Diabetic Foot*, 5th edn. St Louis: Mosby Year Books, 1993: 149–80.
152 Pogonowska MJ, Collins LC, Dobson HL. Diabetic osteopathy. *Radiology* 1967; **89**: 265–71.
153 Stevens MJ, Edmonds ME, Foster AVM, Watkins PJ. Selective neuropathy and preserved vascular responses in the diabetic Charcot foot. *Diabetologia* 1992; **35**: 148–54.
154 Marshall A, Young MJ, Boulton AJM. The neuropathy of patients with Charcot feet: Is there a specific deficit? *Diabetic Med* 1993; **10** (Suppl. 1): 101.
155 McEnery KW, Gilula LA, Hardy DC, Staple TW. Imaging of the diabetic foot. In: Levin ME, O'Neal LW, Bowker JH (eds), *The Diabetic Foot*, 5th edn. St Louis: Mosby Year Books, 1993: 341–64.
156 Johnson JTH. Neuropathic fractures and joint injuries. Pathogenesis and rationale of prevention and treatment. *J Bone Joint Surg* 1967; **49A**: 1–30.
157 Connolly JF, Jacobsen FS. Rapid bone destruction after a stress fracture in a diabetic (Charcot) foot. *Nebr Med J* 1985; **70**: 438–40.
158 Selby PL. Osteopenia and diabetes. *Diabetic Med* 1988; **5**: 423–8.
159 Coburn JW. Renal Osteodystrophy. *Kidney Int* 1980; **17**: 677.
160 Edmonds ME, Clarke MB, Newton S, Barrett J, Watkins PJ. Increased uptake of bone radiopharmaceutical in diabetic neuropathy. *QJ Med* 1985; **57**: 843–55.
161 Carter DR, Hayes HC. The compressive behaviour of bone as a two-phase porous structure. *J Bone Joint Surg* 1977; **59A**: 954–62.
162 Edelman SV, Kosofsky EM, Paul RA, Kozak GP. Neuro-osteoarthropathy (Charcot's joints) in diabetes mellitus following revascularisation surgery: three case reports and a review of the literature. *Arch Intern Med* 1987; **147**: 1504–8.
163 Eichenholtz SN. *Charcot Joints*. Springfield: Charles C Thomas, 1966.
164 Keenan AM, Tindel NL, Alavi A. Diagnosis of pedal osteomyelitis in diabetic patients using current scintigraphic techniques. *Arch Intern Med* 1989; **149**: 2262–5.

165 Close CF, Griffith JF, Krentz AJ, Wright AD, Davies AM, Nattrass M. The evolution of neuroarthropathy in the diabetic foot—a computed tomographic study. *Diabetic Med* 1993; **10** (Suppl. 3): A22.

166 Lesko P, Maurer RC. Talonavicular dislocations and midfoot arthropathy in neuropathic diabetic feet: natural source and principles of treatment. *Clin Orthop* 1989; **240**: 226.

167 Miller DS, Lichtman WF. Diabetic neuropathic arthropathy of the feet. *Arch Surg* 1955; **70**: 513.

168 Tom RK, Pupp GR. Talectomy for diabetic Charcot foot. An alternative to amputation. *J Am Podiatr Med Assoc* 1992; **82**: 447–53.

169 Sanders LJ, Frykberg RG. Diabetic neuropathic osteoarthropathy: The Charcot foot. In: Frykberg RG (ed.), *The High Risk Foot in Diabetes*. New York: Churchill Livingstone, 1991: 297–308.

170 Rehman MTA, Clayson AD, Marsh D, Adams J. Canteril J, Anderson DC. Treatment of reflex sympathetic dystrophy with intravenous pamidronate. *Bone* 1992; **13**: 116.

171 Selby PL, Young MJ, Boulton AJM. Bisphosphonates—a new treatment for diabetic Charcot neuroarthropathy? *Diabetic Med* 1994; **11**: 28–31.

8

Initial Management of Non-insulin-dependent Diabetes Mellitus in the Elderly

ALAN J. SINCLAIR

Department of Geriatric Medicine, University of Birmingham, UK

INTRODUCTION

Previous reports provide ample proof of the economic, social and health burden of diabetes in the elderly[1-3]. Strategies likely to reduce this burden must be initiated at an early stage and include aiming for individual and *realistic* levels of glycaemic control, screening for complications, and involving patients and carers in educational programmes[4].

The present state of diabetic care for the older patient is essentially unstructured, poorly co-ordinated, often inappropriate, and therefore in great need of reorganization[4]. Partly responsible for this unsatisfactory situation is the relative neglect of diabetes in the elderly in the medical literature, for example, published articles dealing with diabetic research involving specific studies in elderly patients account for less than 5% of those published between 1978 and 1988.

There are likely to be many reasons for considering the type of diabetes in old people to be a mild disease and therefore not worthy of attention by doctors. Many patients are of course asymptomatic and have 'lowish' blood glucose levels in the range 8–11 mmol/l. Patients, themselves, may consider that they do not have a problem at all, and if symptoms are present, they are likely to be attributed to ageing. Few may be involved in home blood

Diabetes in Old Age. Edited by P. Finucane and A. J. Sinclair
© 1995 John Wiley & Sons Ltd

glucose monitoring, and since many are not on insulin, it cannot be serious! A large majority are unlikely to have seen a hospital specialist[5].

RATIONALE FOR GOOD QUALITY CARE

Type 2 (non-insulin-dependent) diabetes (NIDDM) accounts for 95% of cases of diabetes in old age[6]. Although Type 1 (insulin-dependent) diabetes (IDDM) can occur *de novo*[7] its true incidence is unknown but probably underestimated. The presentation of diabetes in the older patient is varied (Table 8.1).

Table 8.1. Presentation of diabetes in the elderly

Asymptomatic
Insulin deficiency
Spectrum of vague symptoms:
  depressed mood
  apathy
  mental confusion
Unexplained weight loss/incontinence
Coexisting illness
Diabetic ketoacidosis
Hyperosmolar non-ketotic coma

The insidious presentation may delay diagnosis and partially account for the high prevalence rate of diabetic complications at the time of diagnosis. For example, up to 10% of newly diagnosed elderly diabetics have evidence of retinopathy[8]. Better screening for complications at the time of diagnosis is, therefore, part of the rationale for promoting quality diabetic care for older patients with diabetes (Table 8.2). The Diabetes Control and Complications Trial (DCCT) Research Group have recently reported the effect of intensive treatment of diabetes in a group of young patients with IDDM[9]. This study demonstrated significant reductions in the onset of complications and a reduced progression of established complications in patients whose glycaemic control was 'tight'. This 'prize' in reducing microangiopathy was paid for by a substantial increase in episodes of hypoglycaemia due to treatment, a fact which has important implications in aged diabetic patients who are vulnerable to this acute complication[10]. Extrapolating data from the DCCT to older patients with NIDDM may not be valid although the UK Prospective Diabetes Study (UKPDS), which is a comparative study investigating the effects of various treatments in patients with newly diagnosed NIDDM and due to report in 1996/7[11], may

Table 8.2. Rationale for good quality care of older diabetics

---

Early diagnosis may prevent progression of undetected complications

Better glycaemic control may reduce incidence of complications

Better screening for maculopathy and cataracts will reduce number of blind registrations

Better management and prevention of peripheral vascular disease and foot problems will reduce amputation rates

Prevents escalating costs and use of health service resources

---

provide confirmatory evidence of a beneficial effect of improved glycaemic control. No major studies have yet demonstrated a reduction in macroangiopathic complications, such as peripheral vascular or ischaemic heart disease with improved glycaemia.

Diabetic maculopathy is one of several age-specific complications of diabetes[5] and is an important cause of blindness in older diabetic patients. It is 2.6 times more common than proliferative retinopathy as a cause of diabetic blind registrations among the UK diabetic population of all ages[12]. Delay in diagnosis of this condition results from lack of awareness of its importance, lack of testing for visual acuity, and failure to use mydriasis. This combined with inexperience at fundal examination, even by medically qualified health professionals, creates an unfortunate situation since more than 70% of patients are likely to benefit from laser photo-coagulation[12].

Elderly patients comprise the majority of diabetic amputees and the high level of resulting disability is discussed in more detail in Chapter 7. Screening for early signs of skin damage such as ischaemia or ulceration, is a fundamental requirement to lessen the burden of this complication which results in less than one in 10 patients regaining independent mobility[13] and a mortality of up to 50% at 2 years post-surgery[14].

The high cost of diabetic care in Western societies is discussed in detail in Chapter 1. Since the elderly comprise the majority of patients with diabetes, and elderly diabetic patients have a high usage of hospital services[15], it is clear that health strategies which result in less complications and decreased disability, will also lead to a fall in diabetes-related costs.

INITIAL MANAGEMENT

Until fairly recently it was generally accepted that the main aims of treating elderly diabetics were twofold: (i) to provide relief from symptoms of hyperglycaemia, and (ii) to avoid troubling (and often dangerous) hypoglycaemia in those taking oral hypoglycaemic drugs or insulin. This approach, however, is now inadequate[16]. Increased life expectancy means that many aged diabetics live long enough to suffer from disabling (but potentially preventable) complications such as blindness, lower limb amputation and foot ulceration. Furthermore, some complications are predominantly a feature of the aged (Table 8.3). The essential aims in managing elderly patients with diabetes have been listed in Table 8.4. The relative priority of each needs to be established at an early stage in the management.

ACUTE PRESENTATION

Diabetes in elderly patients with NIDDM may present acutely in several ways: in diabetic ketoacidosis (DKA) or as hyperosmolar non-ketotic coma (HONK), or more commonly, as hyperglycaemia without ketosis or increased osmolality with or without coexisting acute illness, e.g. acute cerebrovascular accident. These metabolic disturbances are covered in more detail in Chapter 5. Seriously ill patients require insulin therapy (especially those with ketones) given either as an intravenous infusion or by regular subcutaneous injections of short-acting insulin.

Table 8.3. Age-specific complications of diabetes in old age

Diabetic maculopathy
Diabetic amyotrophy
Hyperosmolar non-ketotic coma
Diabetic ophthalmoplegia
Malignant otitis externa
Necrotizing fasciitis

Adapted from Tattersall (1984)[1]

Table 8.4. Aims in managing diabetes in the elderly

---

1. To promote freedom from symptoms of hyperglycaemia

2. To assess the impact of coexisting disease, e.g. ischaemic heart disease

3. To prevent undesirable weight loss

4. Avoid hypoglycaemia and other adverse drug reactions

5. To screen for and prevent complications

6. To maintain patient well-being and quality of life

DKA is confirmed by evidence of significant ketosis (3+ ketostix in urine or plasma), and significant acidosis (venous plasma bicarbonate <15 mmol/l or arterial pH below 7.2). Treatment involves insulin (often by use of an insulin pump) and intravenous fluid therapy with normal saline if the plasma sodium level is <155 mmol/l or half-normal saline if the sodium level is >155 mmol/l. Often, 6–8 l are required during the first 24 h and the insertion of a central venous line may be necessary to monitor therapy. The use of intravenous bicarbonate therapy in patients with an arterial pH <7.0 is still advocated[17], although some studies have found little evidence of bicarbonate's efficacy in DKA[18]. Presentation with HONK is associated with a significant mortality in the elderly (>30%)[19]. Various precipitating factors have been identified (Table 8.5). Blood glucose levels are often greater than 50 mmol/l and patients are severely dehydrated (plasma osmolality >350 m osmol/l). Ketosis is usually absent (Table 8.6). Treatment involves administering insulin, intravenous fluid therapy, prophylactic heparin (to prevent thrombotic complications), and usually antibiotics since many cases are precipitated by infection. Survivors frequently do not require long-term insulin therapy. In all severe cases arterial blood gases should be measured to assess acid–base balance.

NON-ACUTE PRESENTATION

The majority of elderly Type 2 diabetic patients are not severely unwell at presentation and the majority should ideally be managed in the community by the general practitioner. At this stage there are four important objectives: (i) satisfy yourself that the patient has diabetes; (ii) screen for complications; (iii) identify who will be responsible for diabetic care, i.e. the patient or someone else; and (iv) initiate treatment.

Table 8.5. Hyperosmolar non-ketotic coma—precipitating factors

1. 50% unknown

2. Infection

3. Operation (surgery)

4. Myocardial infarction

5. Stroke

6. Drugs:
    propranolol
    thiazides
    steroids
    dialysis
    (glucose drinks)

Table 8.6. Hyperosmolar non-ketotic coma

Marked hyperglycaemia (mean value of glucose >50 mmol/l)
Absence of significant ketosis
Absence of severe acidosis
Marked dehydration
Plasma osmolality >350 m osmol/l (NR 285–295)

Making the Diagnosis

The WHO criteria for the diagnosis of diabetes applies equally to elderly subjects as to younger counterparts[20]. This is discussed in greater detail in Chapter 4. It should be appreciated, however, that many patients may not be able to give an accurate history of symptoms; 'classic' symptoms of polyuria and polydipsia due to excessive glycosuria may be absent due to the raised renal threshold found in elderly subjects. A true fasted blood sample is often difficult to obtain, and an oral glucose tolerance test (OGTT) may be thought of as time-consuming and inconvenient. In addition, many patients have elevated plasma glucose levels which are secondary to acute illness, diabetogenic drug therapy, or other stress-inducing disorders. If the physician has any doubt about the diagnosis of diabetes, it is wise not to treat but to retest later and use an OGTT if necessary.

Screening for Complications at Diagnosis

A detailed history may reveal symptoms of a distal sensory diabetic neuropathy such as numbness, paraesthesiae, burning pains, and hyper-aesthesiae from bedclothes at night-time. Symptoms of postural hypotension (especially after treatment for coexisting hypertension with vasodilators has been started), diarrhoea or constipation, and impotence should alert you to the possibility of autonomic neuropathy. Symptoms of claudication should be enquired about. Physical examination requires measurement of lying and standing blood pressure and assessment of peripheral blood vessels. Visual acuities (VA) can be checked using a 3 m Snellen chart. Patients whose VA is worse than 6/6 in either eye should be examined using the pin-hole test which will partially correct a refractive error. Alternatively, they may use their distance glasses if worn. In patients with poor VA which remains unaltered or worsens after the pin-hole test, the retina should be closely inspected for lesions, particularly those of maculopathy.

Direct ophthalmoscopy should start with the lens set at zero and a red reflex obtained. When present, this indicates that there is no significant evidence of a cataract, vitreous haemorrhage, or retinal detachment. By setting the lens at +10 initially, and using a succession of less powerful lenses, a direct inspection of the cornea, anterior chamber and lens is possible. Diabetic retinopathy should be looked for after pupillary dilatation using 0.5–1.0% tropicamide eye drops. Relative contraindications for this include those with previous eye surgery, lens implants, or history of narrow angle glaucoma. The precipitation of previously undiagnosed acute glaucoma, although distressing at the time, may be a service to the patient in the long run since treatment may prevent further visual loss. Patients with scattered microaneurysms and blot haemorrhages require review at 6 months. Diabetic maculopathy (Figure 8.1), which can be sight-threatening requires urgent referral to the ophthalmologist. Other

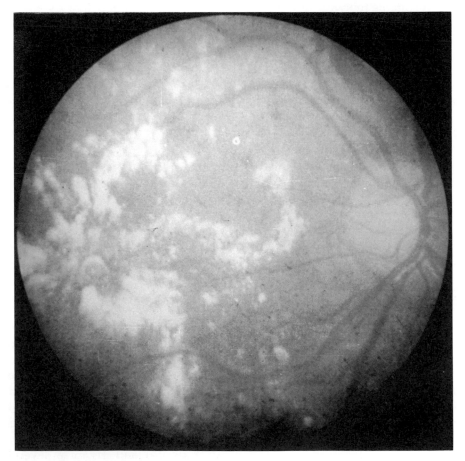

Figure 8.1. Diabetic exudative maculopathy

reasons for referral include the presence of yellow, waxy hard exudates, proliferative retinopathy, severe cataract formation, or rapid decrease in VA, e.g. within previous 3 months (noticed by the patient—subjective; or evidence of a two-line deterioration in VA using a Snellen chart— objective).

Examination of the limbs for sensory neuropathy should include an assessment of knee and ankle reflexes, sensation by testing with pin-prick and cotton wool, vibration sense by 128 c/s tuning fork (bearing in mind the age-associated loss of vibration sense), and proprioception.

Infection, foot ulceration, presence of pressure areas and the presence of sharp, poorly cut nails requires referral to the chiropodist. Management may also include radiology, antibiotic therapy, rest, use of pressure-relieving devices, and even surgery. Effective education including advice about suitable footwear dramatically reduces the risk of new foot lesions[21].

Other investigations include: serum creatinine, glycosylated haemoglobin (HB A$_1$c), lipid profile (triglycerides, total and high-density lipoprotein (HDL) cholesterol) in those aged less than 75 years, especially those with coronary artery disease. In patients who may have had undiagnosed diabetes for some time with marked hyperglycaemia, hyperlipidaemia may be present. In these cases, it is worth rechecking their lipids after 6 months to see whether treatment has reversed the abnormality. An electrocardiogram looking for ischaemia, arrhythmias and ventricular hypertrophy is useful. Urinalysis (in the absence of infection) may demonstrate proteinuria although this is not particularly common at diagnosis in the elderly. Microalbuminuria is also uncommon at diagnosis although we routinely screen for it in our diabetic clinic when the dipstick test is negative for protein. I routinely complete a Barthel scale and mini-mental state examination to assess both physical disability and mental function. Brain failure may make the patient totally dependent on others (spouse, other relative or district nurse) both for treatment and monitoring.

Patient and Carer Responsibilities

In most situations an individual care plan must be adopted and agreed by all concerned. This may be organized by the primary care physician (general practitioner), although diabetes specialist nurses can play an important role in this decision-making. This will consist of identifying the principal carer, setting realistic glycaemic goals, planning the timing and frequency of visits, and being aware of the indications for hospital referral to a specialist (Table 8.7) or admission. Ideally, the health care team should aim to provide written information about diabetes for each newly diagnosed patient (and carer where appropriate) and organize several educational tutorials over the next 6–12 months.

Table 8.7. Indications for referral to hospital specialist for elderly patients with diabetes

---

1. Patients with severe complications, e.g. maculopathy, foot ulceration, peripheral vascular disease.

2. Patients whose metabolic/symptom control is suboptimal irrespective of treatment, e.g. oral agents or insulin.

3. Complex management problems in those with coexisting disease, e.g. patients with chronic pulmonary disease taking steroids.

4. Patients with increasing dependency and immobility, e.g. post-stroke.

5. Patients not adequately cared for in primary care.

Initial Treatment

In patients whose random glucose values lie between 8 and 17 mmol/l and who are not troubled by symptoms an initial 6–12 week course of dietary instruction only is warranted. The British Diabetic Association (BDA) have updated a series of dietary recommendations for diabetic patients, which now includes a small section on the elderly[22]. The main elements include consuming 50–55% of total energy intake as carbohydrate (including a fibre intake of at least 30 g/day), 30–35% fat intake (<10% saturated fat), and 10–15% protein.

Dietetic treatment will depend on several factors but must include the patient's ability to cooperate, physical and mental well-being, and the patient's natural desire to be independent. This process is a form of negotiation and some dietitians are now developing a 'Getting Started' diet sheet for initial management. There is a shift away from traditional 'food exchanges' towards a more generalized plan of healthy eating (provision of 'healthy eating messages'). In those patients who are overweight, a plan of fat restriction may be beneficial. Other practical advice including alcohol consumption and benefits of exercise are often given at this time.

When dietary advice fails to reduce levels of glycaemia or improve patient well-being, or when initial random glucose levels are greater than 17 mmol/l and patients feel unwell, several treatment options are available (Table 8.8), although in most cases, oral agents are then prescribed.

GUAR GUM

Guar is a dietary fibre (polysaccharide) obtained from the seeds of the Indian cluster bean that forms a highly viscous gel when mixed with water. It has been proposed that guar delays gastric emptying and reduces

Table 8.8. Treatment options for diet failures

---

1. Further period of intense dietary therapy requiring inputs from both physician and dietitian.

2. Specified and appropriate exercise programme.

3. Guar gum.

4. Acarbose—alpha-glucosidase inhibitor.

5. Oral hypoglycaemic agents—sulphonylureas or metformin.

6. Insulin therapy—usually considered on a temporary basis in well-defined circumstances only, such as acute illness.

---

intestinal absorption and has been used in diabetes to reduce hyper-glycaemia and in patients with hyperlipidaemia to reduce total and low-density lipoprotein (LDL) cholesterol levels.

Side-effects of therapy with guar include flatulence, gastrointestinal pain, nausea and diarrhoea. Symptoms tend to be most severe at the start of therapy and lessen with continuing therapy. A recent study[23] concluded that guar does not improve glycaemic control in NIDDM. Other investigators have found similar disappointing results, although some studies have observed benefit. The consensus is at the moment that guar has only a marginal effect in lowering blood glucose levels in patients with NIDDM[24].

PHYSICAL ACTIVITY AND EXERCISE

The contribution of exercise to the management of NIDDM is discussed earlier in Chapter 4. Exercise should be recommended as an adjunct to proper diet and weight control and may even be protective against the development of NIDDM[25]. It has several beneficial actions: lowering of hyperinsulinaemia and an improvement in glucose tolerance occurs probably secondary to a reduction in insulin resistance[26]. The lipid profile becomes less atherogenic with a reduction in total plasma cholesterol and triglycerides while increasing HDL-cholesterol. A fall in blood pressure may take place as a direct result of exercise as well as the effect of weight loss. Some patients (especially older patients) are unable to participate in exercise programmes because of decreased joint mobility due to diabetes-related joint stiffness and/or osteoarthrosis, or because of a previous stroke. Limited exercise only is possible in those with poor metabolic control and ketosis or those with ischaemic heart disease, advanced retinal or renal disease.

The importance of promoting weight loss in overweight patients cannot be overemphasized since obese patients with NIDDM pose several unique problems in diabetic management. First, increasing body weight makes the attainment of normoglycaemia by dietary manipulation exceedingly difficult. Secondly, there is clinical and epidemiological evidence linking obesity, and its consequent insulin resistance and hyperinsulinaemia, with the development of, and exacerbation of, NIDDM[27]. Furthermore, there is evidence to suggest that insulin resistance and hyperinsulinaemia promote the development of hypertension and dyslipidaemia, which in turn increases the risk of cardiovascular disease[28]. The term 'syndrome X' has been applied to the clinical association of insulin resistance, hypertension, and increased very low-density lipoprotein and decreased HDL (dyslipidaemia)[29]. Thirdly, treatment with sulphonylureas or insulin is associated with hyperinsulinaemia, which promotes both weight gain and may paradoxically increase insulin resistance. These factors are important and should be considered when antidiabetic therapy is instituted.

ORAL AGENTS

Newer oral hypoglycaemic therapies are being evaluated but at the present time I predominantly use sulphonylureas in the elderly (Table 8.9). In choosing a specific drug several factors need to be considered including renal and hepatic function, coexisting disease, possible drug interactions, and the likelihood of producing significant hypoglycaemia. For this reason, glibenclamide and chlorpropamide, which have prolonged durations of action, can accumulate in renal dysfunction, and have a high associated risk of hypoglycaemia (sometimes with fatal consequences)[10,30], should not be prescribed for diabetic subjects aged 60 years or older. Patients should be warned of the possibility of hypoglycaemia developing and educated with practical advice on how to both avoid and prevent this potentially serious situation developing. In relatively newly diagnosed patients, failure to achieve acceptable glycaemic targets with diet and sulphonylureas after 6 months should lead to a further review of treatment. Up to fairly recently, only two options were tried: addition of metformin or starting the patient on insulin.

Metformin is the main biguanide in clinical use world-wide since its predecessor, phenformin, was withdrawn more than a decade ago in some countries because of its association with lactic acidosis. This metabolic complication has been calculated to be 10–15 times less common with metformin which has a different molecular structure and pharmaco-dynamic profile[31]. Although a small risk of precipitating lactic acidosis (especially in a setting of renal or circulatory failure) is present with metformin, better prescribing habits by physicians have lessened this risk.

Table 8.9. Pharmacokinetics of oral sulphonylurea drugs

	Chlorpropamide*	Glibenclamide*	Tolbutamide	Gliclazide	Glipizide	Glibornuride†	Gliquidone††
Maximum daily dose	300 mg	15 mg	1.5 g	320 mg	30 mg	50–75 mg	60–120 mg
Duration of action(h)	60	16–24	6–12	24	12–24	24	24
Frequency of dosing	Single	Single/DD	Single/DD	Single/DD	Single/DD	Single/DD	Single/DD
Metabolism	Hepatic	Hepatic	Hepatic	Hepatic	Hepatic	Hepatic	Hepatic
Rate of renal excretion	90% in 4 days	50% in 5 days	100% in 24 h	Less than 5% in 24 h	90% in 3 days	70% in 3 days	Less than 5% in 24 h

* Should not be prescribed in the elderly.
† Not usually prescribed in the UK.
†† Not commonly prescribed in the UK.
DD: divided doses.

I do not recommend the use of metformin as monotherapy except in patients who are grossly obese (body mass index >30) since it has an anorectic action. It may also be beneficial in patients with hyperlipidaemia since during therapy, both triglyceride and LDL cholesterol levels may fall. Where sulphonylureas have failed to maintain glycaemic control, addition of metformin may be useful in improving glycaemic control[32,33]. It also has the added advantage that it does not usually lower plasma glucose levels below the euglycaemic range and, therefore, in normal therapeutic doses, does not cause hypoglycaemia. Metformin can be started at a dose of 500 mg twice daily initially. After 2 weeks, the dose can be increased if necessary. The maximum dose I recommend in subjects aged between 60 and 75 years is 2 g daily. As a rule, I do not prescribe metformin in patients older than 75 years, although this practice may be unjustified. Gastrointestinal side-effects such as anorexia, nausea, abdominal discomfort and diarrhoea occur in nearly one-third of patients treated with metformin. These symptoms can be minimized by taking the drug with or after meals and using a low initial dose with subsequent gradual titration of higher doses. Although guidelines issued by the European NIDDM Policy Group do not recommend metformin in subjects aged older than 65 years[34], I feel that as long as patients are closely monitored, age *per se* should not be the primary barrier to the use of metformin.

HYPOGLYCAEMIA WITH SULPHONYLUREAS

Sulphonylureas are metabolized in the liver to metabolites with minimal hypoglycaemic activity, which are cleared via urinary excretion. For this reason sulphonylureas are contraindicated in hepatic and renal disease, both of which increase the risk of hypoglycaemia. Sulphonylurea-induced hypoglycaemia (SIH) is much less common than insulin-induced hypogly-caemia. The incidence of severe SIH with coma has been estimated at 0.19–0.25 per 1000 patient years[35,36] in contrast with insulin-induced hypoglycaemia coma with an incidence of 100 per 1000 patient years[37]. The incidence of less severe symptoms is considerably higher with as many as one in five outpatient diabetic subjects experiencing hypoglycaemia regularly[38].

Prolonged hypoglycaemia with glibenclamide and chlorpropamide is a worrying clinical problem. Glibenclamide-induced hypoglycaemia may be more pronounced because the drug accumulates within beta cells and its metabolites retain some hypoglycaemic activity. Due to the long elimina-tion half-life (35 h) of chlorpropamide, continued dosing results in drug accumulation (steady state being achieved by 7–10 days). In the presence of impaired renal function, further prolongation of hypoglycaemia occurs.

In the elderly, hypoglycaemia is often mistaken for transient neurological or cardiac events, and appears to have a worse prognosis: 10% of those admitted to hospital die and 3% have permanent neurological damage[39], presumably because of an already compromised cerebral circulation.

Most sulphonylureas have caused fatal hypoglycaemia, although this is often associated with chlorpropamide or glibenclamide[40]. Other factors apart from old age which predispose to fatal hypoglycaemia are alcohol consumption, poor food intake, renal impairment, potentiation of hypoglycaemia by other drugs, prescription of sulphonylureas with prolonged actions in patients with only marginal elevations of blood glucose levels[41]. Many if not all these factors are directly relevant in the elderly patient with NIDDM.

TREATMENT OF SIH

SIH (blood glucose level <3.0 mmol/l) may be prolonged (up to a week) and requires hospital admission. A bolus intravenous injection of 20–50 ml of 50% dextrose should be given immediately, followed by an intravenous infusion of 10 or 20% dextrose to maintain the plasma glucose level between 6 and 12 mmol/l until residual hypoglycaemic effects of the drug are minimal. Diazoxide, which has a direct inhibitory effect on insulin secretion, may be used as an adjunct to treatment. In the unconscious patient, diazoxide can be given as a slow intravenous infusion of 300 mg over 30 min, and be repeated every 4 h if necessary, although I do not use this drug.

Glucagon is widely used to reverse hypoglycaemia in insulin-induced hypoglycaemic coma in patients with IDDM. Since glucagon may stimulate insulin secretion, it is usually contraindicated in patients with NIDDM who may have residual beta-cell function.

ACARBOSE

Acarbose is a competitive inhibitor of a group of hydrolytic enzymes called alpha-glucosidases which comprises glycoamylase, sucrase, maltase and alpha-dextrinase and binds to them at the brush border of the intestinal lumen. These enzymes are required to degrade starch, sucrose, and maltose to allow absorption of the resulting monosaccharides (mainly glucose) to take place (Figure 8.2).

Acarbose has a chemical structure similar to natural carbohydrate and has been shown to slow the release of glucose from complex carbohydrates by as much as 80% in the upper part of the small bowel. It does not affect lactase activity and does not influence the absorption of free glucose. The impact of acarbose is thus clearly enhanced if patients consume carbo-hydrates which are rich in poly- and oligosaccharides (rather than monosaccharides). This is part of the current dietary recommendations for patients with diabetes.

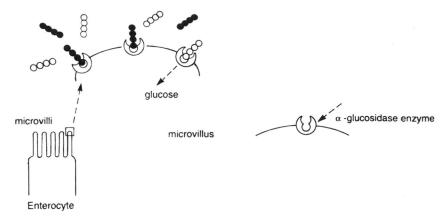

Figure 8.2. Mechanism of action for acarbose[33]. By binding to the enzyme, acarbose prevents immediate digestion of carbohydrates and subsequent release of glucose. ●●●●, Acarbose; OOOO, oligosaccharide from starch. Reproduced by kind permission of PMH Publications Ltd, Chichester

Treatment with acarbose may lead to a cascade of physiological events, which are of advantage in patients with NIDDM: reduction in post-prandial blood glucose increments with a consequent reduced stimulation of insulin release. Falls in both hyperglycaemia and hyperinsulinaemia result in decreased insulin resistance. There is also evidence that postprandial triglyceride synthesis in the liver is reduced after acarbose. Thus, acarbose potentially ameliorates many of the metabolic defects in NIDDM.

Acarbose has been used extensively in patients with NIDDM in several countries including Germany and the Netherlands. A review by Clissold and Edwards[42] has summarized the clinical efficacy of acarbose. In 12 placebo-controlled trials involving 164 patients, acarbose tended to reduce postprandial glucose levels, an effect which was significant in eight of the trials (105 patients). Addition of acarbose to a controlled dietary regimen leads to a fall in postprandial glycaemic peaks (1–3 h) of approximately 3 mmol/l, and accompanying postprandial insulin levels are reduced by 20–25%. As anticipated, fasting glucose levels are only mildly lowered (1 mmol/l) and fasting insulin levels are unchanged. Several studies suggest that addition of acarbose to treatment with sulphonylureas produces a further decrease of postprandial glycaemia of approximately 3 mmol/l and in glycosylated haemoglobin of 0.8–1.0%. This is accompanied by a significant fall in postprandial insulin levels in sulphonylurea-treated patients[33,43,44].

A place for acarbose in the treatment of patients with IDDM requires to be established, although several studies indicate that treatment with acarbose in IDDM results in a reduction of postprandial hyperglycaemia and a reduction of insulin dosage.

Acarbose has recently been granted a licence in the UK for treatment in patients with NIDDM. There are two main indications for use which may be summarized as follows: (i) as monotherapy in patients poorly controlled on dietary therapy alone; (ii) as an adjunct to treatment with diet and oral hypoglycaemic agents when metabolic control remains unsatisfactory. Acarbose may also be useful in patients poorly controlled on sulphonylureas who are unable to tolerate metformin therapy or in elderly patients who should not be prescribed metformin, or in obese diet failures where weight gain with sulphonylureas is undesirable.

The majority of patients do not appear to experience side-effects when acarbose is taken at doses up to 100 mg three times daily, although I usually prescribe 50 mg daily initially and increase the daily dose gradually. When side-effects occur, they are principally gastrointestinal in nature especially flatulence, abdominal distension, diarrhoea and borborygmus. These side-effects, which are more common at higher doses, are attributable to gas formation due to fermentation of unabsorbed carbohydrate in the bowel. Systemic side-effects of treatment with acarbose are infrequent probably reflecting the fact that only about 1% of an oral dose is degraded in the bowel and the absorbed metabolites are excreted by the kidneys[45].

INSULIN THERAPY

Few newly diagnosed elderly diabetics require insulin therapy to sustain life and prevent DKA, although some patients may have a slowly developing form of Type 1 diabetes and will inevitably require insulin in the future. The usual indications to start insulin are: (i) persisting symptoms with poor patient well-being; (ii) continued weight loss; and (iii) failure to achieve satisfactory glycaemic control with diet and oral agents. Other indications are shown in Table 8.10 and a more detailed discussion of insulin therapy is given in Chapter 9.

A common error in managing elderly Type 2 diabetics is undue reluctance to start insulin therapy. This view is often shared by patients until they try insulin. Underlying reasons for patient's attitudes include horror of injections, awful stories of 'hypos', fear of further hospitalization, and the belief that taking insulin will change their lives for the worse[46]. It is imperative that the decision to start insulin is taken after full discussion with the patient (and carers, as appropriate) and although there are no time limits for when this decision should take place I suggest a maximum of 6 months' perseverance with diet and oral agents before insulin is initiated. In practice,

Table 8.10. Some indications for insulin therapy in NIDDM

---

1. Persistent poor metabolic control in patients taking diet therapy and oral hypoglycaemic agents.

2. Severe intercurrent illness.

3. Major surgery.

4. Hyperosmolar non-ketotic coma.

5. Complications such as diabetic amyotrophy or acute painful neuropathy.

6. Evolution of ketosis-prone diabetes (IDDM).

---

this decision may have been delayed for several years. Able patients can begin insulin at home like their younger counterparts with treatment organized by a diabetes specialist nurse[47], in cooperation with the general practitioner. Patients who are unwell, or have other severe medical problems, or where community support is lacking, require to be admitted.

I find that once-daily insulin regimens (e.g. using an intermediate-acting insulin) leads to poor control over the whole 24-h period and in more episodes of hypoglycaemia. I prefer a twice daily preparation containing either an intermediate-acting isophane insulin alone (e.g. Humulin I, Insulatard), or in combination with a short-acting soluble insulin (e.g. Humulin M2 or M3, Mixtard). Usually, treatment can start with about 12–16 units of insulin per day and adjusted thereafter. In certain cases, however, such as those with confusion, visual loss, or arthritis, the technique of insulin administration should be taught to the spouse or to another relative or friend.

The success of insulin may be objectively evaluated by factors such as glycaemic control, patient well-being, episodes of hypoglycaemia, or frequency of hospital admissions due to diabetes.

COMBINATION THERAPY

It remains controversial whether combining insulin with oral agents has any significant advantages in terms of improved metabolic control or beneficial effects on long-term complications[48]. A recent meta-analysis of 17 studies designed to assess the efficacy of combination therapy with insulin and sulphonylurea drugs concluded that the combination results in diabetic control comparable with that achieved with insulin alone, but at lower insulin doses[49]. Another recent study found that the addition of NPH insulin in the evening in NIDDM patients taking sulphonylureas and/or metformin led to improved diabetic control associated with less weight gain and reduced hyperinsulinaemia[50]. Further studies, however, will be required to clarify the role of combination therapy in the treatment of NIDDM, and this is unlikely to be a frequent area of clinical decision-making during the early phase of the disease.

DIABETIC CONTROL/MONITORING

Urine testing for glucose remains a common practice but is inconvenient, messy, and often misleading because of the raised renal threshold of the elderly. Also, both patients and physicians are often uncertain about the significance of glycosuria and I no longer advise its routine use. Testing for the presence of ketones (when poor control is present—persistent values of blood glucose >17 mmol/l, or during severe acute illness) is worth carrying out if patients and carers have been suitably educated about its significance.

Blood glucose monitoring (e.g. using BM reagent strip measurements) should be encouraged in all those able to cooperate. Measurements can be taken twice weekly. Pre-meal and before bedtime estimations are ideal but few patients are this compliant. In other cases, spouses, district nurses or diabetes specialist nurses may monitor control.

Guidelines for reasonable diabetic control in the elderly are as follows: a fasting glucose of 7–9 mmol/l, and a random level of 8–11[30]. These limits should allow patients to remain well and be relatively free of symptoms of hyperglycaemia, and avoid the risk of hypoglycaemia. It should be remembered that even glucose levels of 11 mmol/l can make some patients feel lethargic and these require lowering. A Hb A_1c value less than 2% above the upper range of normal for the laboratory should also be aimed for. However, in many patients, stricter control is feasible and should be aimed for (see Chapter 4—metabolic targets). This is especially so in the light of the findings of the DCCT[9].

CONCLUSIONS

The management of the older diabetic patient represents a major challenge to any physician, whether based in the community or in a hospital setting. Hospital physicians without specialist training in diabetes should seek the advice of a consultant diabetologist for patients whose glycaemic control is persistently unacceptable or those with severe diabetic complications, for example, extensive foot ulceration, autonomic neuropathy or painful neuropathy. Patients with significant diabetic eye disease, for example, proliferative and preproliferative retinopathy or maculopathy require prompt referral to a consultant ophthalmologist. A detailed assessment of other cardiovascular risk factors is beyond the scope of this chapter but the presence of hypertension, ischaemic heart disease, or hyperlipidaemia, may warrant further attention and interventions. The development of local specifications for diabetic care, agreed by all health professionals involved, helps this process of referral to take place efficiently and with the most benefit for each patient.

REFERENCES

1 Tattersall RB. Diabetes in the elderly—a neglected area? *Diabetologia* 1984; **27**: 167–73.
2 Harrower ADB. Prevalence of elderly patients in a hospital diabetic population. *Br J Clin Pract* 1980; **34**: 131–3.
3 Neil HAW, Thompson AV, Thorogood M, Fowler GH, Mann JL. Diabetes in the elderly: the Oxford community diabetes study. *Diabetic Med* 1989; **6**: 608–13.
4 Sinclair AJ, Barnett AH. Special needs of elderly diabetic patients. *Br Med J* 1993; **306**: 1142–3.
5 Sinclair AJ. Diabetes care in the aged—time for reappraisal. *Practical Diabetes* 1994; **11**(No 2): 60–3.
6 Laakso M, Pyorala K. Age of onset and type of diabetes. *Diabetes Care* 1985; **8**: 114–17.
7 Kilvert A, Fitzgerald MG, Wright AD, *et al.* Clinical characteristics and aetiological classification of insulin-dependent diabetes in the elderly. *Q J Med* 1986; **60**: 865–72.
8 Caird FI. Complications of diabetes in old age. In: Evans JG, Caird FI (eds), *Advanced Geriatric Medicine*. London: Pitman, 1982: 3–9.
9 The Diabetes Control and Complications Trial Research Group. The effect of intensive treatment of diabetes on the development and progression of long-term complications in insulin-dependent diabetes mellitus. *N Engl J Med* 1993; **329**: 977–86.
10 Asplund K, Wilholm BE, Lithner F. Glibenclamide-associated hypoglycaemia: a report of 57 cases. *Diabetologia* 1983; **24**: 412–17.
11 UK Prospective Diabetes Study II. Reduction in HbA$_1$c with basal insulin supplement, sulphonylurea or biguanide therapy in maturity onset diabetes. *Diabetes* 1985; **61**: 32–6.
12 Rohan TE, Frost CD, Wald NJ. Prevention of blindness by screening for diabetic retinopathy: a quantitative assessment. *Br Med J* 1989; **299**: 1198–201.
13 Houghton AD, Taylor PR, Thurlow S, Rootes E, McColl I. Success rates for rehabilitation of vascular amputees. *Br J Surg* 1992; **79**: 753–5.
14 Waugh NR. Amputations amongst diabetics. *Diabetic Med* 1986; **3** (Suppl. 1): 71 (586A).
15 Damsgaard EM, Froland A, Green A. Use of hospital services by elderly diabetics: the Frederica Study of diabetic and fasting hyperglycaemic patients aged 60–74 years. *Diabetic Med* 1987; **4**: 317–22.
16 Sinclair AJ. Diagnosis and early management of type 2 diabetes in the elderly: a 1990s perspective. *Care of the Elderly* 1993; **5**: 69–72.
17 Berger W, Keller U. Treatment of diabetic ketoacidosis and non-ketotic hyperosmolar diabetic coma. *Bailliere's Clin Endocrinol Metab* 1992; **6**: 1–22.
18 Morris LR, Murphy MB, Kitabchi AE. Bicarbonate therapy in severe diabetic ketoacidosis. *Ann Intern Med* 1986; **105**: 836–40.

19 Krentz AJ, Natrass M. Diabetic ketoacidosis, non-ketonic hyperosmolar coma and lactic acidosis. In: Pickup J, Williams G (eds), *Textbook of Diabetes*. Oxford: Blackwell Scientific Publications, 1991: 479–94.

20 WHO Expert Committee on Diabetes Mellitus: Second Report. *WHO Tech Rep Ser* 1980; **646**: 1–80.

21 Boulton AJ. Update on long-term diabetic complications. In: Lewin IG, Seymour CA (eds), *Current Themes in Diabetic Care*. London: Royal College of Physicians of London, 1992: 45–53.

22 Nutrition SubCommittee, British Diabetic Association, Dietary recommendations for people with diabetes: an update for the 1990s. *Diabetic Med.* 1992; **9**: 189–202.

23 Tattersall R, Mansell P. Fibre in the management of diabetes. Benefits of fibre itself are uncertain. *Br Med J* 1990; **300**: 1336–7.

24 Nuttall FQ. Dietary fibre in the management of diabetes. *Diabetes* 1993; **42**: 503–8.

25 Helmrich SP, Ragland DR, Leung RW, Paffenbarger RS. Physical activity and reduced occurrence of non-insulin-dependent diabetes mellitus. *N Engl J Med* 1991; **325**: 147–52.

26 Koivisto VA. Exercise and diabetes mellitus. In: Pickup JC, Williams G (eds), *Textbook of Diabetes*. Oxford: Blackwell Scientific Publications, 1991: 795–802.

27 Ferrari P, Weidmann P. Insulin, insulin sensitivity and hypertension. *J Hypertension* 1990; **8**: 491–50.

28 Niskanen LK, Uusitupa MI, Pyorala K. The relationship of hyperinsulinaemia to the development of hypertension in type 2 diabetic patients and in non-diabetic subjects. *J Hum Hypertension* 1991; **5**: 155–9.

29 Reaven GM. Role of insulin resistance in human disease. *Diabetes* 1988; **37**: 1595–607.

30 Frey HMMM, Rosenlund B. Studies in patients with chlorpropamide-induced hypoglycaemia. *Diabetes* 1970; **19**: 930–7.

31 Jenkins C, Sinclair AJ. A frequent clinical dilemma: sulphonylureas or metformin? *Geriatr Med* 1994; **24** (2): 11–12.

32 Campbell IW. Sulphonylureas and metformin: efficacy and inadequacy. In: Bailey CJ, Flatt PR (eds), *New Antidiabetic Drugs*. London: Smith-Gordon, 1990: 33–51.

33 Sinclair AJ. Rational approaches to the treatment of patients with non-insulin-dependent diabetes mellitus (NIDDM). *Practical Diab* 1993; **10** (6): S15–20.

34 Alberti KGMM, Gries FA. Management of non-insulin-dependent diabetes mellitus in Europe: a consensus view. *Diabetic Med* 1988; **5**: 275–81.

35 Berger W. Incidence of severe side-effects during therapy with sulphonylureas and biguanides. *Horm Metab Res* 1985; **15**: 111–15.

36 Campbell IW. Metformin and the sulphonylureas: the comparative risk. *Horm Metab Res* 1985; **15**: 105–11.

37 Gerich JE. Oral hypoglycaemic agents. *N Engl J Med* 1989; **34**: 1231–45.

38 Jennings AM, Wilson RM, Ward JD. Symptomatic hypoglycaemia in NIDDM patients treated with oral hypoglycaemic agents. *Diabetic Care* 1989; **12**: 203–8.

39 Williams G. Management of non-insulin-dependent diabetes mellitus. *Br Med J* 1994; **343**: 95–100.

40 Ferner RE, Neil HAW. Sulphonylureas and hypoglycaemia. *Br Med J* 1988; **296**: 949–50.

41 Seltzer HS. Drug-induced hypoglycaemia: a review of 1418 cases. *Endocrinol Metab Clin North Am* 1989; **18**: 163–83.

42 Clissold SP, Edwards C. Acarbose. A preliminary review of its pharmaco-dynamic and pharmacokinetic properties and therapeutic potential. *Drugs* 1988; **13** (Suppl. 3): 47–52.

43 Sinclair AJ. Therapeutic choices in general practice. *Diabetes Care Today* 1993; **Part 4**: 6–11.

44 Hanefield M. Acarbose efficacy review. *Practical Diabetes* 1993; **10** (6): S21–7.

45 Spengler M. Acarbose safety review. *Practical Diabetes* 1993; **10** (6): S28–31.

46 Taylor R. Use of insulin in non-insulin-dependent diabetes. *Diabetes Rev* 1992; **1**: 9–11.

47 Sinclair AJ. Diabetes specialist nurse: how a specialist nurse can lighten the doctor's load. *Geriatr Med* 1988; **18**: 63–70.

48 Raskin P. Combination therapy in NIDDM. *N Engl J Med* 1992; **327**: 1453–4.

49 Pugh JA, Ramirez G, Wagner ML, *et al*. Is combination sulphonylurea and insulin therapy useful in NIDDM patients? A meta-analysis. *Diabetes Care* 1992; **15**: 953–9.

50 Yki-Jarvinen H, Kauppila M, Kujansuu E, *et al*. Comparison of insulin regimens in patients with non-insulin-dependent diabetes mellitus. *N Engl J Med* 1992; **327**: 1426–33.

51 Sinclair AJ. Is good diabetic control necessary in the elderly? *Modern Med* 1989; **3** (March) (Editorial).

9

Insulin Therapy

ANTHONY H. BARNETT

University Department of Medicine, Birmingham Heartlands Hospital,
Birmingham, UK

The isolation of insulin by Banting and Best in 1922 was the most important milestone in the history of diabetes mellitus[1]. Before this the diagnosis of diabetes for many meant a death sentence from slow starvation, dehydration, acidosis and coma with death often a merciful release. These patients had what we now call Type 1 or insulin-dependent diabetes. It was not until the mid-1950s that oral hypoglycaemic agents came on the scene. Prior to this insulin was the only therapy available, in addition to diet, for the management of the 80–85% of diabetics who have non-insulin-dependent or Type 2 diabetes. Insulin was therefore lifesaving for some diabetics and health preserving for many others.

Even with the advent of oral hypoglycaemics a substantial number of Type 2 diabetics will eventually have to go on to long-term insulin therapy, usually because of problems of control, often in association with symptoms such as tiredness, vulval pruritus, thirst and polyuria. It is now clear that initiation of insulin therapy, even in elderly Type 2 diabetics, is often too long delayed and patients have suffered as a result.

This chapter will consider insulin in the management of both Types 1 and 2 diabetes in elderly patients. This will include an appraisal of the aims of insulin treatment, description of suitable insulin regimens, the importance of patient education, monitoring, prevention of complications and hypo-glycaemia. Insulin delivery devices, such as 'pen' injectors will also be described.

Diabetes in Old Age. Edited by P. Finucane and A. J. Sinclair
© 1995 John Wiley & Sons Ltd

AIMS OF DIABETIC MANAGEMENT

These can be summarized as follows:

1. to keep the patient feeling well
2. to prevent long-term vascular complications
3. to preserve quality of life.

The quality of life issue has been much neglected, but should be a major consideration in the management of any chronic disease.

The therapeutic options available to help fulfil these aims for Type 2 diabetic patients include diet ± oral hypoglycaemic agents or diet + insulin. Dietary advice has been simplified in recent years with much less emphasis on 'portions' and 'exchanges'. Diet is the mainstay of treatment in the management of Type 2 diabetes and needs to be realistic. It is inappropriate to expect someone who has spent 70 years eating a particular range of food to make drastic changes in their eating habits. As already described the recommendations for 'healthy eating' for the whole population should be followed[2]. This means that the diet should be high in unrefined, high fibre carbohydrate (if possible based on 50% of calorie content) and fats should not contribute more than 35% of calories. If the patient is heavily symptomatic on diet alone or adequate control is not established after 2–3 months of dietary treatment then tablet therapy should be considered. The choice has historically been between sulphonylureas and biguanides. A number of other agents have also been introduced in recent years, e.g. Guar gum, because of its high fibre content, and Acarbose, an alpha-glucosidase inhibitor. The latter acts as an enzyme inhibitor reducing the breakdown of complex carbohydrates in the gut and therefore reducing their absorption.

For the elderly, most physicians start with a short-acting sulphonylurea, such as gliclazide, glipizide or tolbutamide, at the manufacturers' lowest recommended dose. These drugs are thought to act by stimulating insulin release from the pancreatic beta cell[3] and perhaps by increasing insulin receptor binding sites[4], decreasing gluconeogenesis and prostaglandin inhibition. Their principal action in the first few months is by promoting insulin release and they cannot work without functioning beta cells. They are efficacious in most Type 2 diabetics, particularly those recently diagnosed and their main side-effect is hypoglycaemia, which can occasionally be profound and dangerous. Significant morbidity and mortality has been reported, particularly with the longer acting drugs[5,6]. These longer acting agents are best avoided in the over 60 age group. Gliclazide and glipizide may be preferable to tolbutamide as short-acting agents as they can be prescribed in a once daily dosage, whereas the latter usually needs to be given three times per day.

Metformin is the only biguanide in therapeutic use. Its action is not dependent on functional beta cells. It may increase glucose uptake by peripheral tissues and increase insulin sensitivity, and possibly impairs glucose absorption and decreases hepatic gluconeogenesis[7,8]. Side-effects are common, e.g. gastrointestinal disturbance, diarrhoea, anorexia, dyspepsia, metallic taste in the mouth, malaise. They do not cause hypoglycaemia and may have an appetite suppressant effect. Potency is limited but they can be used as a first-line drug in those who are grossly obese. It is otherwise used as a second-line agent in combination with a sulphonylurea. The only serious side-effect of metformin is lactic acidosis, which is very rare but has a high mortality[9]. It is normally only seen in association with significant hepatic or renal impairment. For this reason some specialists do not use this drug in the elderly population, although others prescribe it freely even in the over 70 age group.

The only therapeutic option for Type 1 diabetes is diet plus insulin, which is also an option for many Type 2 diabetics in certain circumstances.

AIMS OF INSULIN TREATMENT

The term juvenile-onset diabetes has long since been replaced by the much better and more accurate term Type 1 or insulin-dependent diabetes. Type 1 diabetes can and does occur at any age, although it is more common in younger age groups. In addition, there are large numbers of Type 1 diabetics diagnosed in youth who survive long enough to draw their pensions! Thus, although the great majority of elderly diabetics are Type 2 it is certainly not safe to assume that they all are. The major aim of insulin treatment in elderly Type 1 diabetics is to preserve life and prevent ketoacidosis.

Other aims which apply equally to Types 1 and 2 diabetes are to keep the patient feeling fit and well, to prevent of long-term vascular complications and to preserve quality of life. The aims of insulin treatment are, therefore, exactly the same as the aims of modern diabetic management.

INDICATIONS FOR INSULIN THERAPY

For Type 1 diabetes the indication is clear. Without insulin they will develop ketoacidosis and die. The diagnosis of Type 1 diabetes should be suspected even in an elderly patient where there is an acute onset of diabetic symptoms and the presence of non-fasting ketonuria often in association with significant weight loss. Insulin should be commenced immediately in a twice daily subcutaneous dosage. Indeed, if the patient is acutely sick with nausea or vomiting or in frank ketoacidosis he/she needs emergency hospital admission for intravenous rehydration and continuous insulin infusion (Figure 9.1).

The indications for insulin treatment in Type 2 diabetes are less clear-cut. Most Type 2 diabetics will be adequately controlled on diet, with or without oral hypoglycaemics, for several years, but eventually about half will have to go on to insulin. Table 9.1 outlines the principal indications for insulin therapy in Type 2 disease. Clearly, during acute situations such as serious infection, myocardial infarction, and in the perioperative period, diabetic control may be easily lost and insulin treatment should be instituted. These patients will normally be admitted immediately to hospital and insulin commenced as part of the management of their acute disease.

More controversial is whether insulin will help prevent or retard the long-term vascular complications of the disease (which in this context includes neuropathy). There is a wealth of circumstantial data (reviewed in reference 10) and more recently by data from prospective studies[11-14], which suggest that good glycaemic control will significantly reduce the risks of retinopathy, nephropathy and neuropathy. More recently still the Diabetes Control and Complications Trial (DCCT) has provided firm evidence to support these studies[15]. Glycaemic control is not, however, the

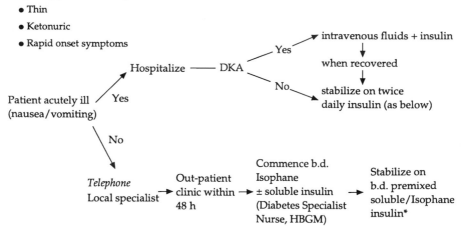

Figure 9.1. Guidelines on insulin treatment for newly diagnosed Type 1 diabetes. DKA, diabetic ketoacidosis; HBGM, home blood glucose monitoring. *Examples include Humulin M3 (Eli Lilly) and Mixtard (Novo/Nordisk). Both contain premixed 70% Isophane and 30% soluble insulins. Various other mixtures for syringes and pens are also available

Table 9.1. Indications for insulin treatment in Type 2 diabetic patients

---

Acute situations, e.g. serious infection, myocardial infarction, surgical operations

Prevention and treatment of long-term vascular complications

Poor control ± symptoms

---

whole answer and those of us who run diabetic clinics will be aware of patients who have survived for many years without any significant clinical evidence of vascular complications, whereas others have developed serious and debilitating vascular disease within say 10 years of diagnosis without any obvious difference in diabetic control[16]. Despite this, there is an excellent argument for trying to achieve as good control as is realistic in order to help prevent or retard development of complications. This view is relevant even in the elderly population. Substantial numbers now live long enough to have a high likelihood of complications developing!

There is little evidence that once severe complications are established, that improving control has a major effect on disease outcome. Insulin treatment is, however, often of symptomatic benefit where the patient has symptoms of acute diabetic neuritis. This may present as shooting pains down the legs, burning feet and weakness and wasting in the leg muscles (usually the quadriceps)[17].

The third relative indication for insulin treatment is the large group of Type 2 diabetics who have persistent poor control sometimes in association with the classical symptoms of diabetes. Many of these patients, however, have poor control but deny symptoms. Careful questioning, however, often reveals that they have 'hyperglycaemic malaise'[18].

THE SYNDROME OF 'HYPERGLYCAEMIC MALAISE'

Many Type 2 diabetics have poor control based on biochemical testing. A high proportion of these patients may deny typical symptoms of thirst or polyuria, but will admit to tiredness, malaise and reduced well-being. In a recent study 15 elderly 'asymptomatic' oral hypoglycaemic treated Type 2 diabetics with fasting blood glucose >9 mmol/l agreed to try insulin[19]. This resulted in an improvement in blood glucose and glycated haemoglobin (Hb A$_1$) over several months. By 8 months all patients were reporting a marked improvement in well-being and when given the opportunity only two wanted to resume tablets. The author concluded that so-called 'asymptomatic' hyperglycaemia, particularly in elderly patients, is often associated with reduced well-being and a trial of insulin is reasonable and often beneficial.

ARGUMENTS AGAINST INSULIN TREATMENT FOR TYPE 2 DIABETES

These include statements such as:

1. 'Obese patients do not notice significant improvement in control with insulin treatment'. Although this is the case in a proportion of obese patients many actually feel better on insulin therapy[19,20].

2. 'Patients are frightened of injections'. Fear of injections is usually easily overcome with careful counselling, particularly from the diabetes specialist nurse.

3. 'Hypoglycaemia may be precipitated and can be dangerous'. This is perhaps the most serious objection to insulin treatment, particularly in elderly patients. Dangerous hypoglycaemia, however, is relatively rare in Type 2 diabetics taking insulin particularly since in most cases targets for control are less stringent than in young Type 1 diabetics. In addition, it is worth remembering that sulphonylureas can also cause severe and devastating hypoglycaemia[5].

4. 'Insulin therapy may exacerbate insulin resistance'. This may be incorrect since enhanced insulin sensitivity is common after a period of insulin treatment[21].

5. 'Hyperinsulinaemia may cause accelerated atherogenesis and even hypertension'. Although this is a theoretical possibility there is no clinical evidence to support it. The author's view is that the reality of poor diabetic control causing ill health and perhaps accelerating the complications of diabetes outweighs these theoretical risks.

All of the above points used as an argument against insulin treatment for Type 2 diabetes apply equally and some more profoundly in elderly patients. The most serious danger is hypoglycaemia but dangerous hypoglycaemia in the elderly is in my experience relatively rare, particularly since in most cases targets for control are less stringent than in young Type 1 diabetics. The point about sulphonylureas causing severe and devastating hypoglycaemia should also be borne in more. Difficulties in administration of insulin, e.g. because of arthritis etc., are important and clearly each case needs to be examined on its own merits. The advent of insulin pens has got over this problem in a proportion of these patients.

INSULIN MANAGEMENT REGIMENS IN DIABETES MELLITUS

TYPE 1 (INSULIN-DEPENDENT) DIABETES

Patients with Type 1 diabetes either newly diagnosed (rare in this age group) or established should normally be on twice daily insulin. This is achieved by either the patient self-mixing a quick acting (soluble) and an intermediate acting (usually Isophane) insulin twice daily or using a fixed mixture of soluble and Isophane insulin twice daily. For fixed mixtures insulin can either be administered by a standard needle and syringe or by using an insulin 'pen' (see later).

For elderly Type 1 diabetic patients a fixed mixture of insulin is easier and given the wide range of fixed mixtures available will usually provide just as good control as self-mixed insulins.

Standard insulin regimens are outlined (Figure 9.1) for patients during acute illness and also for day to day management. As a general rule, about two-thirds of the total daily insulin dose is given in the morning and one-third in the evening. The most commonly used fixed mixtures consist of 70% Isophane and 30% soluble insulin (Humulin M3, Lilly Industries UK or Mixtard, Novo/Nordisk UK). The dose has to be tailored to the requirements of the patient. There are now available fixed mixtures of insulins in different proportions varying from 90% Isophane/10% soluble to 50% Isophane/50% soluble.

INSULINS FOR TYPE 2 DIABETES

As already mentioned approximately 50% of Type 2 diabetics will need to go on to insulin for long-term glycaemic control (Figure 9.2). Health professionals have in the past been reluctant to advise insulin for Type 2 diabetes largely because of the mistaken belief that they are 'preserving' the patient's quality of life by withholding injections. Undoubtedly, however, many patient's feel better on insulin and even the elderly generally cope well[19,20]. The diabetes specialist nurse can have a major role in initiation of insulin therapy and indeed the British Diabetic Association Guidelines indicate that all hospital diabetic clinics should have at least one such person attached to them with a significant percentage of their time also spent in the community. If these nurses are used effectively most patients, even the elderly, can be started on insulin in the community. This may mean fairly frequent visits to the patient's home and usage of the district nurse services at least for some days or occasionally for some weeks. In the author's experience it is rarely necessary to admit patients to hospital purely for the reason of starting them on insulin, although where

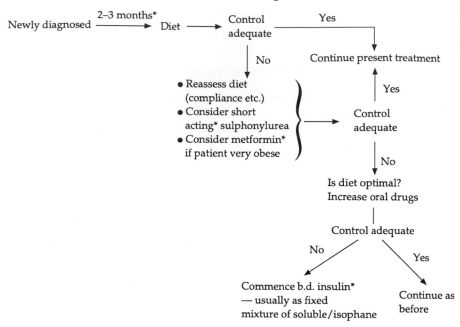

Figure 9.2. Guidelines on insulin treatment for Type 2 diabetic patients. *See text for clarification, and additional information in Chapter 8.

sufficient community support services are not available this may be necessary, particularly for more debilitated patients.

For Type 2 diabetic patients who require insulin it is normally given as twice daily Isophane or a twice daily fixed mixture (e.g. b.d. Humulin M3 or Mixtard). Twice daily Isophane may suffice since these patients still have some endogenous insulin secretion. In addition, many patients will not require the same level of fine control as younger Type 1 diabetic patients.

In the past it was common practice to advise twice daily insulin for Type 1 diabetics and once daily long-acting insulin for Type 2 patients. Single daily injections of insulin are, however, inappropriate for most patients as glycaemic control is unpredictable. This may result in wide swings in blood glucose and increased susceptibility to hypoglycaemia. In certain situations, however, it is much more practical to prescribe once daily insulin, e.g. in patients debilitated from dementia or with serious chronic disease where strict control is unnecessary and it would not be feasible for community nurses to go in twice daily to administer the insulin. Provided the drawbacks to once daily insulin are appreciated this is a perfectly reasonable approach for a small minority of Type 2 diabetic patients.

COMBINED INSULIN AND SULPHONYLUREA THERAPY

This regimen is popular in some European countries, but is not commonly used in the UK. A possible advantage of combined therapy is that endogenous insulin production is enhanced by sulphonylureas and therefore less exogenous insulin is required with (perhaps) better glycaemic control[22]. In practice, most clinicians in the UK perceive little benefit from combined therapy, but possible risks from using yet another (potentially harmful) drug.

INSULIN SPECIES

Over the years available insulins have become much purer with improved production technology. In addition, there has been a move away from the original beef-derived insulin in western Europe and the United States to highly purified pork and more recently human insulin. The human insulin is either manufactured using recombinant DNA technology or by synthesis from porcine insulin.

Human insulin is identical in structure to endogenously produced human insulin. It therefore came as a surprise when largely anecdotal reports appeared in the literature associating loss of awareness of symptoms of hypoglycaemia to the change from pork to human insulin. Several well controlled clinical trials have failed to support these data[23-25]. Reduced awareness of hypoglycaemia is, in fact, common in long-standing diabetics for reasons that are not entirely clear. Where a patient feels, however, that the human insulin is responsible for these problems then he/she should be given the opportunity to switch to pork insulin.

MONITORING OF GLYCAEMIC CONTROL AND PREVENTION OF HYPOGLYCAEMIA

One very important advance in diabetic management over the past two decades has been the 'patient centred approach'. There is now great emphasis on the patient being given sufficient information and help to manage his/her condition. The development of the role of the diabetes specialist nurse and the multidisciplinary approach to diabetes care have both been instrumental in supporting this objective. The availability of home blood glucose monitoring strips has also been a great advance. There are now several types of blood testing strips and blood glucose meters on the market. It is the author's opinion that meters are generally unnecessary for the majority of diabetic patients—visual readouts from properly used blood testing strips are just as useful in long-term management. There are of course exceptions to this, especially where the patient is colour blind or partially sighted.

The principal aims of home blood glucose monitoring include:

1. protection from hypoglycaemia;

2. assessment of the blood glucose profile over the full 24 h;

3. assessment of control during illness.

Protection from hypoglycaemia, particularly in elderly patients, is vital and monitoring enables them to discover for themselves the time of day when they are most susceptible. Measurement at bedtime in those prone to nocturnal hypoglycaemia is valuable and also before driving long distances. Assessment of control during acute illness is also important, particularly since many patients need increased doses of insulin because of the stress of the illness.

A standard regimen for home blood glucose monitoring in the elderly patients would include a full profile (before each meal and at bedtime) initially twice per week reducing to once per week once control is established. Additional testing may be required where there are concerns about hypoglycaemia. Such profiles are very useful for monitoring long-term control and reproducible profiles may be valuable in making sensible adjustments to insulin treatments.

Many patients find that home blood glucose monitoring gives them more control over their disease and in my experience most prefer doing blood tests to urine tests. Urine tests, of course, were the mainstay of monitoring for most elderly Type 2 diabetics until recently but, increasingly, these are being replaced by blood tests. The main problems with urine tests are that they only provide a rough correlation with blood glucose measurements, particularly in elderly patients where renal threshold tends to be high. Some of these patients may show absence of glycosuria even when blood glucose concentration is as high as 15 mmol/l! In addition, urine tests indicate what has been going on in the blood some hours too late!

For each individual patient, particularly the elderly, the level of glycaemic control aimed for must be realistic, taking into account many factors including the possible dangers of hypoglycaemia. For young Type 1 diabetic patients we may wish to try and achieve preprandial blood glucose readings between 4 and 7 mmol/l. In the elderly, a range of 6–10 mmol/l may be more acceptable and safer (and even this may have to be relaxed in certain patients).

In addition to home blood glucose monitoring as an aid to prevention of hypoglycaemia, patients also need to be educated about other ways to avoid this complication. The chances of hypoglycaemia may be reduced by avoidance of delayed meals, taking sufficient carbohydrate (including between meal snacks) and care with exercise. They also need to be aware of the typical symptoms of hypoglycaemia, e.g. shaking, trembling, sweats, anxiety, hunger, which may of course progress further to drowsiness, disorientation and eventually loss of consciousness. Relatives also need to be aware of these symptoms and to know what to do if they occur.

NEW INSULIN DELIVERY DEVICES

Insulin pumps which give soluble insulin by continuous subcutaneous insulin infusion were hailed as a great technical advance in the late 1970s and early 1980s. Their use has fallen greatly because of reports of pump failure, increased incidence of ketoacidosis and hypoglycaemia and occasionally death. They were really marketed for the management of Type 1 diabetics, particularly younger patients, and also for those with problems of control. They are not, at present, a serious option for the management of diabetes in elderly patients.

More recently the insulin 'pen' has improved quality of life for many Type 1 and Type 2 diabetic patients[26,27]. The earliest pen-shaped delivery device was introduced in 1981[28] and the first pen to gain wide acceptance was manufactured by Novo (Novo Pen I) and sold in 1984. At the same time insulin cartridges were developed, which could be loaded into the device in a similar way to loading a fountain pen. The 'pen' was initially marketed as part of a multiple injection regimen[29] giving soluble insulin before each meal by the 'pen' and a longer acting insulin by syringe at bedtime. Thus, it was mainly used for younger Type 1 diabetic patients.

Subsequently, pre-mixed insulins were produced in cartridge form for use in Novo Pen II (Figure 9.3). These had the particular advantage that they could be used in a twice daily dosage and for many patients could replace a standard syringe and needle for administration of fixed mixture insulins.

Other 'pens' have since come on the market. Recently, for example, Eli Lilly has in collaboration with Becton Dickinson produced the B-D pen (Figure 9.4). Both the Novo Pen II and B-D Pen are simple to load and can be operated singlehandedly. The patient simply sets the dose and gives it (Figure 9.5). The cartridge has to be changed every few days depending on the insulin dose.

A number of studies have been done to look at ease of use of the pen and quality of life issues compared with standard syringe and needle. We recently carried out a study of the B-D Pen, which uses Humulin (Eli Lilly) insulin cartridges[26]. The firm conclusion was that the device was

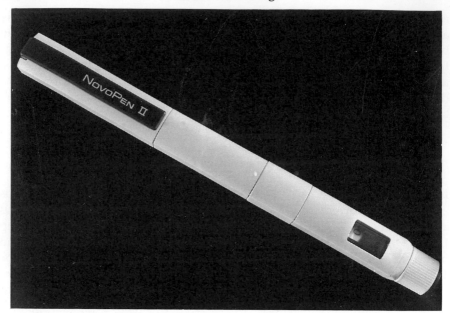

Figure 9.3. Illustrates Novo Pen II

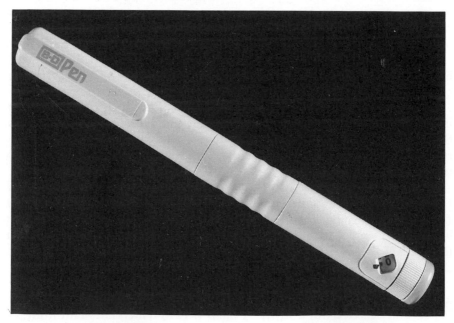

Figure 9.4. Illustrates B-D pen

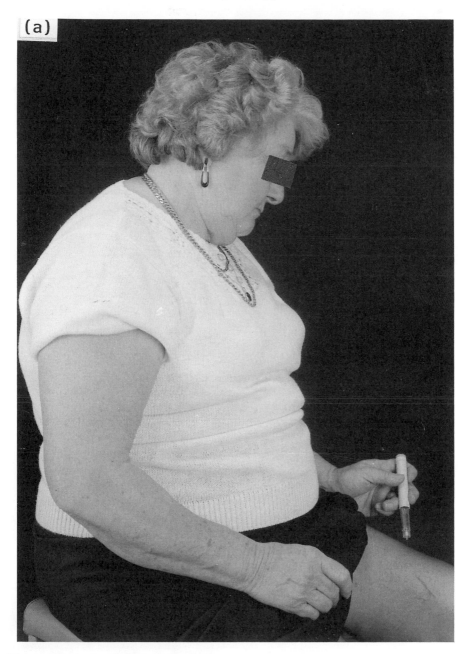

Figure 9.5. An insulin pen device in use

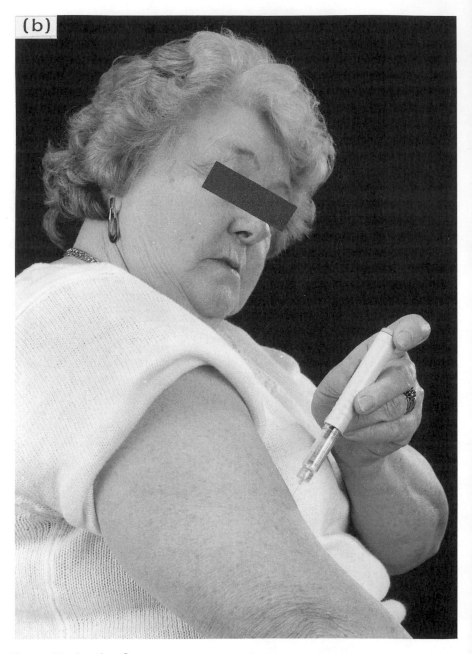

Figure 9.5. (*continued*)

easy to use by most Type 1 and Type 2 diabetics, including the elderly and was preferable to syringes and needles in over 90% of cases. Half of those studied noticed an improvement in quality of life and the rest no change.

'Pens' can also offer independence to those who are dependent on others to draw up their insulin, particularly those with impaired vision. The currently available 'pens' all have click dose mechanisms and the Novo Pen II has a touch sensor for those who have hearing difficulties. The 'pens' are also larger than disposable syringes, which may be an advantage for patients with chronic rheumatic disease such as rheumatoid arthritis. These patients may, however, need help to load new cartridges.

The 'pens' are generally easy to use and are preferred by the great majority of patients who have tried them. They do not suffer from the problems of insulin pumps and no serious problems have been reported with 'pen' injector delivery devices, presumably because mechanical failure is easily noted. It is important, however, that patients are given a back-up device or are taught to use a conventional syringe and needle in case of 'pen' failure.

The availability of 'pen' devices together with advances in patient education and monitoring and simplification of dietary regimens has improved quality of life of many diabetic patients. A wide range of 'pens' and insulin in cartridge form offers more freedom and convenience to a variety of patients, including the elderly.

SUMMARY AND CONCLUSIONS

Insulin is a vital therapy for Type 1 diabetes, but should also be seen as an appropriate therapeutic option in the management of Type 2 disease. Too many patients have suffered as the result of delay in initiation of insulin therapy. They have suffered through years of ill health and difficulty coping with day to day living. Most patients, including the elderly, manage well on insulin. The level of diabetic control should be towards the best standard that can be realistically achieved for each individual. There is no longer any barrier, if there ever was, to starting insulin therapy for most poorly controlled Type 2 diabetics. Indeed, most of these patients once started on insulin would not want to return to tablets! Insulin should be considered as part of a multidisciplinary approach to the provision of care for diabetic patients. The patient should be seen as the central figure, with vital input from other health care professionals, particularly the diabetes specialist nurse as well as the general practitioner, hospital specialists and dietitian. Insulin should always be considered as a serious option for poorly controlled diabetics whatever their age.

REFERENCES

1 Bliss M. *The Discovery of Insulin*. Edinburgh: Paul Harris Publishing, 1983.
2 Mann JI, Lewis-Barned NJ. Dietary management of diabetes mellitus in Europe and North America. In: Alberti KGMM, Defronzo RA, Keen H, Zimmet P (eds), *International Textbook of Diabetes Mellitus*. Chichester: John Wiley & Sons, 1992: 685–700.
3 Hosker JP, Burnett MA, Davies EG, Turner RC. Sulphonylurea therapy doubles beta-cell response to glucose in Type 2 diabetic patients. *Diabetologia* 1985; **28**: 809–14.
4 Feinglos MN, Leboritz HE. Sulphonylureas increase the number of insulin receptors. *Nature* 1978; **275**: 184–5.
5 Asplund K, Wilholm B, Lithner F. Glibenclamide associated hypoglycaemia: a report on 57 cases. *Diabetologia* 1983; **24**: 412–17.
6 Campbell IW. Metformin and the sulphonylureas: the comparative risks. *Horm Metab Res* 1985; **15** (Suppl.): 105–11.
7 Prager R, Schernthaner G, Graf H. Effect of metformin on peripheral insulin sensitivity in non-insulin dependent diabetes mellitus. *Diabetes Metab* 1986; **12**: 346–50.
8 Gawler DJ, Milligan G, Houslay MD. Treatment of streptozotocin diabetic rats with metformin restores the ability of insulin to inhibit adenylate cyclase activity. *Biochem J* 1988; **249**: 537–42.
9 Ryder RE. Lactic acidosis: high dose or low-dose bicarbonate therapy. *Diabetes Care* 1984; **7**: 99–102.
10 Tchrobroutsky G. Relation of diabetic control to development of microvascular complications. *Diabetologia* 1978; **15**: 143–52.
11 Lauritzen T, Larsen HW, Deckert T, Steno Study Group. Two years experience with continuous subcutaneous insulin infusion in relation to retinopathy and neuropathy. *Diabetes* 1985; **34** (Suppl. 3): 74–9.
12 The Kroc Collaborative Study Group. Diabetic retinopathy after two years of intensified insulin treatment. *JAMA* 1988; **260**: 37–41.
13 Brinchmann-Hansen O, Dahl-Jorgensen K, Sandrik L, Hanssen KF. Blood glucose concentrations and progression of diabetic retinopathy: the seven years results of the Oslo Study. *Brit Med J* 1992; **304**: 19–22.
14 Reichard P, Berglund B, Britz A, Cars I, Nilsson BY, Rosenqvist U. Intensified conventional insulin retards the microvascular complications of insulin-dependent diabetes (IDDM): the Stockholm Diabetes Intervention Study (SDIS) after 5 years. *J Intern Med* 1991; **230**: 101–8.
15 Diabetes Control and Complications Trial Research Group. The effect of intensive treatment of diabetes on the development and progression of long-term complications in insulin-dependent diabetes mellitus. *N Engl J Med* 1993; **329**: 977–86.
16 Barnett AH, Pyke DA. The genetics of diabetic complications. *Clin Endocrinol Metab* 1986; **15**: 715–26.
17 Ward JD. Clinical aspects of diabetic somatic neuropathy. In: Pickup J, Williams G (eds), *Textbook of Diabetes*. London: Blackwell Scientific Publications, 1991: 623–34.
18 Taylor R. Use of insulin in non-insulin dependent diabetes. *Diabetes Rev* 1992; **1**: 9–11.
19 Berger W. Insulin therapy in the elderly Type 2 diabetic patient. *Diabetes Res Clin Prac* 1988; (Suppl.): 24–8.

20 Peacock I, Tattersall RB. The difficult choice of treatment for poorly controlled maturity onset diabetes: tablets or insulin? *Br Med J* 1984; **288**: 1956–9.

21 Genuth S. Insulin use in NIDDM. *Diabetes Care* 1990; **13**: 1240–64.

22 Holman RR, Steemson J, Turner RC. Sulphonylurea failure in Type 2 diabetes: Treatment with a basal insulin supplement. *Diabetic Med* 1987; **4**: 457–62.

23 Patrick AW, Bodmer CW, Tieszen KL, White MC, Williams G. Human insulin and awareness of acute hypoglycaemic symptoms in insulin dependent diabetes. *Lancet* 1991; **338**: 528–32.

24 Colagiuri S, Miller JJ, Petocz P. Double-blind cross over comparison of human and porcine insulins in patients reporting lack of hypoglycaemic awareness. *Lancet* 1992; **339**: 1432–5.

25 Editorial. Hypoglycaemia and human insulin. *Drug Ther Bull* 1993; **31** (2): 7–8.

26 Rowe BR, Pizzey M, Barnett AH. A clinical evaluation of the B-D (Becton–Dickinson) pen as a delivery device for human insulin. *Practical Diabetes* 1992; **9**: 138–9.

27 Rowe BR. Insulin pen delivery systems. *Diabetes Rev* 1992; **1**: 2–4.

28 Paton JS, Wilson M, Ireland JT, *et al.* Convenient pocket insulin syringe. *Lancet* 1981; **1**: 189–90.

29 Jefferson IG, Marteau TM, Smith MA. A multiple injection regimen using an insulin injection pen and pre-filled cartridged soluble human insulin in adolescents with diabetes. *Diabetologia* 1985; **2**: 493–7.

10

Managing Surgery in the Elderly Diabetic Patient

GEOFFREY V. GILL

The Diabetes Centre, Walton Hospital and Department of Medicine, University of Liverpool, Liverpool, UK

INTRODUCTION

During their lifetime, most patients with diabetes will require some form of surgery, and the likelihood increases as age advances. Nowadays a considerable amount of major surgery is undertaken in the elderly (e.g. coronary artery bypass grafts, peripheral vascular and aneurysm surgery, removal of malignancies, etc.), of whom more are proportionately likely to have diabetes than at earlier stages of their lives. Though carefully planned and executed surgery is highly successful in the elderly, such patients with diabetes may tolerate metabolic and infective complications less well than younger subjects. Diabetes *per se* should never be a reason to decide *not* to operate on an elderly patient, but it *is* a reason for careful planning and management—both pre-, peri- and postoperatively. In this chapter we will examine the potential problems, the basis of current management systems, and practical methods of treatment.

METABOLIC AND OTHER PROBLEMS INDUCED BY SURGERY

Anxiety, anaesthetic drugs and possibly the underlying disease requiring surgery; may all contribute to metabolic destabilization in the diabetic surgical patient. The most important factors, however, are starvation and

Diabetes in Old Age. Edited by P. Finucane and A. J. Sinclair
© 1995 John Wiley & Sons Ltd

the pathophysiological metabolic and humoral response to trauma. All but the most minor of operations involve some interruption of normal food intake, and this may not infrequently last for several days. This poses obvious practical difficulties for diabetic patients whose tablets or insulin injections must be accompanied by food. Of more sinister note, however, is that starvation leads to catabolism, and in the presence of insulin deficiency (i.e. the diabetic state), ketosis becomes likely and eventually inevitable[1,2].

Such problems are greatly increased by the well-known humoral and metabolic changes associated with trauma, which also greatly enhance catabolism. Surgical trauma disturbs the usual fine balance between

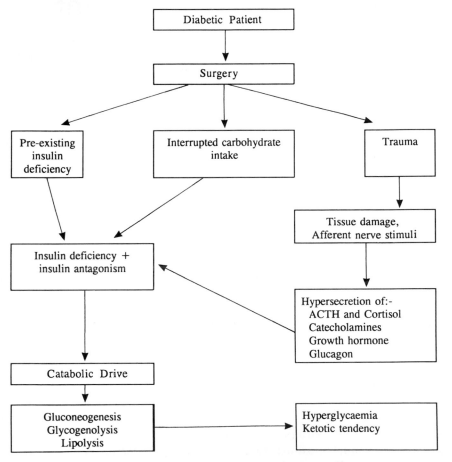

Figure 10.1. Diagram outlining the hormonal and metabolic effects of surgery in the diabetic patient

anabolism (effectively controlled only by insulin) and catabolism (driven by a variety of hormones—notably cortisol, catecholamines, growth hormone and glucagon). These latter hormones are often collectively known as the 'stress' or 'counter-regulatory' hormones, and they are hypersecreted in traumatic states. Cortisol and adrenaline levels in particular rise promptly (within minutes or hours after the initiation of trauma) and often massively (to some extent in proportion to the degree of trauma). In addition insulin secretion is relatively reduced, and a state of insulin resistance ensues[1-3]. Many of these changes are neurally mediated via afferent nerves from the injured tissue (cortisol for example is secreted secondarily to adrenocorticotrophic hormone release)[4]. The result of these changes are a massive catabolic drive (see Figure 10.1), with increased gluconeogenesis and glycogenolysis leading to glucose release into the circulation. Lipolysis and protein breakdown also occur, though in the non-diabetic, even small amounts of insulin ('basal') secretion are sufficient to contain dangerous hyperglycaemia and lipolysis. This of course is not true in the insulin-deficient or diabetic state. The danger of this metabolic scenario to the diabetic depends on its degree (as previously mentioned roughly proportional to the severity of trauma), and to the level of insulin reserves available.

IMPLICATIONS FOR MANAGEMENT

These basic principles can be translated logically into principles of management for diabetic patients undergoing surgery[5]. The major requirement is to ensure adequate insulinization; and the important variables are the degree of surgical trauma and the individual level of endogenous insulin reserves. Practically, patients can be divided into those on insulin treatment and those on diet and/or oral hypoglycaemic agents (OHAs). The insulin-treated group may or may not be truly insulin-dependent (IDDM, Type 1 diabetes), but even if insulin-treated non-insulin-dependent diabetes (NIDDM) patients, they can be assumed to have little or no insulin reserves, to have been deemed to need such treatment. These patients need continuous exogenous insulin treatment for all types of surgery.

Those not on insulin, i.e. NIDDM (Type 2) must have at least limited insulin reserves, and for minor to moderate degrees of surgical trauma can usually be closely observed only. Major surgery, however, will require continuous insulin as for the first group above. These principles are summarized in Figure 10.2.

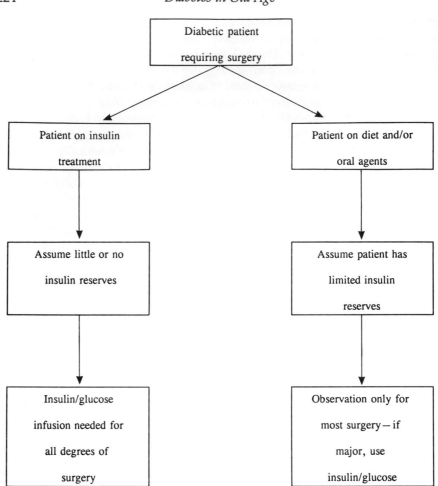

Figure 10.2. Schematic flow chart demonstrating the principles of managing diabetes during surgery

POTENTIAL RISKS OF SURGERY IN DIABETIC PATIENTS

There are surprisingly few studies on postoperative mortality and morbidity comparing diabetic with non-diabetic subjects. Diabetes was certainly considered to be a major risk factor for surgery in past decades. An American study in 1963 reported a 5% mortality postoperatively in a large (487) group of surgical diabetic patients—the major causes of death being ketoacidosis, infection and myocardial infarction[6]. It is likely, however, that methods of management were highly suboptimal compared with modern management principles. A recent study[7], using modern treatment methods, has shown no difference in mortality between diabetic and non-diabetic subjects (2.2% versus 2.7%, respectively).

Turning to morbidity, there is again no conclusive evidence that diabetes *per se* causes increased risk. Diabetics with pre-existing cardiac or renal problems may have increased morbidity, but not if relatively uncomplicated and properly managed[8,9]. Risk of postoperative infection also does not appear definitely increased, contrary to normally accepted clinical dogma[7,9]. In the Danish study of Hjortrup *et al.* for example[7], the wound infection rate was identical among diabetics (13 of 224 or 5.8%) and non-diabetics (12 of 224 or 5.4%).

Overall, critical assessment of the available literature does not support an increased risk for diabetic patients undergoing surgery, in terms of both mortality and postoperative complications.

SPECIAL PROBLEMS IN THE ELDERLY

Increased age is known to increase postoperative morbidity, and possibly mortality, in general. This includes diabetics, but again there is no convincing evidence in the literature that the effect is significantly greater among such patients. In general, however, diabetic surgical patients are frequently older and 'sicker' than their non-diabetic counterparts[9] (e.g. amputees, coronary bypass surgery, etc.), but when these factors are taken into account, any increased morbidity among diabetics becomes insignificant or much less significant.

Later, we will be discussing potential iatrogenic complications of diabetes management during surgery. Elderly diabetics tolerate hypoglycaemia poorly[10], and are less efficient at maintaining water homeostasis than their younger counterparts[11], increasing the risk of fluid and electrolyte imbalance in the postoperative period.

PRACTICAL MANAGEMENT

AIMS OF TREATMENT

Obvious aims of treatment are avoidance of excess mortality and morbidity. As discussed above, with modern management there should nowadays be little or no excess mortality or post-surgical infection risk. Ideally, the period of hospitalization should not be unduly prolonged, though admission a day or two earlier than usual is often required (see later).

Postoperative ketoacidosis should no longer occur, but hypoglycaemia is always a risk with intravenous insulin delivery. Avoidance of hypoglycaemia is very important—the surgical patient may be unable to perceive or report hypoglycaemia, and low blood glucose (BG) levels may therefore be allowed to become profound and serious before detection and treatment. Additionally, there is no evidence that overzealous attempts at achieving normoglycaemia are of benefit in the surgical situation. Indeed, paradoxically Hjortrup and colleagues[7] found that patients with particularly 'good' control appeared to be at greater risk of postoperative complications.

Glycaemic aims should therefore be to avoid hypoglycaemia at all costs, but in addition to not allow excessive hyperglycaemia or to risk ketoacidosis. In numerical terms, blood glucose levels in the region of 6.0–12.0 mmol/l would be a reasonable compromise target.

PREOPERATIVE ASSESSMENT

Preoperative assessment of the elderly diabetic is aimed at checking general fitness for surgery, ensuring that diabetic management is appropriate, and that glycaemic control is reasonable. By 'inappropriate' management is meant potentially hazardous drugs such as the potent and/or long-acting sulphonylureas glibenclamide and chlorpropamide. Regrettably, a number of older diabetics remain on such preparations and treatment may need to be updated prior to surgery. There are theoretical reasons for avoiding metformin also if possible[12].

Assessment of glycaemic control should be by 'bedside' BG monitoring with reagent strips, but the potential inaccuracies of such measurement need to be borne in mind[13], and occasional laboratory BG levels should be checked, and if possible a preoperative glycosylated haemoglobin (Hb A_1). As previously mentioned, 'excellent control' is not necessary, but significant hyperglycaemia (e.g. consistently >10.0 mmol/l) needs action. This may involve moving patients from diet to sulphonylureas, increasing tablet doses if already on oral agents, or perhaps introducing insulin on a temporary basis. If the latter step is required, thrice daily short-acting insulin (e.g. Actrapid, Humulin S), or twice-daily 30/70 premixes (e.g. Humulin M_3, Actraphane, Mixtard) are usually suitable. Such patients will of course need preoperative treatment for 'insulin-requiring' diabetes.

Other preoperative assessment in the elderly should include checking for autonomic neuropathy. This can be done by simple electrocardiographic tests (e.g. R–R ratio standing and lying—the '30:15 ratio'; or during deep breathing)[14]. This is important because autonomic neuropathy (which is more common in the elderly) is associated with sudden perioperative death[15] and also increased intraoperative morbidity[16]. Anaesthetists need to be aware of such information, so that patients can have close cardiac monitoring.

It can be appreciated that much of the standard preoperative assessment can be done prior to admission, either by liaison with the patient's physician or at a pre-admission anaesthetic clinic. Though this has been advocated for many years[5], regrettably it rarely occurs, and patients continue to need admission at least a day or two earlier than usual. Moreover, surgery may need to be further delayed if unforeseen problems are discovered following admission.

Finally, Table 10.1 gives a summary checklist for preoperative diabetic assessment. Note the important final step of liaising with the anaesthetist.

MANAGEMENT IN NIDDM

There is general agreement that diabetic patients *not* on insulin treatment, undergoing surgery of less than major severity, can be managed conservatively by observation only[1,17-20]. Surprisingly, there has been very little critical evaluation of this presumed optimal therapy, though what information that is available does support a conservative approach. Thus Thompson and colleagues[21] measured BG and metabolite responses to three groups of male patients undergoing transurethral surgery to the bladder or prostate gland. The groups were non-diabetics, NIDDM patients treated with intravenous glucose and insulin ('GKI infusion'[22]), and NIDDM patients treated conservatively. There was no significant difference between the two diabetic groups in terms of peri- and postoperative BG levels. Serum insulin and blood metabolite levels were actually closer to the non-diabetic group in the diabetics *not* treated with insulin. The authors concluded that 'GKI' in this situation induced an abnormal metabolic state with no overall glycaemic benefit. This study is of general importance, but is especially so for those caring for elderly diabetics requiring surgery. The

Table 10.1. Checklist for preoperative diabetic assessment

1. Assess as out-patient and/or admit 2–3 days earlier than usual.
2. Full medical assessment. Chest X-ray and electrocardiogram, electrolytes, serum creatinine, etc.
3. Full diabetic assessment. Four times daily bedside blood glucose levels, Hb A_1, autonomic function, etc.
4. Optimize diabetic management; avoid excessively long-acting hypoglycaemic agents.
5. Ensure reasonable glycaemic control.
6. Liaise closely with the anaesthetist.

patients studied had a mean age of about 65 years, and had NIDDM—by far the commonest type of diabetes in the elderly.

Guidelines for the conservative management of diabetes in surgery for NIDDM patients are shown in Table 10.2. It must again be emphasized that *major* surgery in NIDDM (e.g. opening the abdominal or thoracic cavity) should be treated as for insulin-treated patients. Note the importance of avoiding glucose-containing intravenous solutions, which can greatly destabilize glycaemic control. Lactate-containing fluids (e.g. Ringer lactate and Hartmann's) should also not be used as they can have hyperglycaemic effects[23]. Close BG monitoring is of course essential, and again liaison with the anaesthetist important (it is often in theatre that the dextrose or Ringer's drip is erected!). Surgery in the morning is advisable for all types of diabetes—there are no special metabolic reasons for this, but from a practical point of view it is much easier (and safer) to manage postoperative control problems in the afternoon rather than the middle of the night!

These simple management principles are successful in almost all NIDDM patients. Very rarely excessive postoperative hyperglycaemia may occur. This should be managed by subcutaneous short-acting insulin with meals; or if the patient cannot tolerate food, a 'GKI' infusion.

MANAGEMENT IN IDDM

In this section, the term 'IDDM' includes true insulin-dependent patients, patients with NIDDM on insulin treatment, and patients with NIDDM requiring temporary perioperative insulin because of poor glycaemic control or planned major surgery. Historically, a confusing number of systems have been advocated at various times; including early bizarre systems such as complete omission of insulin, or insulin with no subsequent glucose[12,24]. Not surprisingly, these systems did not work well! Later systems involved subcutaneous insulin with subsequent intravenous glucose infusions. Many such systems were complex, with widely varying

Table 10.2. Guidelines for surgical care in diabetics *not* on insulin treatment*

---

1. Operate in the morning if possible.
2. Frequently monitor bedside blood glucose levels (e.g. 2-hourly).
3. If on oral agents, omit on morning of surgery, and restart with first postoperative meal.
4. Avoid glucose and lactate-containing fluids intravenously.
5. Liaise with anaesthetist.

---

* Unless surgery is of major severity, or preoperative control poor—in which case GKI infusion is advisable.

types, amounts and proportions of insulin, and equally varied concentrations and rates of glucose infusion[11]. Results with such methods were variable, though in good hands they were comparable with more modern methods[25,26].

Subcutaneous methods of insulin delivery have, however, now been generally abandoned because they are awkward and inflexible. Continuous intravenous insulin and glucose delivery was introduced in the late 1970s[27], and became rapidly popular because of its flexibility and simplicity. There are two major methods of use.

The 'Separate-Line' System (see Figure 10.3)

Here, insulin is infused continuously via a syringe pump, with glucose infused separately (though the two separate lines can be 'piggy backed', e.g. via a 'Y connector' or 'traffic light'). The glucose infusion is usually 10% dextrose, delivered at a rate of 100 ml/h (10 g/h) via an electric drip counter. Insulin is usually delivered via a 50 ml syringe driver—50 units soluble insulin (e.g. Actrapid, Humulin S) in 50 ml 0.9% saline. Thus 1 ml/h

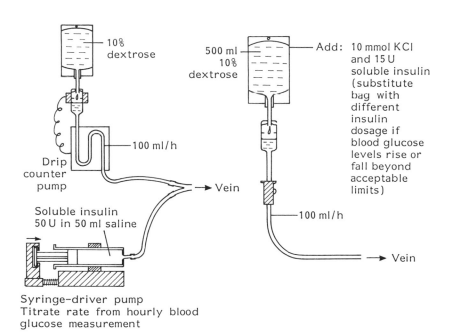

Figure 10.3. The 'separate line' (left) and 'GKI infusion' (right) systems of delivering intravenous insulin and glucose to diabetic patients undergoing surgery[26]. Reproduced by kind permission of Blackwell Scientific Publications Ltd

is equivalent to 1 unit/h. An average starting infusion rate is 3 units/h. The glucose infusion rate is kept constant throughout, and the insulin rate varied according to frequent (e.g. 1–2 hourly) bedside BG measurements, aiming to maintain BG levels in the range of 6–12 mmol/l.

It can be appreciated that this system is highly flexible and simple. However, it is very 'high tech', and requires expensive equipment, which may not always be available. There is also a potential for metabolic 'disaster' if one of the lines comes adrift—thus interruption of glucose will lead to dangerous hypoglycaemia and cessation of insulin will conversely lead to hyperglycaemia and possibly ketosis.

The 'GKI' Infusion (see Figure 10.3)

A simpler and more 'user-friendly' version of the above method is to combine glucose and insulin in the same infusion bag, and give them together. A small amount of potassium is added to avoid hypokalaemia— hence the term 'GKI' (glucose–KCl–insulin). Interestingly, this method was first advocated in 1963[6] by Galloway and Shuman, but did not become popular until redescribed by Alberti and Thomas[24] in 1977, and modified by the same group in 1982[22]. The present most widely used 'mix' is 500 ml in 10% dextrose with 15 units soluble insulin and 10 mmol KCl, delivered at 100 ml/h. This gives 3 units of insulin and 10 g glucose per hour, as does the 'separate-line' technique described above, but without the need for pumps and drip counters. Because the insulin and glucose are delivered together, the potential metabolic problems of rate alterations, line blockages, etc. do not exist. The main disadvantage of GKI is that if dose changes are needed, the whole bag has to be discarded and a fresh one made up and erected. In practice this only occurs in 10–20% of cases[22].

These methods of delivering glucose and insulin are shown in Figure 10.3. Of these two methods there is no right or wrong. Which is adopted in any particular hospital depends on facilities, equipment, staff and experience. Many hospitals use GKI in the general ward situation, and 'separate lines' in high dependency or intensive care situations. The GKI system certainly works well in practice and is supported by a study of 85 episodes of surgery using GKI, in which mean BG levels ranged from 8.3 to 10.2 during the operative and first two postoperative days[28]. Figure 10.4 shows a summary algorithm for the management of the surgical diabetic patient, including a suggested scheme for altering GKI infusions if necessary according to bedside BG monitoring. Note that electrolytes should be measured daily in patients on GKI infusion, in case hyponatraemia develops. Finally, it should be noted that both systems described here can be used with 5% dextrose if desired, halving the insulin dose delivered appropriately. Similarly, if infused volume needs to be reduced—as may be the case in elderly patients with cardiac problems—20% dextrose at

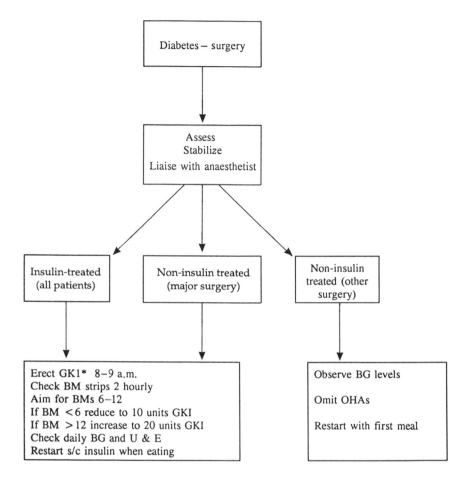

Figure 10.4. Summary chart for managing diabetes in surgery. *Standard GKI: 500 ml 10% dextrose + 15 units soluble + 10 mmol KCl infused at 100 ml/h

half the volume can be used, or a standard 10% GKI system used at 50 ml/h rather than 100 ml/h (this would be equivalent to a 5% dextrose system).

SPECIAL SURGICAL SITUATIONS

Emergency Surgery

Truly urgent surgery is fortunately relatively rare in diabetic patients, but it does occur, and is perhaps more common in the elderly: examples are peripheral and mesenteric embolization, ruptured aneurysms and trauma.

Urgent blood glucose, urea and electrolyte estimates are of course mandatory, and if the glycaemic and metabolic status is adverse it is best to correct this as far as possible prior to surgery. The urgency of the surgical situation will of course need to be assessed carefully in each case, and no 'blanket' rules can be made. Similarly, as regards the method of perioperative glycaemic control, this too has to be decided individually. Generally, a GKI system will be advisable in these unplanned situations, but the amounts of insulin needed cannot always be predicted. For example, if the patient requiring urgent surgery has had a sulphonylurea drug or insulin injection within the last 12 h, the amount of insulin in the GKI infusion may need to be reduced. Each situation needs to be judged individually and very frequent bedside BG monitoring is necessary. In many cases, it may be judged that a 'separate line' system of delivery may be indicated to give extra flexibility.

Open Heart Surgery

Cardiac surgery is now very common and coronary artery bypass grafting in particular is well established as a symptom-relieving and sometimes life-prolonging operation of low mortality. As such it is now being offered to many relatively elderly patients. Compared with other forms of surgery, coronary artery bypass grafting is unusual. It is a long and unusually traumatic operation and patients are also rendered hypothermic and later given large doses of inotropic agents after restoration of cardiac activity. All these factors will promote increased insulin demands. Additionally, however, it was traditional to use a dextrose 'priming solution' to fill the cardiopulmonary pump, often amounting to a glucose load of about 75 g at the start of surgery[29]. Not surprisingly, initial results using standard GKI systems in this situation were poor[29,30]. However, changing to a non-glucose priming solution greatly improved perioperative glycaemic control[30,31]. A 'separate line' system for glucose and insulin provision is essential, with frequent BG monitoring. Relatively large insulin doses are needed[32], but results are good and algorithms have been produced to aid insulin delivery decisions[33]. Using modern systems such as these, the results of open heart surgery in diabetics are comparable with non-diabetic counterparts[34,35], thus fulfilling the most important aims of diabetes management during surgery—acceptable glycaemic control by a simple and logical system without excess mortality or morbidity.

CONCLUSIONS

Though few centres are currently researching practical and theoretical aspects of the operative care of the diabetic patient, the subject continues to be a popular topic for review articles[36,37]. Perhaps this is not surprising. As a clinical problem it is very common, and though current management procedures are well accepted, their detailed application continues to cause confusion.

Safe and effective perioperative diabetic care requires the acceptance of hospital-based agreed protocols of care which must be widely distributed. Transferring these protocols to safe and effective patient treatment, depends on a team approach by physician, surgeon and anaesthetist.

REFERENCES

1 Allison SP, Tomlin PJ, Chamberlain MJ. Some effects of anaesthesia and surgery on carbohydrate and fat metabolism. *Br J Anaesth* 1979; **41**: 588–93.
2 Elliott MJ, Alberti KGMM. Carbohydrate metabolism—effects of preoperative starvation and trauma. *Clin Anaesthesiol* 1983; **1**: 527–50.
3 Nordenstrom J, Sannenfield J, Arner P. Characterization of insulin resistance after surgery. *Surgery* 1989; **105**: 28–35.
4 Hume DM, Egdahl RH. The importance of the brain in the endocrine response to injury. *Ann Surg* 1959; **150**: 697–712.
5 Gill GV, Alberti KGMM. Surgery and diabetes. *Hosp Update* 1989; **15**: 327–36.
6 Galloway JA, Shuman CR. Diabetes and surgery. *Am J Med* 1963; **34**: 177–91.
7 Hjortrup A, Sorenson C, Dynemose E, Hjortso NC, Kehlet H. Influence of diabetes mellitus an operative risk. *Br J Surg* 1985; **72**: 783–5.
8 MacKenzie CR, Charlson ME. Assessment of perioperative risk in the patient with diabetes mellitus. *Surg Gynaecol Obstet* 1988; **167**: 293–9.
9 Sandler RS, Maule WF, Baltus ME. Factors associated with post-operative complications in diabetics after biliary tract surgery. *Gastroenterology* 1986; **91**: 157–62.
10 Jennings AM, Wilson RM, Ward JD. Symptomatic hypoglycaemia in NIDDM patients treated with oral hypoglycaemic agents. *Diabetes Care* 1989; **12**: 203–8.
11 Faull CM, Holmes V, Baylis PH. Water balance in elderly people: is there a deficiency of vasopression? *Age Ageing* 1993; **22**: 114–20.
12 Gill GV, Alberti KGMM. The care of the diabetic patient during surgery. In: Alberti KGMM, De Fronzo RA, Keen H, Zimmet P (eds), *International Textbook of Diabetes Mellitus*. Chichester: John Wiley & Sons Ltd, 1992: 1173–83.
13 Hutchison ASA, Shenkin A. BM strips: how accurate are they in general wards? *Diabetic Medicine* 1984; **1**: 225–6.
14 Ewing DJ, Martyn CN, Young RJ, Clarke BF. The value of cardiovascular autonomic function: 10 years experience in diabetes. *Diabetes Care* 1985; **8**: 491–8.
15 Page MM, Watkins PJ. Cardiorespiratory arrest with diabetic autonomic neuropathy. *Lancet* 1978; **i**: 14–16.
16 Burgos LG, Ebert TJ, Asiddao C, *et al.* Increased intraoperative cardiovascular morbidity in diabetics with autonomic neuropathy. *Anaesthesiology* 1989; **70**: 591–7.
17 Podolsky S. Management of diabetes in the surgical patient. *Med Clin North Am* 1982; **66**: 1361–72.
18 Hirsch IB, McGill JB, Cryer PE, White PF. Perioperative management of surgical patients with diabetes mellitus. *Anaesthesiology* 1991; **74**: 346–59.
19 Alberti KGMM, Marshall SM. Diabetes and surgery. In: Alberti KGMM, Krall LP (eds), *The Diabetes Annual*. Amsterdam: Elsevier, 1988: 248–71.

20 Schade DS. Surgery and diabetes. *Med Clin of North Am* 1988; **72**: 1531–43.
21 Thompson J, Husband DJ, Thai AC, Alberti KGMM. Metabolic changes in the non-insulin dependent diabetic undergoing minor surgery: effect of glucose–insulin–potassium infusion. *Br J Surg* 1986; **73**: 301–4.
22 Alberti KGMM, Gill GV, Elliott MJ. Insulin delivery during surgery in the diabetic patient. *Diabetes Care* 1982; **5**: 65–77.
23 Thomas DJB, Alberti KGMM. The hyperglycaemic effects of Hartmann's solution in maturity-onset diabetes during surgery. *Br J Anaesth* 1978; **51**: 693–710.
24 Alberti KGMM, Thomas DJB. The management of diabetes during surgery. *Br J Anaesth* 1979; **51**: 603–710.
25 Thomas DJB, Platt HS, Alberti KGMM. Insulin-dependent diabetes during the peri-operative period. *Anaesthesia* 1984; **39**: 629–37.
26 Gill GV. Surgery and diabetes mellitus. In Pickup J, Williams G (eds), *Textbook of Diabetes*. London: Blackwell Scientific, 1991: 820–8.
27 Taitelman U, Reece EA, Bessman AN. Insulin in the management of the diabetic surgical patient. Continuous intravenous administration versus subcutaneous administration. *JAMA* 1977; **237**: 658–60.
28 Husband DJ, Thai AC, Alberti KGMM. Management of diabetes during surgery with glucose–insulin–potassium infusion. *Diabetic Med* 1986; **3**: 69–74.
29 Gill GV, Sherif IH, Alberti KGMM. Management of diabetes during open heart surgery. *Br J Surg* 1981; **68**: 171–2.
30 Stephens JW, Krause AH, Petersen CA, *et al.* The effect of glucose priming solutions in patients undergoing coronary artery bypass grafting. *Ann Thorac Surg* 1988; **45**: 544–7.
31 Crock PA, Ley CJ, Martin IK, *et al.* Humoral and metabolic changes during hypothermic coronary artery bypass surgery in diabetic and non-diabetic subjects. *Diabetic Med* 1988; **5**: 47–52.
32 Elliott MJ, Gill GV, Home PD, *et al.* A comparison of two regimens for the management of diabetes during open-heart surgery. *Anaesthesiology* 1984; **60**: 364–8.
33 Watson BG, Elliott MJ, Pay DA, *et al.* Diabetes mellitus and open heart surgery. A simple practical closed loop insulin infusion system for blood glucose control. *Anaesthesia* 1986; **41**: 250–7.
34 Lawrie GM, Morris GC, Glaeser DH. Influence of diabetes mellitus on the results of coronary bypass surgery. Follow-up of 212 diabetic patients 10 to 15 years after surgery. *JAMA* 1986; **256**: 2967–71.
35 Devinen R, McKenzie FN. Surgery for coronary artery disease in patients with diabetes mellitus. *Can J Surg* 1985; **28**: 367–70.
36 Hirsch IB, McGill JB, Cryer PE, White PF. Perioperative management of surgical patients with diabetes mellitus. *Anaesthesiology* 1991; **74**: 346–59.
37 Hughes TAT, Borsey DQ. The management of diabetic patients undergoing surgery. *Practical Diabetes* 1994; **11**: 7–10.

11

Rehabilitating the Elderly Diabetic Patient

PAUL FINUCANE

Flinders University of South Australia, Bedford Park, Adelaide, Australia

INTRODUCTION

Earlier chapters of this book have documented the catastrophic events which can complicate the course of diabetes mellitus. For anybody, the onset of either a stroke, a myocardial infarct, an ischaemic limb requiring amputation, or significant loss of vision is potentially devastating. The process of rehabilitation aims to minimize the consequences of such catastrophes. For people young or old, diabetic or otherwise, the principles of rehabilitation are broadly similar. However, special considerations arise when the patient happens to be elderly and diabetic, as problems tend to be complex and more difficult to address.

IMPAIRMENT, DISABILITY AND HANDICAP

An understanding of the terms impairment, disability and handicap greatly facilitates an appreciation of the process of rehabilitation. Impairment refers to a defect in an organ, i.e. a pathological process. Disability refers to the loss of function resulting from the impairment, and handicap to the social disadvantage resulting from the disability. Take for example, a woman with a thrombotic stroke resulting in hemiplegia. The impairment is the cerebral infarct, indirect evidence of which is found by neurological examination and more direct evidence by computerized tomography or

Diabetes in Old Age. Edited by P. Finucane and A. J. Sinclair
© 1995 John Wiley & Sons Ltd

magnetic resonance imaging scanning. Resulting disability may take the form of inability to perform activities of daily living because of a motor deficit, hemianopia and sensory inattention. Consequently, she may be handicapped, and unable to continue with her former pastimes of reading, golfing and playing the organ at church.

Every impairment has the potential to trigger the onset of disability and handicap. While many definitions of rehabilitation have been advanced, it can simply be regarded as a process which minimizes the disability and handicap resulting from impairment. To understand this process, it is essential to have an understanding of the determinants of disability and handicap.

FACTORS INFLUENCING THE DEVELOPMENT OF DISABILITY AND HANDICAP

It is remarkable how people with similar underlying impairments differ in the extent of their resulting disability and handicap. For example, some people are fully independent and have resumed a normal life-style within a few weeks of having an ischaemic leg amputated, while others are left permanently incapacitated, following months in hospital. Some of the major determinants of disability and handicap (summarized in Table 11.1)

Table 11.1. Factors influencing the extent of disability and handicap

---

The impairment
  Severity
  Site
  Reversibility
  Chronicity
Intrinsic patient factors
  Physical status
    coincidental pathology
    premorbid health
    physiological reserve
  Mental and psychological status
    mood
    ability to adjust
    motivation
Extrinsic patient factors
  Health care
  Social supports
    spouse/family/friends/pets
    housing
  Financial status

---

need to be recognized. In an individual patient, all these factors interact, and they should not therefore be considered as discrete.

THE IMPAIRMENT

It is a truism that the greater the severity of an impairment, the greater the likelihood of disability and handicap. The site of the impairment may also be important. For instance a small cerebral infarct involving the internal capsule may cause profound disability, while a much larger lesion involving a 'silent' region of the brain may go unnoticed. Some impairments may spontaneously resolve, be halted or be reversed by therapeutic intervention, while others inexorably progress. The chronicity of the impairment may also be important. For some people, long-standing impairment promotes familiarity and the development of adaptive skills, which limit disability. Thus the diabetic person with angina learns to avoid exercise likely to precipitate chest pain and/or use nitrate prophylaxis. In other situations, people become gradually worn down by continuing impairment, consequently fail to develop or lose adaptive skills and so become disabled and handicapped.

INTRINSIC PATIENT FACTORS

People with long-standing diabetes, irrespective of their chronological age, may well have a number of active impairments at any one time. Thus, retinopathy and nephropathy commonly coexist, and macrovascular disease may involve the coronary, cerebral and peripheral vasculature simultaneously. Furthermore, elderly patients, diabetic or otherwise, often have coincidental diseases which are not necessarily linked aetiologically. For example, a person with chronic chest disease may also have an arthropathy and prostatic hyperplasia.

The elderly diabetic patient tends to have the worst of both worlds, with multiple impairments both related and unrelated to diabetes. Thus, visual impairment may be as much a consequence of macular degeneration as diabetic retinopathy and autonomic neuropathy as much a consequence of Parkinson's disease as diabetes. The presence of multiple impairments is of particular importance in a rehabilitation setting where it can prevent the achievement of goals. Take for example, the patient recovering from a lower limb amputation whose exercise tolerance is limited by angina and/or chronic chest disease, or whose mobility is limited by osteoarthritis and/or peripheral neuropathy involving the remaining leg.

The physical status of the patient prior to the onset of the impairment therefore has a major impact on the extent of subsequent disability and handicap. Other things being equal, the person who was fit and active prior to onset of the impairment has a better prognosis than another with pre-existing disease. Unfortunately, the life-styles of many old people do not promote cardiorespiratory or neuromuscular fitness. In a Canadian study, for example, less than half of people with non-insulin-dependent diabetes mellitus (NIDDM) participated in any form of exercise programme, either formal or informal[1].

A decline in cardiorespiratory and neuromuscular function with ageing means that an older person with impairment is more likely to develop disability and handicap than a younger person with similar impairment[2]. This lack of 'physiological reserve' to meet the challenge of a new impairment was given undue emphasis in the past, leading to nihilistic and ageist attitudes in the area of rehabilitation as elsewhere. In practice, advanced chronological age *per se* is no barrier to successful rehabilitation.

As will be discussed later (cf. 'Psychological aspects of rehabilitation'), psychological factors have an enormous impact on the extent of disability and handicap resulting from impairment. Thus the person who rapidly comes to terms with an impairment, perceives it as a challenge rather than as a negative event and is well motivated, is likely to fare better than another with a different attitude.

EXTRINSIC PATIENT FACTORS

As discussed in Chapter 3, access to high quality health care can do much to prevent impairment. Even if impairment develops, medical intervention can retard the progression to disability and handicap. For example, vascular reconstructive surgery can reverse limb ischaemia and laser photocoagulation can retard the development of visual loss in diabetic retinopathy. As will later be explained, even when disability and handicap have resulted, a multidisciplinary rehabilitation team can work to restore function and social competence.

Reduced social supports are a particular problem for the elderly diabetic patient. In the UK, for example, over 50% of women and 25% of men aged over 65 years have no living spouse[3]. As a result, one-third of this age group and an even greater proportion of older groups live alone. The vast majority of such people live full and independent lives, even if they happen to be diabetic. However, for those who struggle to cope with illness, the physical and emotional support which a partner, family members or friends can provide is a major asset in preventing disability and handicap. The important role that pets play in the lives of some people should also be recognized. The author well remembers a woman who was making a good recovery following a major stroke. On learning that a well-meaning relative had had her dog put down following her admission to hospital, she lost motivation and died shortly after.

Financial resources or their lack can further determine the extent to which impairment results in disability and handicap. Access to personal care, and to appropriate housing and technology can be expensive and in all societies is influenced to some extent by one's ability to pay. Here again, elderly people are disadvantaged. In Australia, for example, 78% of older people are reliant on an age pension the equivalent of 25% of the average adult working wage, and 85% of pensioners are eligible for means-tested supplementary benefits[4].

COMMON CONDITIONS NECESSITATING REHABILITATION IN NIDDM

The chronic complications of diabetes (Table 11.2) have been described in Chapter 6. All of these impairments can result in significant disability and handicap. At a glance, it can be seen that some impairments can result in a number of disabilities, and that some disabilities can be due to a number of different impairments. Before going on to deal with some specific rehabilitation issues, some general points about rehabilitation should first be understood.

Table 11.2. Common impairments and resulting disabilities in people with NIDDM

Impairment	Disability
Neuropathy	
Peripheral	Impaired mobility
	Impaired manual dexterity
Autonomic	Impaired mobility
	Incontinence
	Impotence
Retinopathy	Visual impairment, blindness
Nephropathy	Reduced exercise tolerance
Coronary artery disease	Reduced exercise tolerance
Cerebrovascular disease	Communication problems
	Impaired cognition
	Visual problems
	Impaired mobility
	Incontinence
Peripheral vascular disease	Impaired mobility

REHABILITATION: SOME GENERAL POINTS

THE PROCESS

The principles of rehabilitation are broadly similar, irrespective of the problem with which one is dealing. An understanding of impairment, disability and handicap as explained above, helps to explain the process, and the need for a multidisciplinary team approach. A properly resourced rehabilitation team will have input from medical and nursing staff, physiotherapists, occupational therapists, speech pathologists, clinical psychologists and social workers. Diabetic patients in particular benefit from access to dietitians and podiatrists.

All rehabilitation programmes must be planned. The first step is to accurately assess the patient's current level of impairment, disability and handicap. Diagnostic skills and the appropriate use of investigative technology are required to define the impairment. A plethora of assessment scales are available to assess disability; the Barthel scale[5] is most widely used and despite its limitations, has stood the test of time. While several 'quality of life' scales have been devised, the extent of handicap has proved difficult to quantify due to their subjective nature. It is also important to formally assess cognitive function, even in patients who appear alert and orientated. At the very least this will establish a baseline, which may later prove useful. The 30-point Mini Mental Status Examination[6] has become popular, perhaps because it best combines sensitivity with ease of administration.

Following assessment, the second step is to identify goals and a time frame within which to achieve them. All team members must be involved in these initial steps and it is essential that consensus is achieved. Otherwise cohesion gives way to chaos. The patient is an important (though often forgotten) member of the team. It is crucial that he or she be involved in establishing goals, as any goal that is not shared by the patient is unlikely to be achieved. For goals to be realistic, the patient's level of function prior to the new impairment must be taken into account. As a general rule, it is unrealistic to aim for greater than the premorbid level of function, though there may be exceptions to this.

Having established goals, the combined talents of the team are brought to bear in meeting them. A detailed description of the skills used by individual team members when dealing with various impairments and disabilities is beyond the scope of this chapter and is well dealt with elsewhere[7]. Medical staff are mainly responsible for the identification and management of impairment. In a rehabilitation setting, they must focus on the current impairment, coincidental impairments, underlying risk factors and potential complications. Thus in a diabetic patient who has had a limb amputation, they may be called upon to supervise the wound, treat phantom limb pain, monitor diabetic control, and manage coexisting angina and hypertension.

Remedial therapists are best equipped to manage disability. Occupational therapists primarily assess problems encountered with activities of daily living and help the patient to devise strategies to overcome them. Physiotherapists plan and implement physical therapies which target specific problems, and enhance cardiorespiratory and neuromuscular function. Speech pathologists have particular expertise in the area of communication difficulties and swallowing disorders. For some patients, the main disability may be psychological rather than physical and input from a clinical psychologist can be invaluable in addressing this. Social workers have particular expertise in helping patients to deal with handicap, the social disadvantage resulting from disability. They can harness the support needed to maintain a disabled person in the community, as well as provide information, advice and practical help with financial and legal matters.

While multidisciplinary team members have discrete areas of expertise, it is essential that each also has a global perspective which spans impairment, disability and handicap. Each must understand what the other is doing. For example, the speech pathologist must have a knowledge of neuroanatomy and the medical practitioner must understand the need for home modifications and meals on wheels provision. Nurses are arguably the most holistic of the health professionals, as their role encompasses impairment, disability and handicap. In a hospital rehabilitation setting, they ensure continuity of patient care while other team members tend to be available only during 'office hours'. In this regard, they are the true linchpins of the rehabilitation process.

For such a disparate group to function cohesively, there must be effective communication. When team members are co-located in a specific area (e.g. a rehabilitation unit), exchange of information occurs regularly and informally. In addition, most teams have regular formal meetings to review the progress of individual patients and revise the rehabilitation goals. A leader or chairperson is required to ensure that all perspectives are aired and that consensus is reached. Team meeting should also be used for discharge planning and to organize follow-up following discharge from the unit.

WHEN TO REHABILITATE

To be most effective, rehabilitation should start as soon as possible, so as to prevent further impairment and minimize the risk of disability. This implies that the initial impairment can be compounded if managed inappropriately. Take for example, the patient with a flaccid hemiplegia and therefore at risk of shoulder subluxation. Inappropriate handling, as might occur when helping the patient to move in bed or to transfer to a chair can result in serious and persistent shoulder damage[8]. Such a problem is less likely to develop in a rehabilitation setting where staff are sensitized and trained in its prevention.

Selection of appropriate patients for rehabilitation is important and can sometimes be difficult. On the one hand it is unfair to subject a patient who will not benefit to a demanding rehabilitation programme and in the process to raise false expectations. This is also wasteful of resources. On the other hand, those who can benefit, even to a limited extent should not be denied access to rehabilitation. In certain situations, it is appropriate to set modest goals, such as helping a hemiplegic patient to regain sitting balance or an amputee patient to become wheelchair independent. The quality of the person's life can be greatly improved if such goals are achieved.

Patients are most likely to benefit from a rehabilitation programme if they are able to actively participate and if they are well motivated. For those who do not benefit, there is usually an identifiable reason, such as an overwhelming physical impairment, cognitive impairment, depression or a personality disorder. A small minority of patients simply lack the motivation to combat their impairment. As explained later, strategies exist to help such people.

WHERE TO REHABILITATE

This is largely determined by the nature and extent of the impairment. With some conditions, such as an uncomplicated myocardial infarction, only a few days of in-hospital treatment is required and an out-patient rehabilitation programme is most appropriate. Other impairments, such as major strokes and limb amputations generally require hospital-based rehabilitation, at least in the early stages. In large centres of population, rehabilitation of elderly diabetic patients is often carried out in units specializing in specific impairments. This has the advantage of allowing high levels of expertise to be developed together with complementary facilities such as workshops for artificial limbs and appliances. Having people with similar impairments in a single unit provides opportunities for patient education, the training of health professionals and for research. Specialized units have a role in setting standards of excellence and in the design, implementation and evaluation of new therapeutic tools and techniques. However, the principles of rehabilitation can be provided in any setting if staff with the necessary knowledge, skills and attitudes are available.

With the proliferation of geriatric day hospitals in the 1960s, much rehabilitation is now undertaken in an out-patient setting, often after an initial period of more intensive in-patient treatment. Alternative community-based or domiciliary-based rehabilitation programmes are increasingly being developed and may have some advantages over traditional day hospital programmes[9].

PSYCHOLOGICAL ASPECTS OF REHABILITATION

The onset of impairment is usually associated with some emotional disturbance, particularly if the event is catastrophic, e.g. a major stroke or loss of a limb. There may be a feeling of loss with regard to one's physical and/or mental faculties, to relationships with others or to inanimate objects such as one's home or other possessions. Normally, a grief reaction occurs, with phases of denial, anger and depression leading to a level of acceptance sufficient to allow a relatively normal life to be resumed. However, adjustment to impairment is sometimes abnormal. For example, 20% of people have severe and often persistent depression following acute myocardial infarction[10]. Several studies have documented high levels of psychosocial dysfunction in people following a stroke[11,12], even despite participation in a rehabilitation programme[9].

The manner in which people adapt to impairment greatly influences the development of disability and handicap. Some people seem to be inherently more adaptable than others in responding positively to an adverse situation. Such 'highly motivated' people are keen to participate in a rehabilitation programme, and work hard to achieve their goals. At the other end of the spectrum are those who appear to succumb to impairment, disengage, surrender power and autonomy and adopt a 'sick role'.

There are psychological theories to explain such different responses. An excellent model is proposed by Kemp[13] who explains motivation as a dynamic process, determined by four elements: the person's wants; beliefs; the rewards for achievement; and the costs to the patient. Thus if a person really wants something, believes it to be attainable and if attainment is likely to bring reward, they will strive to achieve it, provided the cost (in terms of pain and effort) is acceptable. On the other hand, a lack of achievement can occur of the goal is not strongly wanted, if the person believes that it cannot be attained, if there is little or no reward for attaining the goal or if the perceived cost of achievement is too high. By using this framework, the rehabilitationist can help individual patients in a number of ways.

First, a patient can be helped to identify wants or, in other words, to establish goals. In a rehabilitation setting, failure to achieve goals is often attributable to their being set by rehabilitationists without reference to the patient. The role of therapists is to ensure that the goals which patients set themselves are realistic; if goals are unrealistic, the patient should be encouraged to modify them. Secondly, the patient's beliefs should be explored and important misconceptions should be corrected. Thirdly, having established what goals are important to the patient, the rehabilitationist should ensure that he or she is appropriately rewarded when goals are achieved. Interim goals as well as final goals should be set and rewarded. For example, a patient who has regained a certain level of independence might have some weekend leave from hospital, the time spent at home increasing as new goals are met. When progress is gradual, patients will need to be reminded of their achievements. It is often useful to have concrete evidence of progress, as when a hemiplegic patient compares their current status with a video of themselves taken shortly after the onset of impairment. Finally, the patient's perception of the cost of rehabilitation needs to be explored, and any misconceptions should be addressed.

It follows that an understanding of individual patients is a prerequisite for successful rehabilitation. This can only be achieved by listening, not only to the people concerned, but to others who know them intimately. Health professionals should consistently demonstrate a positive approach to patients as well as to their progress at rehabilitation. Respecting patients as people fosters a sense of self-worth and among other things, further enhances motivation. While providing positive feedback is important, honesty and sincerity should never be compromised, and false expectations should not be generated.

By acting as a 'self-help group' or 'therapeutic community' patients on a rehabilitation unit can provide each other with support and encouragement. The rehabilitation team should endeavour to create an atmosphere conducive to this and should structure the ward and organize ward activities so as to promote camaraderie. On the other hand, relationships between patients are occasionally destructive and staff may need to intervene if the rehabilitation programme is to be salvaged. For example, sleeping and dining arrangements may need to be reviewed so that some people are kept apart.

It is worth while remembering that for many patients with diabetes, concerns about the future may be just as significant as concerns about the present. The onset of one disability may trigger justifiable apprehension of further loss in the future. Thus, the onset of angina pectoris may raise fears of a fatal myocardial infarct and calf claudication fears of limb amputation. Indeed anxieties about future morbidity and premature mortality can be an important source of 'dis-ease' in people with 'uncomplicated' diabetes. Again, listening to the patient is the key to identifying and addressing the problem. Unless concerns for the future surface spontaneously, they should be sought by direct questioning.

All members of the multidisciplinary rehabilitation team should at least have a basic understanding of the psychology of loss and motivation and some practical skills to overcome those problems that commonly surface. More complex problems may require input from a clinical psychologist and having access to such expertise is a valuable resource. Psychologists also have an educative role in helping other team members to understand their own feelings and behaviour. They can also help to resolve conflict, whether arising within or between patients, within or between team members or between patients and team members.

SPECIFIC REHABILITATION PROBLEMS IN DIABETIC PATIENTS

For reasons given earlier, rehabilitation problems seldom exist in isolation in the elderly diabetic patient. Thus, the person whose immediate concern is a lower limb amputation may also have a residual hemiparesis from a previous stroke, together with angina and visual impairment. Efforts to regain mobility can be influenced as much by the remote as the recent problems. It is therefore somewhat artificial to discuss specific problems as if they existed in isolation. In the clinical setting it is essential to have a holistic approach, particularly as attempts to relieve one problem may exacerbate another. Thus, mobilizing an amputee patient may provoke an acute myocardial infarct, while drug therapy for angina may exacerbate peripheral vascular disease, heart failure or renal failure. These considerations should be kept in mind when considering specific rehabilitation problems.

THE PATIENT WITH STROKE

For the person with diabetes, a stroke is undoubtedly the impairment with the greatest potential to cause disability and handicap. About half of stroke victims are dead within 6 months of onset and one-third of survivors have severe residual disability[14]. Motor and sensory deficits, gait disorders, cognitive deficits, visual field defects, communication disorders, dysphagia and incontinence are all potentially devastating and all too common sequelae. Some patients will have a number of these disabilities. A detailed description of the rehabilitation process following stroke is beyond the scope of this text. Readers are referred to the admirably concise and informative paper on the topic by Reding and McDowell[8].

A few points are worthy of emphasis, however. For the individual, it is often difficult to predict outcome in the immediate aftermath of a stroke and in the process to decide on the utility or futility of a rehabilitation programme. Epidemiological evidence indicates that previous health status, the extent and severity of the stroke, and the level of consciousness, cognition and continence following the stroke are the best pointers[15]. However, most survivors of the acute stage improve to some extent. Having a range of rehabilitation options to choose from is the ideal, with those most likely to improve being admitted to the more intensive programmes. For some people, rehabilitation goals must be modest. They are none the less valid, as helping people to recover their ability to swallow, to transfer from bed to chair more easily or to become wheelchair independent can greatly enhance the quality of life. The role of the various members of the multidisciplinary rehabilitation team is described elsewhere[8]. As with all rehabilitation situations, the role which the patient's family has to play should not be forgotten.

THE PATIENT WITH MYOCARDIAL INFARCTION

Not only are diabetic patients more susceptible to myocardial infarction, they are also at greater risk from its consequences in both the short-term and long-term. For example, one-quarter of diabetic patients admitted to hospital with acute infarction do not survive to discharge[16], the risk of in-hospital death being greatest in diabetic women[17]. Overall, more than 50% of diabetic patients admitted to hospital with myocardial infarction are dead by 1 year. This excess short-term and long-term mortality is some 50% greater in diabetics than non-diabetics[17]. Poor pre-infarction cardiac status and greater damage resulting from the infarct, together with the diabetic state itself all seem to contribute to the relatively poor prognosis in diabetics. Fatal reinfarction is a particular concern, being over twice as common in diabetic than in non-diabetic people[16].

Rehabilitation programmes which aim to improve the long-term prognosis for people post myocardial infarction have been described and evaluated. They tend to be exercise-based, though some also aim to reduce or eliminate risk factors for coronary artery disease. Though most studies have been too small to detect any meaningful benefit, a meta-analysis of 4554 patients enrolled in 22 randomized trials detected a 20% reduction in total and cardiovascular mortality[18]. The benefits were apparent 1 year after randomization and persisted for at least 3 years. Almost all studies excluded elderly subjects and provided no data on the subgroup of subjects with diabetes so that there is no evidence of the efficacy of postinfarction rehabilitation programmes for elderly diabetic patients. However, because of the relatively poor prognosis of myocardial infarction, this group has potentially most to gain. At the very least, exercise programmes enhance self-esteem, feelings of autonomy and self-confidence[19].

Before embarking on any exercise-based rehabilitation programme, it is important to establish that exercise is safe and to quantify the level of cardiorespiratory reserve. An exercise stress test under the supervision of a trained health professional clarifies these issues. Assessing functional reserve allows exercise programmes to be tailored to the individual and allows progress to be measured. It is also important to identify factors which limit the ability to exercise, as some of these, for example foot deformities or unsuitable footwear, can be rectified. Aerobic exercise (in which muscular effort is sustained by oxygen) and not anaerobic exercise should be engaged in. In practice, exertion which leads to muscular aches and pains on the following day should be avoided. Ideally, exercise should cause the heart rate to rise to between 70 and 85% of maximum for at least 30 min, three to four times each week[20]. As a rule of thumb, maximal heart rate approximates 220 minus the patient's age in years. If the patient experiences angina during or following exercise, this regimen must be revised. Exercise in the context of primary prevention in diabetes is discussed in more detail in Chapter 3 and the principles of exercise prescribing for elderly people are summarized in Table 3.2.

Assuming that medications (e.g. beta blockers) which control heart rate are not being prescribed, individual patients should aim to maintain heart rate within a predetermined range when exercising. To this end, the pulse rate should be monitored regularly, and the degree of exercise modified accordingly. An adequate warm-up and cool-down regimen should begin and end every exercise session. Running, swimming, cycling, tennis and gym work-outs are examples of suitable exercise. Exercise which the person finds enjoyable is best. For some people, group exercise has the added benefit of promoting social interaction. Those struggling to psychologically adjust to a recent myocardial infarction for example may find it helpful to meet with others who are similarly affected.

THE AMPUTEE PATIENT

As peripheral vascular disease is now the main cause of lower limb amputations in Western countries, the majority of amputee patients are elderly and many are diabetic. In the UK, 80% of people undergoing lower limb amputation are aged over 60 years[21]. In the United States 45% of all patients undergoing lower limb amputation in the late 1970s were diabetic[22]. Furthermore, the incidence of lower limb amputation is some 15 times higher in diabetic than in non-diabetic people[22].

The process of rehabilitating the elderly diabetic amputee goes through a number of overlapping stages[21]. Getting the stump to heal is the first step and to this end, an adequate blood supply is crucial. Surgeons aim to preserve as much of a limb as possible without compromising the viability of the stump. Whether the initial procedure should be a below-knee amputation (BKA) or an above-knee amputation (AKA) is a crucial and often difficult decision. On the one hand, there is a particular advantage in preserving the knee joint, as following a BKA people regain and retain mobility far more effectively than those with an AKA. On the other hand, if the stump fails to heal following a BKA, an AKA will be required. The need for a second more radical operation after a prolonged and futile effort to heal the stump delays the rehabilitation process and often demoralizes the patient.

Once the suture line has healed, the patient can be mobilized on a temporary device such as a pylon or on a pneumatic post-amputation mobility (PPAM) aid. When the stump wound is soundly healed, a permanent prosthesis is fashioned. Initially, the stump will be oedematous, with the swelling gradually resolving over a number of weeks. The socket which interfaces between the stump and prosthesis will therefore need to be modified or recast as the swelling reduces. The prosthesis needs to be customized for the individual patient. While in the past, it was necessary to strike a balance between durability and weight, strong and lightweight materials are increasingly available. The cosmetic appearance is also important, though many people cover their prosthesis with trousers. Depending on need, the ankle section of the prosthesis can be either fixed or dynamic.

Peripheral vascular disease in the diabetic patient is usually a bilateral condition, so that following amputation, the remaining leg may be critically ischaemic. Over 50% of diabetics will have lost their remaining leg within 4 years of the first amputation[23]. This highlights the need to monitor the remaining leg carefully and to educate the patient about optimal diabetic control and foot care. Arteriography and vascular reconstruction should also be considered[24]. Mortality rates among diabetic amputees are also high; survival rates of only 50% 3 years following amputation have been quoted[25]. The patient's general medical condition must be considered; coincidental cerebrovascular and coronary artery disease should be suspected and appropriately managed.

Pain is sometimes a problem, particularly in the early phase of amputee rehabilitation. Stump pain can be due to infection, ischaemia, a bony spur or a neuroma. Appropriate management requires an accurate diagnosis. Phantom limb pain is common and sometimes debilitating. Carbamazepine is often effective and the pain tends to resolve with time.

THE PATIENT WITH DIABETIC RETINOPATHY

Diabetic retinopathy is a significant cause of visual impairment in elderly people. In the Framingham Study, 3% of all people aged 65–74 years had diabetic retinopathy, with 7% of 75–85 year olds being affected[26]. The duration of diabetes is the critical risk factor in the development of retinopathy; those with NIDDM have a similar risk to those with insulin-dependent diabetes mellitus[27].

Strategies to prevent or retard the development of diabetic retinopathy are described in Chapter 6. Even if visual impairment does result, much can be done to minimize resulting disability and handicap. Ophthalmology departments usually have affiliated units specializing in the provision of low vision aids and other appliances. An array of products are also available to help the visually impaired with blood sugar monitoring and insulin administration[28]. In many countries, those registered as visually impaired or blind are eligible for special services and benefits, which help to reduce the impact of visual impairment.

OTHER COMPLICATIONS IN THE DIABETIC PATIENT

Diabetic patients with end-stage renal disease (ESRD) and who are dependent on renal dialysis are obliged to be physically inactive for long periods of time and tend to lose cardiorespiratory and neuromuscular fitness. Tiredness resulting from uraemia and chronic anaemia limits exercise capacity and leads to further loss of fitness. Renal osteodystrophy is an early complication of renal failure and the loss of bone mass is exacerbated by lack of exercise. Exercise programmes can reduce disability and handicap in patients with ESRD[29], and therefore qualify as valid rehabilitation tools.

Sensory neuropathy sometimes limits the exercise options available to the elderly diabetic patient and loss of fitness can result. For those who do exercise, trauma to the foot can result in blistering and ulceration of the skin, muscular sprains and fractures. Muscles and tendons are at risk from overstretching. Neuropathic weight-bearing joints are easily traumatized, and a Charcot joint can result. For these reasons, exercises such as swimming and cycling which minimize weight-bearing are best. Sensory loss also makes some patients dependent on vision when performing motor skills and visual aids may need to be incorporated into the exercise programme.

Between 20 and 40% of all diabetic patients have some degree of autonomic dysfunction[30]. Exercising can be hazardous for the person with diabetic autonomic neuropathy as essential cardiovascular responses and endocrine responses may be blunted or absent[31,32]. Not only is the capacity for exercise reduced, there is also a risk of silent myocardial ischaemia and infarction, together with sudden cardiac death. It is therefore essential that simple tests of autonomic function[30] are performed on all diabetic patients before they embark on an exercise-based rehabilitation programme and that those with abnormalities undergo a formal exercise test. For those with autonomic dysfunction, intensive exercise and activities which require rapid changes in posture must be avoided. For such people exercises in water or while sitting or lying help to maintain blood pressure and are particularly suitable[33].

AIDS AND ADAPTATIONS

Technology has much to offer in minimizing disability and handicap. A large variety of aids can assist with such activities of daily living as dressing, toiletting and housework as well as with recreational pursuits. Those in common use have been described by Mulley[34]; they range from the simple and inexpensive to the sophisticated and costly. Mobility can be enhanced by a variety of walking aids, wheelchairs and motorized vehicles. Communication difficulties can be reduced with a range of devices, both simple and complex. Some elderly diabetic people also benefit from low-vision, continence and memory aids. The environment in which the person functions can also be adapted so as to reduce disability and handicap. Requirements can range from the provision of a simple hand rail which helps with toilet use to major structural changes to one's home.

It is crucial that aids and adaptations are tailored to meet the needs of the individual. An assessment of need is therefore the preliminary step; the premorbid level of functioning, degree of current disability and aspirations for the future must all be considered. The most important perspective is that of the patient, though it is important to differentiate between the patient's perceived needs and actual needs. If the patient's perception of need conflicts with that of the health professional, agreement should be reached through negotiation. It should be kept in mind that the inappropriate use of aids or the use of inappropriate aids can promote rather than relieve disability and handicap. For this reason, advice on the suitability of aids and adaptations is best left to occupational therapists or others with particular expertise in this area. Physiotherapists can give advice on the selection of mobility aids, speech pathologists with communication aids and audiologists with hearing aids.

For the diabetic patient with retinopathy or other causes of visual impairment, a number of assistive devices can enhance vision. Most large centres of population have access to a 'low vision clinic' or other centre where specialized advice and equipment is available. These usually work hand in hand with ophthalmology services with patients regularly being referred from one service to the other. Where stroke has left the patient with a visual field defect, the use of prisms fitted to spectacles can enlarge the field of binocular vision[35].

METABOLIC CONTROL IN THE DISABLED DIABETIC PERSON

While this chapter has focused on disability and handicap resulting from diabetic complications, it should be appreciated that the onset of disability and handicap can have implications for diabetic control. Thus the person with hemiplegia or visual impairment may have difficulty with self-monitoring of glycaemia and with self-administration of insulin. Reduced mobility may lead to weight gain and/or loss of good metabolic control. As part of the rehabilitation programme, the ability of the person to manage their diabetes should be assessed and when necessary, remedial action taken.

EDUCATION AND REHABILITATION

Rehabilitation is essentially an educational activity, in which the patient acquires the knowledge, skills and attitudes (the key components of any educational package) to minimize the disability and handicap resulting from impairment. As far as possible, patient education should be integrated into the rehabilitation programme and should be acknowledged as an essential component, which requires time and other resources. It is important that all rehabilitation team members acknowledge their role as educators, preferably to the extent of acquiring formal education skills. If educational resources directed at the diabetic population (e.g. a diabetes educator or education team) are available, their input into a rehabilitation programme can be invaluable.

Education can have a number of objectives relevant to rehabilitation. It promotes good metabolic control and behaviours that prevent further impairment and minimize disability and handicap (cf. Chapter 3: Secondary and Tertiary Prevention). Furthermore, participation in education programmes can foster autonomy, improve self-esteem and coping skills and reduce anxiety and depression[36]. In other words, education can reduce the psychological handicap resulting from diabetes. Support groups or self-help groups can also have a major impact on psychological rehabilitation, though it is valuable to have input from a health professional, preferably one with some training in psychotherapy[37].

Of the three components of an educational package, attitudinal learning is more difficult to attain than is knowledge or skills acquisition. For example, the difficulty in getting people to modify their diet, level of exercise and other life-style factors is well recognized, even in people with knowledge about what constitutes a healthy life-style[1]. Health professionals who fail to understand the value of rehabilitation also require education, to counteract nihilistic attitudes. It is important that such people come to understand that neither old age nor diabetes are barriers to successful rehabilitation. As stated eloquently by Roald Dahl[38]: 'It is possible for anyone, given a lot of guts and a bit of luck, to overcome gigantic misfortunes and terrible illness'.

REFERENCES

1 Searle MS, Ready AE. Survey of exercise and dietary knowledge and behaviour in persons with Type II diabetes. *Can J Pub Health* 1991; **82**: 344–8.
2 Seymour DG. The physiology of ageing. In: Pathy MSJ, Finucane P (eds), *Geriatric Medicine, Problems and Practice*. Berlin: Springer-Verlag, 1989: 3–13.
3 Hine D. Demography and epidemiology of old age. In: Pathy MSJ, Finucane P (eds), *Geratric Medicine, Problems and Practice*. Berlin: Springer-Verlag, 1989: 15–30.
4 Australian Institute of Health. *Australia's Health 1990*. Canberra: Australian Government Publishing Service.
5 Mahoney FI, Barthel DW. Functional evaluation: Barthel Index. *MD State Med J* 1965; **14**: 61–5.
6 Folstein M, Folstein S, McHugh P. Mini-mental state: A practical method for grading the cognitive state of patients for clinicians. *J Psychiatr Res* 1975; **12**: 189–98.
7 Andrews K. *Rehabilitation of the Older Adult*. London: Edward Arnold, 1987.
8 Reding MJ, McDowell F. Stroke rehabilitation. *Neurol Clin* 1987; **5**: 601–30.
9 Young JB, Forster A. The Bradford community stroke trial: results at six months. *Br Med J* 1992; **304**: 1085–9.
10 Leng GC. Depression following myocardial infarction. *Lancet* 1994; **343**: 2–3.
11 Ahlsio B, Britton M, Murray V, Theorell T. Disablement and quality of life after stroke. *Stroke* 1984; **15**: 886–90.
12 Schmidt SM, Herman LM, Keonig P, Leuze M, Monahan MK, Stubbers RW. Status of stroke patients: a community assessment. *Arch Phys Med Rehabil* 1986; **67**: 99–102.
13 Kemp BJ. Motivation, rehabilitation, and aging: A conceptual model. *Top Geriatr Rehabil* 1988; **3**: 41–51.
14 Sacco RL, Wolf PA. Kannel WB, McNamara PM. Survival and recurrence following stroke. The Framingham study. *Stroke* 1982; **13**: 290–4.
15 Flicker L. Rehabilitation for stroke survivors—a review. *Aust NZ J Med* 1989; **19**: 400–6.
16 Malmberg K, Ryden L. Myocardial infarction in patients with diabetes mellitus. *Eur Heart J* 1988; **9**:259–64.
17 Sprafka JM, Burke GL, Folsom AR, McGovern PG, Hahn LP. Trends in prevalence of diabetes mellitus in patients with myocardial infarction and effect of diabetes on survival. *Diabetes Care* 1991; **14**: 537–43.
18 O'Connor GT, Buring JE, Yusuf S, *et al.* An overview of randomized trials of rehabilitation with exercise after myocardial infarction. *Circulation* 1989; **80**: 234–44.
19 Fentem PH. Benefits of exercise in health and disease. *Br Med J* 1994; **308**: 1291–5.
20 Penhall RK. Wasting away of the old: can it and should it be prevented. *Modern Med* 1994; **37**: 16–26.

21 Chadwick SJD, Wolfe JHN. Rehabilitation of the amputee. *Br Med J* 1992; **304**: 373–6.

22 Most RS, Sinnock P. The epidemiology of lower extremity amputations in diabetic individuals. *Diabetes Care* 1983; **6**: 87–91.

23 Ebskov B, Josephsen P. Incidence of reamputation and death after gangrene of the lower extremity. *Prosthet Orthotics Int* 1980; **4**: 77–80.

24 LoGerfo FW, Coffman JD. Vascular and microvascular disease of the foot in diabetes. *N Engl J Med* 1984; **311**: 1615–19.

25 Bild DE, Selby JV, Sinnock P. Browner WS, Braveman P, Showstack JA. Lower-extremity amputation in people with diabetes. *Diabetes Care* 1989; **12**: 24–31.

26 Kini MM, Leibowitz HM, Colton T, Nickerson RJ, Ganley J, Dawber TR. Prevalence of senile cataract, diabetic retinopathy, senile macular degeneration, and open-angle glaucoma in the Framingham eye study. *Am J Ophthalmol* 1978; **85**: 28–34.

27 Nathan DM, Singer DE, Godine JE, Harrington CH, Perlmuter LC. Retinopathy in older Type II diabetics. *Diabetes* 1986; **35**: 797–801.

28 Petzinger RA. Diabetes aids and products for people with visual and physical impairment. *Diabetes Educ* 1992; **18**: 121–38.

29 Painter P. Exercise in end-stage renal disease. *Exerc Sport Sci Rev* 1988; **16**: 305–40.

30 Ewing DJ, Clarke BF. Diagnosis and management of diabetic autonomic neuropathy. *Br Med J* 1982; **285**: 916–18.

31 Hilsted J, Galbo H, Christensen NJ. Impaired responses of catecholamines, growth hormone, and cortisol to graded exercise in diabetic autonomic neuropathy. *Diabetes* 1980; **29**: 257–62.

32 Hilsted J, Galbo H, Christensen NJ, Parving HH, Benn J. Haemodynamic changes during graded exercise in patients with diabetic autonomic neuropathy. *Diabetologia* 1982; **22**: 318–23.

33 Graham C, Lasko-McCarthey P. Exercise options for persons with diabetic complications. *Diabetes Educ* 1990; **16**: 212–20.

34 Mulley GP. *Everyday aids and appliances*. London: British Medical Journal, 1989.

35 Roper-Hall G. Effect of visual fields defects on binocular single vision. *Am Orthop J* 1976; **26**:74–82.

36 Rubin RR, Peyrot M, Saudek CD. Effect of diabetes education on self care, metabolic control, and emotional well-being. *Diabetes Care* 1989; **12**: 673–9.

37 Toth EL, James I. Description of a diabetes support group: lessons for diabetes caregivers. *Diabetic Med* 1992; **9**: 773–8.

38 Dahl R. In: Griffith VE (ed.), *A Stroke in the Family*. London: Wildwood House, 1975.

12

The Role of the General Practitioner in the Care of the Elderly Diabetic Patient

PETER R. W. TASKER

King's Lynn, Norfolk, UK

INTRODUCTION AND PRINCIPLES OF MANAGEMENT

One of the most exciting changes that has taken place in the management of diabetic patients during the last decade, is the change in clinical management responsibility from the hospital-based service to that based in general practice. This is particularly true for the elderly patient since careful follow-up is essential. Hospital-based clinics could not cope with the work-load of all these patients and it is therefore very important that the primary care is thoughtfully and carefully organized. However, the hospital-based service does have a vital role and the shared-care model may be the most beneficial to elderly patients.

However, there is a real risk that sharing care means duplication of care with advice being conflicting and thus very clear protocols of care must be devised. A model of care has to be evolved and must meet the needs of the individual patient within the specific locality. In some localities the patient's needs may be best met by the caring family doctor and practice nurse, while in others the ideal continuing management may be provided by the local hospital-based diabetic service.

Diabetes impinges on almost all branches of medicine, this is particularly true in the elderly population with important implications for therapy and

Diabetes in Old Age. Edited by P. Finucane and A. J. Sinclair
© 1995 John Wiley & Sons Ltd

the informed general practitioner is very well placed to manage elderly diabetic patients.

It is important in the elderly group of patients that treatment goals be clearly defined. The overriding principle of management must be maintaining or improving the quality of life while controlling the diabetes. Symptom relief is important but it must be stressed that some symptoms may be quite elusive and include vague signs, such as non-specific mental deterioration and general reduced mobility. Individual treatment goals should be defined and it should be remembered that biological as opposed to chronological age be considered. Considerable care with regard to tight control of blood sugar should be taken and treatment side-effects, particularly hypoglycaemia which can be devastating in this group of patients, should be avoided. However, some carers feel that since the elderly are at risk of developing complications and poor control increases this risk then the standard of control should not be relaxed. This is not practical in many cases and the effect of severe hypoglycaemia on patients and the carers is so devastating that it should be regarded as acceptable practice to be slightly more flexible when controlling elderly diabetic patients.

PREVALENCE

If the primary health care team is to accept the challenge of diabetic management then it is vital to predict the work-load that will be generated and therefore the prevalence of diabetes must be recognized. The combined prevalence of diagnosed insulin-dependent diabetes and non-insulin-dependent diabetes (NIDDM) is between 1 and 2% of the white British population. This means that between 500 000 and 750 000 people in the UK have clinically proven diabetes. Allowing for those undiagnosed patients, and there will always be a small percentage of these, the total number of people with diabetes in Britain must be approximately 1 000 000. This means that every general practitioner in the UK with an average list size will have 25–35 diabetic patients under his or her care.

Five of the six population-based studies published in the 1980s in Britain confirm these figures. The results from three of these are tabled and it is clear from them that the prevalence also increases with age. The population in Western society is ageing. Minaker stated that in 1920 only 4.6% of the population of the USA was over 65 years, but by the year 2020, 20% of the population will be in this age group with a substantial number over the age of 85 years. Thus the number of elderly people with diabetes will significantly increase over the next few decades[1].

In our King's Lynn (UK) practice of 18 740 patients we have 487 patients with diabetes giving us a prevalence of 2.5%, 29% of insulin-requiring patients and 63% of non-insulin-dependent patients are 65 years of age or over. It is now recognized that the two population characteristics that most strongly influence the prevalence of diabetes are: first, the age and sex structure of the population; and second the ethnic mix particularly the proportion of people from Asian and Afro-Caribbean origin[2]. The King's Lynn population is almost entirely Caucasian.

DIAGNOSIS

The World Health Organisation criteria for the diagnosis of diabetes applies without age modification (see Chapter 4). It is essential that the diagnosis is accurate—there is no place for flexibility in view of the patient's age. It is also essential that diagnosis is based on the presence of hyperglycaemia, although glycosuria is an indicator of the underlying abnormal metabolic state.

It is very important that diagnosis is accompanied by appropriate education; the elderly group of patients are often worried and confused about diabetes. They may be fearful, having previously known others who have developed devastating complications. It is extremely important for education to take place in easy slow stages since the ability to absorb information may be limited. It is desirable that a friend or younger relative accompany the patient at diagnosis. Reassurance is an extremely vital part of education at this point.

POPULATION SCREENING

In view of the significant morbidity and indeed mortality associated with diabetes, particularly NIDDM, population screening can be very rewarding. Insulin-dependent diabetes is not a condition suitable for population screening since the patient usually presents with acute symptoms. However, for screening tests to be accurately performed and reliably interpreted it is essential that expertise is available. The general practice is an ideal context in which this service can be carried out, since practice nurses can reliably carry out the estimation, interpret the results (having previously been educated with regard to the diagnosis), and probably most important of all provide immediate reassuring education that I have eluded to previously. The place of charitable and pharmaceutical screening has to be questioned, since the follow-up may not be available.

In the UK, a British Diabetic Association Working Party[3] has published recommendations for safe and careful screening practice as follows:

1. Screening should be restricted to those between the ages of 40 and 75 years.

2. Recommended screening procedures are:
   (i) blood glucose 2 h after 75 g oral glucose load:
       capillary plasma glucose >8.8 mmol/l
       capillary whole blood glucose >8.0 mmol/l
       venous plasma glucose >8.0 mmol/l = *positive*
   (ii) fasting blood glucose
       plasma glucose >6.6 mmol/l
       whole blood glucose >6.0 mmol/l = *positive*
       plasma glucose 5.5–6.6 mmol/l
       whole blood glucose 5.0–6.0 mmol/l = *equivocal*
   (iii) urine glucose (urine sampled 2 h after main meal)
       any glycosuria = *positive*.

The choice of screening methods should be made on the basis of local circumstances such as the availability of staff, methods of follow-up, etc. It is not recommended that more than one test be performed on each subject.

3. For screening results to be reliable the equipment and technique of the screener must be regularly checked.

4. Full details of the screening method and result should be given to the person being screened.

5. No diagnosis should be made or treatment started on the basis of screening results. Subjects with a positive or equivocal screening result should be referred to their family doctor.

6. It is recommended that screening needs to be performed only every 5 years in people without symptoms or risk factors. Screening every 3 years would be appropriate for patients over the age of 75 and those in high risk groups—subjects with a family history of diabetes, obese subjects (greater than 120% of ideal body weight) and black subjects.

7. Diabetes screening is best undertaken in a general practice setting, in parallel with other health screening initiatives.

Other views on screening are presented in Chapter 4.

SYMPTOMATOLOGY

Elderly people with diabetes vary as to their mode of presentation. Most elderly patients have NIDDM, which denotes that they can survive long-term without insulin therapy, although it may be used to improve glycaemia control (insulin requiring). A small but significant percentage of patients (possibly 10%) over the age of 65 are insulin dependent presenting with classical signs and symptoms[4].

The classical signs of insulin-dependent diabetes are thirst, passing large quantities of urine, extreme fatigue and weight loss over the course of 2–3 weeks. There are other minor symptoms such as recurrent skin infection, genital pruritus and muscular cramps. Acute hyperosmolar non-ketotic pre-coma or even coma may be a presenting feature in the elderly, frequently having been precipitated by infection or drug therapy. Diuretics and beta blockers have been implicated[5-7]. This metabolic state may sometimes present in unusual and confusing ways, such as neurological signs and seizures[8]. Clinical signs other than weight loss, dehydration and skin sepsis are not usually evident.

NIDDM represents the majority of the elderly group of patients. A community-based study of 640 patients with NIDDM showed the mean age to be 67 with the age at diagnosis being 59 years[9]. Within this group of patients are two subgroups: namely, obese and non-obese. Obesity is a major problem in NIDDM; some 54% of men and 73% of women are over 120% of their ideal body weight at presentation[10]. The aetiological factors in these two groups are probably very different with insulin resistance being very important in the obese patients and reduced insulin secretion in the non-obese.

The classical symptoms of NIDDM are those caused by the osmotic effect of hyperglycaemia, namely thirst and polyuria. However, these symptoms are not always as intense as in the insulin-dependent patient and occur over a longer period of time. Weight loss is not a pronounced feature. However, only 53% of NIDDM patients present with diabetic symptoms[10]. Many patients are discovered during the investigation of other conditions, such as leg ulceration, eye disease or recurrent infection. Indeed many 'asymptomatic' patients are discovered during routine analysis during hospital admission, out-patient clinic attendances, driving/medical insurance medical examinations or the 'over 75' health check which takes place in the UK.

In order that care can be structured and organized, identification of patients with diabetes is one of the first steps in overall management. This will enable practice registers to be formulated. In the absence of a disease index this can be achieved by relying on receptionist memory, doctor's memory and requests for repeat prescriptions of diabetic products.

PRINCIPLES OF MANAGEMENT

It is important in the elderly group of patients that treatment goals be clearly defined. The quality of life must be taken into consideration when controlling their diabetes. An assessment of disability is essential in the management plan. This should include the effect of coexisting physical conditions such as osteoarthritis, heart disease and visual impairment. The patient's mental state must also be taken into consideration, bearing in mind the memory changes associated with normal ageing, as well as depression, a diagnosis frequently missed in the elderly patient. Social deprivation is important—many elderly patients live alone with low incomes—both situations that are far from ideal when struggling with diabetes.

Symptom relief is extremely important in those patients who actually present with symptoms, but it must be stressed that some symptoms may be quite elusive and can include such vague signs as non-specific mental deterioration and generalized reduced mobility. When defining treatment goals biological as opposed to chronological age is most important.

Considerable care with regard to tight control of blood sugar should be taken, side-effects, particularly hypoglycaemia, which can be devastating in this group of patients should be avoided.

WHERE SHOULD MANAGEMENT TAKE PLACE?

The appropriate setting for various elements of the programme of care will vary for any particular patient and between different geographical areas. It is for the general practitioner in consultation with members of the hospital-based team to define protocols that determine where a particular patient receives the various elements of care. It has been clearly shown that general practice-based care can be as good as that based in hospital, as judged by biochemical parameters, as long as the care is structured and organized[11,12]. However, it is broadly agreed that certain groups of patients will need to be followed-up by the hospital team. These may include insulin-treated patients and patients who have developed complications (as well as children, adolescents and women considering or undergoing pregnancy.

The advantages of a general practice-based clinic (Table 12.1) are that the patients are usually seen by the same staff; waiting time is reduced to a minimum and the doctor and nurse are easily accessible. However, a practice-based system is dependent upon the practitioner having an enthusiastic interest in the condition and there being a large enough number of patients to acquire the necessary expertise in dealing with the range of symptoms and problems as they are encountered. A potential

Table 12.1. Advantages of GP-based clinic

Regular doctor
Regular practice nurse
Easy access to primary health care team
Savings of patient time/money

criticism is the fact that general practitioners not involved in diabetic care may lose inherent skills in dealing with diabetic emergencies, as they arise. There is also capital expenditure, general practitioners having to pay for blood glucose meters, record cards as well as secretarial, nursing and dietetic time.

However, for the patient the obvious advantages of being looked after in a general practice setting are usually savings of time and travel and thus probably there is a financial advantage. The close continuity of care that develops between the primary health care team and the patient contributes to better compliance and more confidence in discussing management problems as they arise.

There are three basic models of care in most chronic diseases. These are particularly well exemplified by diabetes. Care can be organized so that it is entirely hospital-based and indeed this should probably be the case for most insulin-treated diabetics and those with severe complications, or it can be organized entirely at primary care level. However, a shared care scheme is probably the most beneficial to all parties, since it combines the expertise of the hospital diabetic specialist and specialist nurse with the general practitioner's detailed knowledge of the patient's general health and social well-being. Shared care of the elderly group must take into account their specific needs such as mobility, multiple drug regimens and chiropody and thus hospital-based care should include experts in the care of the elderly. An evaluation of shared care has concluded that with adequate support from and communication with hospital-based diabetic services, general practitioners are capable of providing care appropriate to the needs of uncomplicated diabetic patients[13].

There are some basic requirements for the successful running of a shared-care scheme (Table 12.2). It is vital from the onset that formulation of policies and protocols include all involved parties cooperating fully. Devising these is a very useful educational exercise and many policies and guidelines have been published. These should be used as a basis but not a substitute for discussion[14,15]. It must be decided which elements of care are the responsibility of the primary health care team and which are those of

Table 12.2. Requirements of successful shared-care scheme

Practice register and recall system

Trained practice nurse — trained in diabetes and trained as an educator

Comunity-based ancillary staff — dietitian/chiropodist

Regular meetings between hospital-based and practice-based teams

Instant access to hospital team and clear guidelines for urgent referrals

Access to hospital-based education system

Laboratory facilities

---

the hospital clinic team. Patients must be able to identify a specific person in the practice team who is able to provide consistent continuity of care—a role that the practice nurse fills very adequately. The practice nurse can be responsible at primary care level for patient education, maintenance of the diabetic register and manage, with secretarial help, an effective recall system. It is vitally important that community-based dietetic and chiropody services are available. There should be regular meetings between the hospital-based and practice-based teams defining their roles and formulating management policies and protocols. These meetings must concern professional education and as such will maintain interest in the shared-care scheme.

Where the patients are looked after within shared-care scheme or entirely at general practice level there are some basic general practice requirements that are needed to ensure success (Table 12.3). Motivated, educated and interested staff are essential for the success of the service. There has been much discussion in a variety of forums as to the need for protected time. It is desirable that diabetic care which involves education, manipulation of

Table 12.3. Requirements to run a GP-based diabetic service

Interested/enthusiatic GP

Practice Sister/Health Visitor

Regular clinic session

Specialized record card

Secretarial facilities

Cooperation with biochemistry department

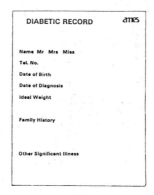

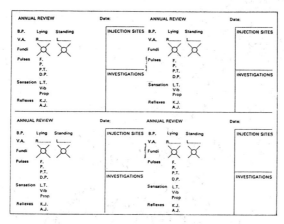

Figure 12.1. Picture of diabetic record card

drugs and multisystem pathology be focused in a single clinical session. It is difficult and time-consuming to 'slot' diabetic patients into a general consulting session. It is important that protocols of care are defined with the full cooperation of patients. These protocols should include such issues as initial management, frequency of follow-up appointments, annual review, initiation of insulin therapy and emergency care. This latter point must include 'sick day rules' with information relating to the treatment changes during acute illness, as well as hypoglycaemic management. While specific issues relating to diabetes can be addressed within a general practice consulting session, it is extremely difficult for all these areas of care to be addressed in a general practice surgery. Protected time, where ancillary staff are focused upon diabetes is the ideal general practice model. It is important that clinical progress be efficiently and adequately documented. Some general practitioner groups have found that specifically designed record cards are helpful (Figure 12.1), while others found duplicated computer records more applicable. Within the general practice secretarial help is essential and close cooperation with a local biochemistry department is highly desirable.

CLINICAL MANAGEMENT

Having established protocols of care, either in conjunction with the hospital service or within general practice, a specific clinic, in protected time, needs to be established. The mechanism of the clinic operation should be decided locally, but certain issues need to be addressed.

First, the length of the consultation needs to be adequate for certain procedures to be carried out, namely, the issue of a prescribed treatment and the opportunity for patients to discuss feelings and problems. Within general practice a review appointment should be not less than 15 min. Within that time the procedures needed to be carried out include weighing the patient, an estimation of biochemical control, blood pressure, foot examination and arrangements for annual review, including fundoscopy should be made. An isolated blood glucose estimation has limited value giving only an indication of immediate control and not reflecting the long-term situation. Glycosylated haemoglobin or fructosamine estimation can be performed a few days before the clinic, so that the result is available to discuss with the patient. If it is carried out within the clinic then arrangements to inform the patient of the result must be made. It is very important particularly in this elderly group of patients for a foot inspection to be carried out and chiropody to be arranged if necessary. Review appointment frequency should be mutually decided upon, but insulin treated patients should be reviewed at least 3 monthly—all other patients should be assessed at least 6 monthly.

The annual review appointment needs to be about 30 min long and should include a careful examination of the peripheral vascular and neurological systems. A detailed foot examination preferably by a chiropodist including suitability of foot wear should be carried out, arrangements for fundal examination through dilated pupils should be made, a dietary review by a dietitian and a biochemical estimation of renal function should be performed. Specific patient and carer concerns should be discussed.

SPECIFIC ISSUES OF MANAGEMENT OF OLDER DIABETIC PATIENTS

MONITORING

Methods of monitoring control do not differ with age but certain other factors do limit the frequency and type of monitoring. The renal threshold for glucose rises with age and thus urine testing may have limited value. However, many elderly patients can adequately carry out the skills necessary to perform self-monitoring of blood glucose. However, the technique needed may be affected by finger dexterity, due to arthritis or tremor, low visual acuity and impaired cognitive function. Community-based nursing staff and personal carers can, however, help this group of patients. Intermittent estimation of glycosylated haemoglobin is extremely helpful in the control of the elderly diabetic patient.

COEXISTING MEDICAL CONDITIONS

The presence of other medical conditions has an important effect on the elderly patient with diabetes, and more information relating to this area is available in Chapter 13.

An increasing number of elderly diabetic patients have visual impairment. There is a high incidence of diabetic retinopathy, cataract, senile macular degeneration and open-angled glaucoma in diabetes[16]. This impairs the patient's ability to read tablet bottle labels, to accurately assess testing strips, to read monitor results and syringe markings. However, many of the problems can be resolved using carers, community nurses and specific visual aids. Elderly diabetic patients should be encouraged to have other ophthalmic conditions treated in order to enhance visual acuity.

Peripheral vascular disease affects many elderly patients. Diabetic peripheral neuropathy renders the elderly foot extremely susceptible to minor trauma. Once traumatized, healing is very slow; ulceration and infection may occur which may result in the need for amputation. Thus it is extremely important that elderly patients are effectively educated and socks should be removed for foot inspection, as patients may not be aware of minor trauma. Elderly arthritic patients, especially those with visual impairment, may not be able to effectively inspect their feet or trim their nails and thus regular chiropody from a registered practitioner is essential.

Assessment of mental function is extremely important when dealing with elderly patients. Impaired memory leads to poor compliance of treatment and thus inadequate control.

CLINICAL AUDIT—EVALUATION OF DIABETES CARE

This area will also be covered later in Chapter 13.

Clinical audit of diabetes care must be carried out regularly. The St Vincent Declaration has enabled identification of meaningful data to be collected. Specific outcomes are set out; however, most of these have 5-year time-scales and thus may not seem to be relevant to the care of the elderly diabetic patient. However, the general goals for people with diabetes include the sustained improvement in health experience and a life approaching normal expectations in quality and quantity. This statement is particularly true in relation to the elderly group of patients and must be a goal that we strive towards in general practice.

CONCLUSIONS

Diabetes mellitus in the elderly poses a specific challenge for general practice. It must be remembered that the organization of care is basically the same as general diabetes care, but there are specific difficulties which need to be addressed. The patients and their carers need specific education and skills in dealing with many of the items discussed in this chapter. Goals of therapy must be realistic and not cause disabling side-effects. Frequently, patients are taking many other drugs and thus one diabetic therapy should preferably be used, and drug interactions must be considered. Above all when dealing with the elderly their biological as opposed to their chronological age must be remembered.

The issues discussed in this chapter highlight the challenge of diabetes in old age, which can be an extremely rewarding experience for doctors working in primary care settings.

REFERENCES

1 Minaker KL. What diabetologists should know about elderly patients. *Diabetes Care* 1990; **13** (Suppl. 2): 34–46.

2 Williams DRR. *Epidemiologically Based Need Assessment—diabetes mellitus*, 2nd edn. University Department of Community Medicine, Addenbrooke's Hospital, Cambridge, 1992.

3 Report of BDA Screening Working Party, British Diabetic Association, London, 1992.

4 Kilvert A, FitzGerald MG, Wright AD, Nattrass M. Newly diagnosed, insulin-dependent diabetes mellitus in elderly patients. *Diabetic Med* 1984; **1**: 115–18.

5 Podolsky S, Pattavina CG. Hyperosmolar non-ketotic diabetic coma. A complication of propranolol therapy. *Metabolism* 1973; **22**: 685–93.

6 Fonseca V, Phear DN. Hyperosmolar non-ketotic diabetic syndrome precipitated by treatment with diuretics. *Br Med J* 1982; **284**: 36–7.

7 Tasker PRW, Mitchell-Heggs PF. Non-ketotic diabetic precoma associated with high dose frusemide therapy. *Br Med J* 1976; **1**: 626–7.

8 Askenasy JJ, Streifler M, Carosso R. Moderate non-ketotic hyperglycaemia—a cause of focal epilepsy. *Eur Neurol* 1977; **16**: 51–61.

9 Gatling W, Muller M, Hill R. General characteristics of a community based diabetic population. *Practical Diabetes* 1988; **5**: 104–7.

10 Multi-centre study. UK Prospective Diabetes Study. iv. Characteristics of newly presenting type 2 diabetic patients: male preponderance and obesity at different ages. *Diabetic Med* 1988; **5**: 154–9.

11 Singh BM, Holland MR, Thorn PA. Metabolic control of diabetes in general practice clinics—comparison with a hospital clinic. *Br Med J* 1984; **289**: 726–8.

12 Day JL, Humphreys H, Alban-Davies H. Problems of comprehensive shared diabetes care. *Br Med J* 1987; **294**: 1590–2.

13 Hoskins PL, Fowler PM, Constantino M, *et al.* Sharing the care of diabetic patients between hospital and general practitioners: Does it work? *Diabetic Med* 1993; **10**: 81–6.

14 *Recommendations for the Management of Diabetes in Primary Care*. British Diabetic Association, London, 1993.

15 Waine C. *Diabetes in General Practice*. London: Royal College of General Practitioners, 1992.

16 Framingham Eye Study. The four major diseases and blindness. *Surv Ophthalmol* 1985; **92**: 1191–6.

13

Modern Perspectives and Recent Advances

CHRISTOPHER J. TURNBULL and ALAN J. SINCLAIR*
Arrowe Park Hospital, Wirral, UK and *Department of Geriatric Medicine,
University of Birmingham, UK

INTRODUCTION

Diabetes in old age is a challenge—not just to obtain a cure or to prevent the condition as these seem unlikely to be achieved in the foreseeable future—but in order to manage the condition effectively and prevent complications.

Despite relative neglect in the past, a number of recent developments in diabetic care for the elderly provide optimism that overall management of this large group of patients is improving (Table 13.1). A recognition of new aims of care is now apparent[1] and tailored oral hypoglycaemic therapy is increasingly being adopted. These latter aspects of care along with the more widespread use of insulin are discussed in Chapters 8 and 9.

The St Vincent Declaration, which evolved from a meeting of representatives of the World Health Organisation and the International Diabetes Federation, held in St Vincent, Italy in 1989, sets targets for the improvement in care of people with diabetes[2]. In the UK, a joint Task Force has been set up involving the British Diabetic Association (BDA) and Department of Health which aims to translate these targets into improved care. It is hoped that many physicians who are concerned with diabetic care of older people become involved in similar strategies in order for the special needs of this group of patients to be recognized and catered for[3].

Diabetes in Old Age. Edited by P. Finucane and A. J. Sinclair
© 1995 John Wiley & Sons Ltd

Table 13.1. Recent developments in diabetic care for the elderly

Recognition of new aims of care
Tailored oral hypoglycaemic therapy
Increased use of insulin
St Vincent Declaration
Special Interest Group in Diabetes, British Geriatrics Society (UK)

In 1992, in the UK, a Special Interest Group in Diabetes was formed under the umbrella of the British Geriatrics Society. This group, which consists of more than 100 specialists in geriatrics, is committed to improving diabetes care for the elderly as well as promoting research in this area. Similar interest groups should be encouraged to form in other countries where professional bodies of geriatricians exist.

This chapter will focus on areas that we regard as important advances in diabetes care for older patients. Although we report many aspects of the British experience, the basic principles should be international in perspective. The following areas will be discussed: diabetes education, role of diabetes specialist nurses, self-monitoring, annual review process, audit and computerization, role of the geriatric service, institutional care, diabetic complications and disability.

DIABETES EDUCATION OF OLDER PEOPLE WITH DIABETES

Education of older people with diabetes is a relatively neglected area, though 40% of all new diabetic patients are over 60 years of age and more than 50% of current diabetic patients are over 65 years of age[4]. Research has shown that older people with diabetes do have poorer knowledge of diabetes as compared with the young[5]. There is good evidence that older people are less well informed about hypoglycaemia symptoms and this may be due to lack of education[6,7].

It is generally believed that older people are less likely to comply with dietary modifications, although the reason for this may be lack of educational input by health professionals. Elderly people are in fact, often quite willing to make the necessary dietary changes[8]. A community dietitian who visits the elderly person at home and speaks to both relatives and carers is more likely to be effective than a hurried few minutes at the end of a clinic consultation.

Up to fairly recently, little educational material about diabetes for the elderly has been available. In the UK, the BDA, however, has now published an educational booklet specifically aimed at the older person with diabetes: *Diabetes and You—A guide for the older person*. This may also assist diabetic clinic staff in providing advice for patients. Video cassettes, which can be obtained from several national diabetes organizations and some pharmaceutical firms, are an alternative learning aid but are often unpopular with the elderly. As foot ulceration and gangrene are the most important preventable cause of deterioration for the older person with diabetes, education on footwear is especially important. It is also necessary to include the carer as it has been shown that older people with diabetes have great difficulty with personal foot care[9].

DIABETES SPECIALIST NURSING

Without doubt, diabetes specialist nurses (DSNs) have made an enormous contribution to improving the care of patients with diabetes including the elderly. In one UK district it was shown that only 11% of DSNs' time was spent with over 75-year-old patients. Although DSNs are an important source of general diabetes education[10] their ability to start older patients on insulin within the patient's home is a major step forward in diabetic care. This is more convenient for the patient and relatives, and may also aid education; it also avoids costly hospital admissions. It many cases, patients are also taught how to use pen devices for insulin administration.

DSNs also have an important role of instructing patients about self-monitoring of blood glucose. For disabled patients, e.g. those with visual loss, a variety of methods and equipment for self-monitoring are now available, such as those with an electronic memory or talking meters. These invariably improve self-confidence especially for patients on insulin who are fearful of hypoglycaemia.

Table 13.2. The role of the diabetes specialist nurse for the elderly

---

1. Teach, advise and counsel patients and carers both in the clinic and in the patient's home.
2. Where possible, educate patients to achieve self-care.
3. Teach self-monitoring of blood glucose (or urinalysis, if appropriate) and instruct in the use of special monitoring techniques for patients with physical problems, partial-sightedness or blindness.
4. Teaching and advising on insulin administration.
5. Liaison with and referring to other health professionals, chiropodists, community nurses, general practitioners, etc.
6. Commencement of insulin treatment in the patient's home.
7. Advising and guiding residential and nursing home staff to manage patients with diabetes.
8. Provide continuing support and advice to patients and carers when specific problems relating to diabetes arise.

DSNs have several other important roles in managing elderly patients with diabetes[11] and these have been summarized in Table 13.2. In the UK, we feel strongly that DSNs should be part of the district diabetes service rather than linked directly with the District Nursing Service. This avoids organizational and managerial difficulties, which often arise in the latter situation.

Primary care-based (practice) nurses are increasingly providing advice for older people with diabetes and in these situations the role of the specialist nurse may be less clear[12]. Practice nurses can receive specific training in diabetes management which should be encouraged since elderly people with diabetes often do not attend or wish to attend hospital clinics[13,14].

SELF-MONITORING

Patients with insulin-dependent diabetes mellitus (IDDM) usually readily accept home blood glucose monitoring (HBGM). Reasons given to younger patients by physicians for the importance of tight control are the prevention of long-term vascular complications, to allow normal gestation with an improved outcome for the fetus, and a lower risk of hypoglycaemia. For patients with non-insulin-dependent diabetes mellitus (NIDDM) the situation is far less clear and the 'reward' for good glycaemic control is not immediately obvious.

It has been shown, however, that elderly patients on oral hypoglycaemic agents using HBGM have better control[15], although one study showed that improved control does not necessarily lead to improved well-being[16], and may actually lead to a state of learned helplessness[17].

Although HBGM has been shown in one study to be no more effective than urine monitoring[18], it nevertheless provides a more accurate picture of the prevailing level of glucose. Many patients feel that urine tests are inconvenient and unpleasant, and they may not know how to interpret the significance of the presence or absence of glycosuria. Others, however, find the use of urine monitoring to be quite adequate for patients with NIDDM[19], and it must be accepted that it is cheap and simple to perform. For elderly patients on insulin instruction in performing HBGM should be offered to the patient or carer as appropriate; patients who are subject to hypoglycaemia or variable control are most likely to benefit[20].

THE ANNUAL REVIEW

The annual review is seen as an important part of diabetes management in the 1990s. This is discussed in relation to primary care in Chapter 12. In the

UK, the contents of the annual review are clearly stated by the BDA in its standards leaflet *Diabetes Care. What you should expect*[21]. The review should include the same items whether performed in a primary care or secondary care setting (Table 13.3).

Inspection of the feet and footwear is particularly important in older people who are liable to have deformities, peripheral vascular disease and neuropathy. Because of the age-related changes in vibration sense and reflexes, inspection of the feet for the typical deformity and changes of neuropathic feet such as claw feet and red shiny feet are more valuable than neurological testing[22].

Examination of the eyes should include an assessment of visual acuity using a Snellen chart and an inspection of the fundus through dilated pupils to detect maculopathy. Retinopathy increases in prevalence with age in NIDDM affecting more than 25% of patients over 75 years of age[23].

It is helpful for some patients if the carer or spouse comes with them to the clinic and further enquiries about symptoms can be made. The carer can also be advised of the necessary dietary changes and help can be enlisted with self-monitoring. As many elderly people cannot touch their toes and only a few are capable of visualizing and responding to lesions on the plantar aspects, carers can be taught recognition and basic management of foot care problems[9]. Advice can also be given about coexisting disease and social service provision where appropriate. Where state benefits exist, the elderly patient can be advised to apply for them, e.g. attendance allowance (UK).

Table 13.3. Components of the annual review

Nurse-led	Physician-led
Discuss/check:	Assess:
Dietary principles	General health
Home blood/urine glucose monitoring	Adverse drug reactions
Medication history and compliance with treatment	Disability
Insurance/travel advice	Coexisting medical conditions
	Diabetic complications
Measurement of:	
Weight (kg)	Inspect:
Body mass index	Feet
Blood pressure	Fundi
Visual acuity	Peripheral blood vessels
Hb A_1c and serum creatinine	
Urinalysis:	
Protein	

AUDIT AND COMPUTERIZATION

AUDIT

The primary aim of audit activity must be to improve the quality of care delivered to patients. A common approach in audit is to examine current practice against agreed standards, and if inadequacies in care are identified to suggest and implement ways of improving care. After a suitable period, a re-audit is used to measure the effects of the new proposals.

Diabetes care is an ideal area to audit. The prevalence rate of blindness or amputation, or the average glycosylated haemoglobin (Hb A_1c) value can be measured in patients attending a diabetic clinic and these data can be compared with those derived from patients receiving other forms of medical follow-up. These represent outcome audits. Management protocols can be changed and measures repeated to see if there is improvement.

Process audit can be carried out, for example, by checking how many patients attending a diabetic clinic have a full annual review and whether certain items are missed out or not performed satisfactorily. Patients' satisfaction with the organization of clinics could also be audited.

The results of several diabetic audits have been published. One of the authors (CJT) evaluated his own diabetic clinic for the elderly and found disappointing results[24]. General practitioners have also reported their findings[25-27].

COMPUTERIZATION

Many diabetic clinics are now computerized or have a register of patients. The ability to help improve and standardized management of a large population of people with diabetes by computerization has been well shown[28].

Computerization can also be very helpful in the collection and analysis of data. It can provide information about patients who require their blood pressure to be checked more regularly than the annual review (for example, those with severe renal failure) or those who require more frequent assessment of other coexisting medical conditions such as patients on steroids who have chronic obstructive airways disease. Identification of subgroups of patients with particular characteristics is also facilitated by computerization. For example, one author (CJT) wished to identify all patients on human insulin attending his diabetic clinic when the national press published concerns about the possible loss of warning of hypoglycaemia with human insulin. As a result, all patients on human insulin were identified from the computer records and were circulated with an information leaflet produced by the BDA. The database can also be used to identify defaulters from the clinic or to send out reminders to patients to attend for blood tests or to visit their general practitioners for an annual review. Reliable data can permit comparison of a clinic's performance on control of diabetes, eye care offered, screening for complications or development of complications with amazing speed and accuracy.

Finally, the benefits of establishing a district-wide diabetes database have been reported in North London recently and may lead to other UK districts adopting this method of computerization of data[29].

THE ROLE OF THE SPECIALIST GERIATRIC SERVICE

Diabetes is often one of many other coexisting diseases which lead to substantial disability requiring admission to a department of medicine for the elderly. These conditions include stroke, visual loss, ischaemic heart disease, peripheral vascular disease and amputation[24]. One survey in a typical district hospital showed that 17.2% of patients on elderly care wards were diabetic compared with 12.2% on medical wards[30].

These data suggest the need for geriatricians to be familiar with the management of diabetes as well as disability. The potential roles of geriatricians in diabetes care are given in Table 13.4. Patients are likely to benefit from multidisciplinary assessment and management, and need to have access to nurses, physiotherapists, occupational therapists, chiropodists, dietitians, orthotists and social workers. There should also be ready access to vascular, surgical, orthopaedic and ophthalmic advice as required.

Because of the rehabilitative nature of managing many elderly diabetics, attendance at a geriatric day hospital may be beneficial[31]. Educational advice can also be given, glycaemic control checked, and review of complications such as leg or foot ulcers can be undertaken. In some health districts in the UK, special review clinics for elderly diabetic patients have

Table 13.4. Role of geriatricians in elderly diabetic care

Assessment of coexisting disease which impacts on diabetes management

Management of increasing dependency and disability

Recognition and management of cognitive impairment

Assessment and treatment of urinary incontinence

Liaison between hospital and community support services

Provide respite programmes for spouses and carers

Member of hospital diabetic clinic team

---

been established, often organized by a geriatrician with a special interest in diabetes. One model of care for the future would be to involve a geriatrician in the Diabetes Centre (or Adult Diabetic Clinic) to work alongside a diabetologist[3]. This arrangement prevents resources for diabetic care from being divided (and diluted) and concentrates the expertise of both types of physician in managing patients of a wide age range including those with severe disability or increasing dependency[3]. Efforts to establish this approach need to be maintained bearing in mind that in a survey of diabetic clinics in 1983, no clinics recording cooperation with a geriatrician were reported though over 50% had joint clinics with obstetricians and paediatricians[32].

INSTITUTIONAL CARE OF THE DIABETIC ELDERLY

In the UK, there has been a rapid expansion in residential and nursing home care for elderly people with a corresponding reduction in long-term hospital admissions[33]. Many patients are disabled and a large percentage are likely to have diabetes although accurate information is not available.

There is evidence at least in some parts of the UK that these diabetic patients do not get good care of their diabetes[34]. This is partly because patients may not be well enough to attend hospital clinics or general practitioner surgeries, and partly because of inadequate medical review. It is also likely that many patients slip through the net after admission to institutional care. Diabetic complications may thus remain undetected until a late stage with a consequent high morbidity and mortality. For example, in one study, older people with severely uncontrolled diabetes had a mortality rate of 43% compared with 3.4% in those under the age of 50 years[35]. In addition many nursing and residential homes are small and may have only a few diabetic patients at any one time. This provides little practical experience for staff and in some situations, fully trained nurses may not be available.

Common problems making diabetes management more complex in institutionalized patients include the following.

1. The presence of confusion and poor appetite due to concurrent illness making dietary intake unreliable.

2. Recurrent urine, chest and other infections rendering the diabetic person liable to ketosis and poor control.

3. Difficulty in swallowing associated with stroke or other neurological disorders making it difficult to ensure a regular calorific intake, which can be particularly difficult for insulin-treated patients.

4. Leg ulcers and pressure sores, which may rapidly deteriorate in diabetic patients.

5. Aphasia, dysarthria, or deafness and blindness, which may make it difficult to communicate: needs are thus unrecognized and unmet.

It is our clinical experience that patients in institutional care have special needs and the following are suggestions on how this care can be improved.

1. Increased community support from experienced health professionals, such as DSNs. Ready access to patients and educational advice given to care staff are essential.

2. Establish diabetes educational and training programmes for staff working in residential and nursing homes. Topics to be covered include screening for and prevention of complications, principles of treatment, and HBGM.

3. Establish standards of diabetes care for patients within institutions. This will require close cooperation between primary care (general practitioners) physicians and hospital consultants (geriatricians with a special interest in diabetes; diabetologists) and input from other health professionals involved in the care of these patients. The BDA has recently given strong support and encouragement to undertake diabetic review in institutions in the UK. In residential and nursing homes in South Wales, both a survey of care and an educational package for social services care staff is in the process of being established by one of the authors (AJS).

4. Ensure that diabetic patients living in residential and nursing homes should have ready access to chiropody and dietetic advice.

Along with these initiatives, there is also an important need for both research and audit in institutional diabetic care. Hopefully, this may lead to an improvement in the delivery of care to this vulnerable group of patients as well as a corresponding increase in their quality of life.

COMPLICATIONS AND CONSEQUENCES OF DIABETES IN THE OLDER PATIENT

HYPOGLYCAEMIA

This acute metabolic complication is discussed in detail in several chapters of this book (Chapters 5, 8, 9) but its importance in elderly patients prompts us to provide additional comments.

Hypoglycaemia can be very disturbing for older people who find the unpredictability of funny turns, faints and falls shatters their self-confidence and may result in them giving up their homes and moving into residential care. Patients may be admitted to hospital with serious symptoms such as hypoglycaemic coma of sudden onset or even chronic confusion due to hypoglycaemia. Occasionally, there is delay in making the diagnosis.

Seventy per cent of all hypoglycaemic episodes are due to sulphonylurea use. The most common precipitating factor is a restricted carbohydrate intake[36]. All patients on sulphonylureas should therefore be encouraged to have a regular carbohydrate intake spread throughout the day. Other precipitating factors are alcohol intake and diarrhoea[37]. Drug interactions, such as the use of sulphonamides with first-generation sulphonylureas can also cause hypoglycaemia. Older people are particularly at risk because of poor renal function which results in reduced excretion of these drugs. Again, it must be emphasized that sulphonylureas with a shorter biological half-life, such as tolbutamide or gliclazide appear to be less likely to cause hypoglycaemia than the longer-acting drugs, glibenclamide or chlorpropamide[38], and should be preferentially prescribed in elderly diabetic patients.

Patients who are taking insulin are at least four times more likely to suffer hypoglycaemia compared with those on sulphonylureas—a fact which must be considered when recommending insulin for the older Type 2 diabetic person[39]. Hypoglycaemia is less common in Type 2 diabetes but some elderly people on insulin are subject to unpredictable control with recurrent hypoglycaemia. There is often associated cognitive impairment[40]. Other factors that predispose the elderly to hypoglycaemia is their inaccuracy of insulin injection[41] and the frequent use of once-daily insulin preparations, which often lead to unacceptable glycaemic control and increase the number of 'hypos' in the late afternoon or at night.

Elderly people appear to have a poor knowledge of the symptoms of hypoglycaemia[6]. In a recent study of older people with diabetes, hypoglycaemic symptoms such as episodes of confusion, sweating, palpitations, and headaches relieved by sugar are frequent among patients taking sulphonylureas[42]. It remains to be demonstrated that these symptoms in the elderly are due to hypoglycaemia. Older people are also less aware of the development of hypoglycaemia and are therefore more likely to sustain severe hypoglycaemia with the consequence of unexplained falls and faints[42].

All patients who are taking sulphonylureas or insulin should be educated about the symptoms of hypoglycaemia, correct self-management, and advised on the need for a regular carbohydrate intake. All patients on insulin should carry a card or medic-alert badge stating that they are diabetic and what their treatment is. These patients should always carry a source of quick-acting carbohydrate such as dextrose tablets and should have access to further carbohydrate within a few minutes, e.g. carry biscuits with them. For insulin-treated patients who are subject to frequent hypoglycaemia, a competent carer can be taught how to administer a glucagon injection.

AGE-SPECIFIC COMPLICATIONS

There are a number of complications which are particularly common in older diabetic patients and a number of these have been discussed in Chapters 5 and 6. Periodontal disease is very common in those with remaining natural teeth, especially if there is poor diabetic control[43]. In addition many other conditions prevalent in the elderly are especially common in patients with diabetes, e.g. hypothermia, osteoporosis, magnesium deficiency and other infections such as candidiasis and tuberculosis[23].

SPECIFIC INFECTIVE COMPLICATIONS

It is common clinical experience that infections are common in older people with diabetes. It is advised, for example, that all older people with diabetes should be offered influenza vaccination because of the additional risk of staphylococcal pneumonia[44]. Renal papillary necrosis can present with an insidious onset of renal failure and general ill health without the high fever and loin pain that are seen in younger non-diabetic patients. Malignant otitis externa caused usually by *Pseudomonas aeruginosa* infections results in osteomyelitis of the base of the skull and associated complications such as fifth and seventh nerve and other cranial nerve palsies. It has a high mortality rate and treatment entails giving large intravenous doses of several antibiotics[45]. Synergistic necrotizing fasciitis is another condition which occurs particularly in the elderly. It is caused by organisms such as *Bacteroides*, *Staphylococcus aureus* and *Pseudomonas* and is characterized by a rapidly spreading, life-threatening necrosis of the skin and subcutaneous tissues. Treatment involves both surgery and intravenous antibiotics in high doses.

IMPOTENCE IN OLDER PEOPLE WITH DIABETES

This important and often neglected diabetic complication is also discussed in Chapter 6. Impotence is more common with advancing age such that 55% of men over 60 years of age who have diabetes are affected[46]. This is a major cause of concern for many older patients as studies have shown that

75% of men of 60 years of age and over engage in regular coitus[47]. Although only 15% of men over 80 years engage in sexual intercourse[48], 50% remain interested in sexual activity[49]. Assessment of patients with impotence requires skill and training and cannot be left to a brief conversation at the end of a clinic appointment. Impotence in older men with diabetes is probably due to a mixture of vascular and neuropathic causes, although vasoactive drugs, depression, alcohol and psychotropic drugs should always be considered as aggravating or even precipitating factors. In view of underlying microangiopathy, vascular surgery is rarely helpful[50]. Treatment with androgens is associated with minimal benefit only but intracavernous therapy with alpha 1-blockers such as phentolamine and phenoxybenzamine, or smooth muscle relaxants, such as papaverine are helpful in highly motivated and competent patients. In selected cases, vacuum devices to promote erection are a useful form of therapy. However, many elderly patients may find these expensive to purchase, and as a normal erection is not produced, may soon discard them[50]. Surgical insertion of a rigid prosthesis is well-established in some centres, but the take-up rate in elderly patients is small.

PSYCHOLOGICAL FUNCTION AND DIABETES IN THE ELDERLY

The prevalence of depression in elderly diabetic patients increases with duration of diabetes[51], and diabetic patients are more commonly depressed than non-diabetic controls[52]. There is evidence that older diabetic people especially those with poor control of diabetes and peripheral neuropathy have cognitive deficits in psychomotor performance, learning and memory tasks[53,54]. There is some correlation of poor control with deteriorating cognitive function but the correlation with duration of diabetes is not linear[55]. In contrast, in a recent study employing more than 12 measures of neuropsychological assessment, elderly patients with NIDDM of 10 years duration showed no significant change in cognition compared with an age- and sex-matched group of community controls[56].

Another important factor in older diabetic patients is the frequency of cerebrovascular disease and stroke, which results in an increase in the frequency of arteriosclerotic dementia and associated behavioural disorders and focal mental deterioration with development of frontal lobe syndrome, apraxia or agnosia. Deteriorating cognitive function is especially important in the insulin-treated older diabetic because diabetes control becomes much more difficult and can result in the syndrome of brittle diabetes[40]. In these situations, the role of a spouse or principal carer is essential in maintaining an effective level of glycaemic control to prevent hyperglycaemic symptoms and hypoglycaemia. Other important aims in managing diabetes in the elderly are consequently less of a priority.

PHYSICAL AND SOCIAL DISABILITY IN THE ELDERLY

A recent survey has confirmed the widespread clinical impression that an elderly diabetic patient's life-style may be severely limited by angina, claudication, poor eyesight, blindness or stroke[24]. Combined with the other common problems associated with advancing age such as bereavement, separation from a growing family and financial difficulties, diabetes can make life for older people restricted and unpleasant.

Neuropathy, foot ulceration and amputation are common problems which can cause pain, restrict mobility and decrease the quality of life an elderly patient experiences. Sexual problems due to depression or autonomic neuropathy often compound the situation. Where established, support groups can be of help in dealing with these disabilities and handicaps. Entering long-term residential or nursing care can be a depressing and worrying experience. Institutions (including hospitals) seem particularly bad at coping with the special needs of people with diabetes—meals are delivered at unusual times, which are incompatible with good diabetic control and dietary choices may be inadequate. The ability to regulate and administer insulin independently may be denied as well as the facility to self-monitor diabetes. Some of this is a result of lack of knowledge but often it is the lack of the will to make necessary adjustments to an institutional regime.

Although diabetes is now less of a social stigma, it can still restrict an enjoyable life-style. Loss of a driving licence, the constant fear of hypoglycaemia for an elderly person on sulphonylureas or insulin living alone or dictary and alcohol restrictions when eating out may all contribute to a decreased quality of life. Insurance premiums are often higher and with the necessary dietary changes may result in the person not being as well off financially.

Some older people adapt much better than others to the restrictions of diabetes or other disabilities arising with age. They accept readily restrictions and the resulting loss of independence. Occasionally, a newly diagnosed patient has a catastrophic reaction and is unable to accept the diagnosis and the required dietary changes. As a consequence, they may just give up altogether the struggle for independent existence and become morose and totally dependent. Considerable judgement needs to be used when informing patients that they have a disabling disease. For many older people with recently diagnosed diabetes reassurance should be provided that a healthy diet and taking part in regular exercise is all that is required to maintain adequate glycaemic control and freedom from symptoms.

Finally, spouses of older people with diabetes are also often disabled themselves. It is thus crucial that the social environment of the older person with diabetes is taken into consideration when making care plans for them.

CONCLUSIONS

Better organized and more effective management of older people with diabetes will inevitably lead to an increase in the quality of care delivered.

Primary care physicians, diabetologists and geriatricians should liaise and cooperate in developing appropriate strategies of care, but to do this they require an appreciation of the special needs of this large and vulnerable group of patients.

An increasing role of other health professionals including DSNs, chiropodists and community dietitians is paramount to the success of these initiatives.

REFERENCES

1 Sinclair AJ. Diagnosis and early management of Type 2 diabetes in the elderly: a 1990s perspective. *Care of the Elderly* 1993; 5: 69–72.
2 World Health Organisation Europe and European Region of International Diabetes Federation. *The St Vincent Declaration.* Copenhagen: WHO Europe and the European Region of IDF, 1989.
3 Sinclair AJ, Barnett AH. Special needs of elderly diabetic patients. *Br Med J* 1993; 306: 1142–3.
4 Knight PV, Kesson CM. Educating the elderly diabetic. *Diabetic Med* 1986; 3 (Education Suppl.): 170–2.
5 Lockington TJ, Farrant S, Meadows KA, Dowlatski D, Wise PH. Knowledge profile and control in diabetic patients. *Diabetic Med* 1988; 5: 381–6.
6 Mutch WJ, Dingwall-Fordyce I. Knowledge of symptoms of hypoglycaemia in elderly diabetic patients. *Diabetologia* 1982; 23: 472.
7 Thomson FJ, Masson EA, Leeming JT, Boulton AJM. Lack of knowledge of symptoms of hypoglycaemia by elderly diabetic patients. *Age Ageing* 1991; 20: 404–6.
8 Bates A. Diabetes in old age. *Practical Diabetes* 1986; 3: 120–3.
9 Thomson FJ, Masson EA. Can elderly persons co-operate with routine foot care? *Age Ageing* 1992; 21: 333–7.
10 Clarke P. Role of the diabetes nurse specialist. *Practical Diabetes* 1986; 3(5): 229.
11 Sinclair AJ. Diabetes specialist nurses: How a specialist nurse can lighten the doctor's load. *Geriatr Med* 1988; 5: 15–18.
12 Carr EK, Kirk BA, Jeffcoate WJ. Perceived needs of general practitioners and practice nurses for the care of diabetic patients. *Diabetic Med* 1991; 8: 556–9.
13 Burrows PJ, Gray PJ, Kinmonth A-L, Payton DJ, Walpole GA, Walton RJ, Wilson D, Woodbine G. Who cares for the patient with diabetes? Presentation and follow-up in seven Southampton practices. *J R Coll Gen Pract* 1987; 37: 65–9.
14 Tasker PRW. Is diabetes a disease for general practice? *Practical Diabetes* 1984; 1(1): 21–4.
15 Martin BJ, Young RE, Kesson KM. Home monitoring of blood glucose in elderly non-insulin-dependent diabetics. *Practical Diabetes* 1986; 3(1): 37.
16 Dornan TL, Peck G, Dow J, Tattersall RB. Wellbeing does not correlate with blood glucose control in the diabetic elderly? *Diabetic Med* 1990; 7 (Suppl. 1): 24A.

17 Dunn SM. Psychological issues in diabetes management: Blood glucose monitoring and learned helplessness. *Practical Diabetes* 1987; 3: 108–10.

18 Titus Allen B, DeLong ER, Feussner JR. Impact of glucose self-monitoring on non-insulin-treated patients with type II diabetes mellitus. *Diabetes Care* 1990; 13: 1044–50.

19 Gatling W. Home monitoring of diabetes: Urine testing. *Practical Diabetes* 1989; 6(3): 100–1.

20 Self monitoring of blood glucose: Consensus statement. *Diabetes Care* 1990; 13 (Suppl. 1): 41–6.

21 *Diabetes Care. What you should expect.* British Diabetic Association, London, 1993.

22 Thomson FJ, Masson EA, Boulton AJM. Quantitative vibration perception testing in elderly people: An assessment of variability. *Age Ageing* 1992; 21: 171–4.

23 Morley JE, Mooradian AD, Rosenthal MJ, Kaiser FE. Diabetes mellitus in elderly patients. *Am J Med* 1987; 83: 533–44.

24 Turnbull CJ. A geriatric diabetic clinic reviewed. *Practical Diabetes* 1991; 8(4): 154–6.

25 Burrows PJ, Gray PJ, Kinmonth A-L, Payton DJ, Walpole GA, Walton RJ, Wilson D, Woodbine G. Who cares for the patient with diabetes? Presentation and follow-up in seven Southampton practices. *J R Coll Gen Pract* 1987; 37: 65–9.

26 Koperski M. How effective is systematic care of diabetic patients? A study in one general practice. *Br J Gen Pract* 1992; 42: 508–11.

27 Chesover D, Tudor-Miles P, Hilton S. Survey and audit of diabetes care in general practice in south London. *Br J Gen Pract* 1991; 41: 282–5.

28 Hill TD. Community care service for diabetics in the Poole area. *Br Med J* 1976; i: 1137–9.

29 Burnett SD, Woolf CM, Yudkin JS. Developing a district diabetic register. *Br Med J* 1992; 305: 627–30.

30 Lewis F, Jones J, Jones H, Child DF. An audit of diabetic inpatient care. *Practical Diabetes* 1991; 8(5): 171–2.

31 Potter JM. Diabetes in the day hospital. *Care Elderly* 1990; 2: 11–13.

32 Spathis GE. Facilities in diabetic clinics in the UK: Shortcomings and recommendations. *Diabetic Med* 1986; 3: 131–6.

33 Laing W. Living environments for the elderly. 3: The mixed economy in long-term care. In: Wells N, Freer C (eds), *The Ageing Population Burden or Challenge?* Basingstoke: Macmillan Press, 1988: 235–48.

34 Benbow S. Disability in residential and nursing home patients with diabetes. Presentation at the Third Annual Meeting of the Special Interest Group in Diabetes, British Geriatrics Society, Oxford, UK, 13–14 May 1994.

35 Gale EAM, Dornan TL, Tattersall RB. Severely uncontrolled diabetes in the over fifties. *Diabetologia* 1981; 21: 25–8.

36 Seltzer HS. Drug induced hypoglycaemia—a review of 1418 cases. *Endocrinol Metab Clin North Am* 1989; 18: 163–83.

37 Asplund K, Wilholm B-E. Lithner F. Glibenclamide-associated hypoglycemia: A report on 57 cases. *Diabetologia* 1983; 24: 412–17.

38 Campbell JW. Sulphonylureas and metformin: efficacy and inadequacy. In: Bailey CJ, Flatt PR (eds), *New Antidiabetic Drugs*. London: Smith-Gordon, 1990: 33–51.

39 Klimt CR, Knatterud GL, Meinert CL, Prout TE. The University Group Diabetes Program: a study of the effects of hypoglycaemic agents on vascular complications in patients with adult onset diabetes. II. Mortality results. *Diabetes* 1970; 19 (Suppl. 2): 747–830.

40 Griffith DNW, Yudkin JS. Brittle diabetes in the elderly. *Diabetic Med* 1989; **6**: 440–3.

41 Puxty JAH, Hunter DH, Burr WA. Accuracy of insulin injection in elderly patients. *Br Med J* 1983; **287**: 1762.

42 Brierley EJ, Broughton DL, James OFW, Alberti KGMM. Awareness of hypoglycaemia in the elderly. Paper presented to the British Geriatrics Society Spring 1993.

43 Morrow LA, Herman WH, Halter JB. Diabetes. In: Grimley Evans J, Franklin Williams T (eds), *Oxford Textbook of Geriatric Medicine*. Oxford: Oxford University Press, 1992: 135.

44 Department of Health. *Immunisation against Infectious Disease*. London: HMSO, 1992; 95–9.

45 Vernham GA, Robinson D, Resouly A, Shaw KM. Malignant otitis externa—a serious complication of diabetes mellitus. *Practical Diabetes* 1988; **5**(4): 177–9.

46 Smith AD. Causes and classification of impotence. *Urol Clin North Am* 1981; **8**: 79–89.

47 Masters WH. Sex and aging—expectations and reality. *Hosp Pract* 1986; **21**: 175–7, 182–92, 197–8.

48 Pearlman CK, Kobashi LI. Frequency of intercourse in men. *J Urol* 1972; **107**: 298–301.

49 Verwoerdt A, Pfeiffer E, Wang HS. Sexual behaviour in senescence. Patterns of sexual activity and interest. *Geriatrics* 1969; **24**: 137.

50 Whitehead ED, Klyde BJ. Diabetes related impotence in the elderly. In: Froom J (ed.), *Diabetes Mellitus in the Elderly. Clin Geriatr Med* 1990: **6**(4): 771–95.

51 Palinkas LA, Barrett-Connor E, Wingard DL. Type 2 diabetes and depressive symptoms in older adults: a population based study. *Diabetic Med* 1991; **8**: 532–9.

52 Wing RR, Marcus MD, Blair EH, Epstein LH, Burton LR. Depressive symptomatology in obese adults with type II diabetes. *Diabetes Care* 1990; **13**: 170–2.

53 Reaven GM, Thompson LW, Nahum D, Haskins E. Relationship between hyperglycemia and cognitive function in older NIDDM patients. *Diabetes Care* 1990; **13**: 16–21.

54 Perlmuter LC, Hakami MK, Hodgson-Harrington C, *et al*. Decreased cognitive function in aging non-insulin dependent diabetic patients. *Am J Med* 1984; **77**: 1043–8.

55 Tun PA, Nathan DM, Permuter LC. Cognitive and affective disorders in elderly diabetics. In Froom J (ed.), *Diabetes Mellitus in the Elderly. Clin Geriatr Med* 1990; **6**(4): 731–46.

56 Atiea J, Moses J, Sinclair AJ. Neuropsychological function in older patients with non-insulin-dependent diabetes mellitus. *Diabetic Med* 1995; in press.

Index

Index compiled by Jill Halliday